Clinical Cases in
Pediatric Dentistry

WU 480

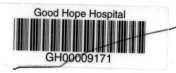

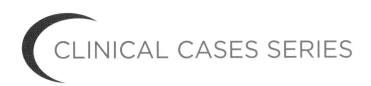

CLINICAL CASES SERIES

Clinical Cases in
Pediatric Dentistry

Editor:

Amr M. Moursi, DDS, PhD

Associate Professor and Chairman
Department of Pediatric Dentistry
New York University College of Dentistry
New York, NY
USA

Associate Editors:

Marcio A. da Fonseca, DDS, MS

Law-Lewis Professor and Director
Pediatric Dentistry Graduate Program
School of Dentistry
University of Washington
Seattle Children's Hospital
Seattle, WA
USA

Amy L. Truesdale, DDS

Clinical Assistant Professor
Department of Pediatric Dentistry
New York University College of Dentistry
New York, NY
USA

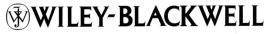

WILEY-BLACKWELL

A John Wiley & Sons, Inc., Publication

Registered office: John Wiley & Sons Ltd, The Atrium, Southern Gate, Chichester, West Sussex, PO19 8SQ, UK

Editorial offices: 2121 State Avenue, Ames, Iowa 50014-8300, USA
The Atrium, Southern Gate, Chichester, West Sussex, PO19 8SQ, UK
9600 Garsington Road, Oxford, OX4 2DQ, UK

For details of our global editorial offices, for customer services and for information about how to apply for permission to reuse the copyright material in this book please see our website at www.wiley.com/wiley-blackwell.

Library of Congress Cataloging-in-Publication Data
Clinical cases in pediatric dentistry / editor, Amr M. Moursi; associate editors, Marcio A. da Fonseca, Amy Truesdale.
     p. ; cm. – (Clinical cases uncovered)
  Includes bibliographical references and index.
  ISBN 978-0-8138-0761-4 (pbk. : alk. paper)
  I. Moursi, Amr M.   II. Da Fonseca, Marcio A.   III. Truesdale, Amy.   IV. Series: Clinical cases uncovered.
  [DNLM: 1. Dental Care for Children–methods–Case Reports.   2. Child.   3. Infant.   4. Oral Surgical Procedures–Case Reports.   5. Tooth Diseases–Case Reports.   WU 480]
  617.6'45–dc23

                                                                                                    2011044218

A catalogue record for this book is available from the British Library.

Wiley also publishes its books in a variety of electronic formats. Some content that appears in print may not be available in electronic books.

Set in 10/13 pt Univers Light by Toppan Best-set Premedia Limited
Printed and bound in Singapore by Markono Print Media Pte Ltd

1 2012

To our students, past, present, and future, and to our patients who teach us so much.

TABLE OF CONTENTS

Chapter 3   Complex Pulp Therapy   89

Chapter 4   Orofacial Trauma   137

LIST OF CONTRIBUTORS

Editor

Amr M. Moursi, DDS, PhD
Associate Professor and Chairman
Department of Pediatric Dentistry
New York University College of Dentistry
New York, NY
USA

Associate Editors

Marcio A. da Fonseca, DDS, MS
Law-Lewis Professor and Director
Pediatric Dentistry Graduate Program
School of Dentistry
University of Washington
Seattle Children's Hospital
Seattle, WA
USA

Amy Truesdale, DDS
Clinical Assistant Professor
Department of Pediatric Dentistry
New York University College of Dentistry
New York, NY
USA

Contributors

Omolola Adetona, DDS
Private Practice
San Antonio, TX
USA

Farah Alam, DDS
Director, Special Care Dentistry
Rose F. Kennedy Center
Children's Evaluation and Rehabilitation Center
University Center for Excellence in Developmental
Disabilities
Albert Einstein College of Medicine
Bronx, NY
USA

Homa Amini, DDS, MPH, MS
Associate Professor of Clinical Dentistry
Postdoctoral Program Director, Pediatric Dentistry
Division of Pediatric Dentistry and Community Oral
Health
College of Dentistry
The Ohio State University
Columbus, OH
USA

**Richard Balmer, BDS, MDent Sci, FDS (Paed Dent),
RCPS (Glasgow)**
Consultant and Lecturer in Paediatric Dentistry
Leeds Dental Institute
University of Leeds
Leeds, United Kingdom

**Angus C. Cameron, BDS (Hons), MDSc, FRACDS,
FDSRCS(Eng), FICD**
Clinical Associate Professor and Head
Department of Paediatric Dentistry
Westmead Hospital
The University of Sydney
Sydney, Australia

Lina M. Cárdenas, DDS, MS, PhD
Private Practice
San Antonio, TX
USA

Paul Casamassimo, DDS, MS
Professor and Chair
Division of Pediatric Dentistry and Community Oral
Health
College of Dentistry
The Ohio State University
Columbus, OH
USA
Chief of Dentistry
Nationwide Children's Hospital
Columbus, OH
USA

Claudia Isabel Contreras, DDS
Assistant Clinical Professor
Department of Developmental Dentistry
University of Texas Health Science Center at San
Antonio
San Antonio, TX
USA

Etty Dayan, DMD
Instructor
Department of Pediatric Dentistry
Hadassah School of Dental Medicine
Hebrew University
Jerusalem, Israel

Jeffrey A. Dean, DDS, MSD
Ralph E. McDonald Professor of Pediatric Dentistry
Professor of Orthodontics
Executive Associate Dean
Associate Dean for Faculty Affairs
Indiana University School of Dentistry
Indianapolis, IN
USA

Kevin J. Donly, DDS, MS
Professor and Chair
Department of Developmental Dentistry
University of Texas Health Science Center at San
Antonio
San Antonio, TX
USA

Nancy Dougherty, DMD, MPH
Clinical Associate Professor
Director, Advanced Education in Pediatric Dentistry
Program
New York University College of Dentistry
New York, NY
USA

Zvia Elazary, DMD
Clinical Instructor
Department of Endodontics
Hadassah School of Dental Medicine
Hebrew University
Jerusalem, Israel

Paddy Fleming, BDentSc, FDS, MS, FFD
Consultant and Senior Lecturer in Paediatric Dentistry
Our Lady's Children's Hospital and Dublin Dental
University Hospital
Trinity College
Dublin, Ireland

Anna B. Fuks, DMD
Professor Emeritus
Department of Pediatric Dentistry
Hadassah Faculty of Dental Medicine
Hebrew University
Jerusalem, Israel

Maria Minerva Garcia, DDS
Clinical Assistant Professor
Department of Developmental Dentistry
University of Texas Health Science Center at San
Antonio
Laredo Regional Campus
Laredo, TX
USA

**Sam Gue, BDS, MDSc, FRACDS, FRACDS(Paed),
FICD**
Associate Professor
Head, Department of Paediatric Dentistry
Division of Paediatric Surgery
Women's and Children's Hospital
Head, Discipline of Paediatric Dentistry
University of Adelaide
Adelaide, South Australia
Australia

Kerrod B. Hallett, MDSc, MPH, FRACDS, FICD
Director of Dentistry
Royal Children's Hospital
Clinical Associate Professor
University of Melbourne
Melbourne, Victoria
Australia

Ilana Heling, DMD, MSc
Clinical Associate Professor
Department of Endodontics
Hadassah School of Dental Medicine
Hebrew University
Jerusalem, Israel

Timothy B. Henson, DMD
Associate Professor
Pediatric Dentistry Postdoctoral Program Director
Department of Developmental Dentistry
University of Texas Health Science Center at San
Antonio
San Antonio, TX
USA

Diane L. Howell, CRNA, MSNA
Affiliate Assistant Professor
Department of Nurse Anesthesia
Virginia Commonwealth University
Richmond, VA
USA

Royana Lin, DDS
Clinical Assistant Professor
Department of Developmental Dentistry
University of Texas Health Science Center at San
Antonio
San Antonio, TX
USA

Jeffrey C. Mabry, DDS, MS
Associate Professor
Department of Developmental Dentistry
The University of Texas Health Science Center at San
Antonio
San Antonio, TX
USA

Evelyn Mamber, DMD
Clinical Instructor
Department of Pediatric Dentistry
Hadassah School of Dental Medicine
Hebrew University
Jerusalem, Israel

Eleanor McGovern, BDS, MFD, MDentCh (Paediatric Dentistry)
Clinical Fellow in Paediatric Dentistry
Our Lady's Children's Hospital
Crumlin, Dublin, Ireland

Dennis J. McTigue, DDS, MS
Professor
Division of Pediatric Dentistry and Community Oral
Health
College of Dentistry
The Ohio State University
Columbus, OH
USA

Moti Moskovitz, DMD, PhD
Clinical Senior Lecturer
Department of Pediatric Dentistry
Hadassah School of Dental Medicine
Hebrew University
Jerusalem, Israel

Eyal Nuni, DMD
Clinical Instructor
Department of Endodontics
Hadassah School of Dental Medicine
Hebrew University
Jerusalem, Israel

Diana Ram, DMD
Clinical Associate Professor
Department of Pediatric Dentistry
Hadassah School of Dental Medicine
Hebrew University
Jerusalem, Israel

Hugo A. Rivera, DDS, MEd
Private Practice
San Antonio, TX
USA

Barbara Sheller, DDS, MSD
Affiliate Professor
Department of Orthodontics
Department of Pediatric Dentistry
School of Dentistry
University of Washington
Seattle Children's Hospital
Seattle, WA
USA

Iris Slutzky-Goldberg, DMD
Post Graduate Program Director
Department of Endodontics
Hadassah School of Dental Medicine
Hebrew University
Jerusalem, Israel

S. Thikkurissy, DDS, MS
Assistant Professor
Division of Pediatric Dentistry and Community Oral Health
The Ohio State University College of Dentistry
Columbus, OH
USA
Director, Inpatient Dental Services
Nationwide Children's Hospital
Columbus, OH
USA

Michael D. Webb, DDS, MEd
Pediatric Dentist/Dental Anesthesiologist
The Center for Pediatric Dentistry and Sedation
Richmond, VA
USA
Adjunct Associate Professor
Virginia Commonwealth University School of Dentistry
Department of Pediatric Dentistry
Richmond, VA
USA

Farhad Yeroshalmi, DMD, FAAPD
Program Director, Pediatric Dental Residency
Department of Pediatric Dentistry
Jacobi Medical Center
Bronx, New York
USA
Assistant Clinical Professor of Dentistry
Albert Einstein College of Medicine
Bronx, New York
USA

ACKNOWLEDGMENTS

The editors would like to thank all of the chapter authors and case contributors for compiling such wonderful teaching cases. We would also like to thank those who helped, in countless ways, to create this book, from inception to completion: Ms. Yan Zhao, Ms. Johanna Rosman, Dr. Enas Othman, Dr. Neal Herman, Dr. Linda Rosenberg, Dr. Scott Sachs, and Dr. Marcia Daronch.

On a personal note I would like to thank my associate editors, Drs. Marcio da Fonseca and Amy Truesdale, for their long hours and perseverance.

Thanks also goes to all of the faculty, students, and residents of the NYU Department of Pediatric Dentistry. My deepest gratitude goes to my family for their sacrifice, patience, and understanding, without which this book would not exist.

And finally, we are all indebted to the many patients, and their parents, who consented to appear in this book.

Amr M. Moursi, DDS, PhD

PREFACE

The scope of pediatric dentistry has evolved to include all aspects of wellness that may influence oral and craniofacial health. Likewise, the education of pediatric dentistry has also evolved to include case-based teaching to better reinforce this more holistic approach. Traditional textbooks are a wonderful resource but by necessity present information in artificially constrained topic groupings. Pediatric dentistry is a discipline in which a whole host of issues need to be addressed simultaneously to properly make a diagnosis and manage a patient's care. A case-based approach to education allows one to use foundational knowledge obtained from reference texts and didactic courses to learn strategies for providing patient-centered care.

The clinical cases included in this book were conceived to provide case studies for a wide array of learning situations. Pre-doctoral students can use the cases as they are introduced to pediatric dentistry and as a study guide for case-based curricula and exams. Post-doctoral students and residents can use these cases as they prepare for case-based exams during their training and board certification. This book will also be a useful tool for educators who will now have a ready collection of clinical cases, covering the essentials of pediatric dentistry, to discuss with their students.

Each case emphasizes a particular topic. Each topic contains one or more fundamental points, which are highlighted in designated blue boxes within the text. Fundamental points address issues that are of importance to the diagnosis, treatment plan, and management of the case. In addition to fundamental points, each case has one or more areas of background information, designated in orange boxes. Issues addressed in background information may include a more in-depth discussion of a particularly

important element of the topic. This element may not necessarily be fully illustrated in the case history.

To use this book as a study guide it is recommended that the reader initially read only the information provided on patient presentation and history, and then determine what additional diagnostic information is necessary and how it would be best obtained. After reading the diagnostic information provided, the reader should then compile a differential diagnosis and problem list. This can then be compared with that provided in the case. Following this, a treatment plan can be proposed which should then also be compared to that listed in the text. Questions and answers are also listed for each case. These can be used to review the key elements of the topic or as a study guide for self-evaluation in preparation for written or oral exams.

Although each clinical case in this book was designed to focus on a particular oral health issue, we were also eager that each case stand alone. Therefore, the reader will encounter some repetition from case to case. The editors have tried to minimize this as much as possible but it will be evident, particularly in the areas of history gathering and the discussion of clinical guidelines and prevention recommendations.

We have selected contributors with an international perspective to make the content universally relevant. However, for consistency we have chosen to use U.S. nomenclature and when referring to clinical guidelines we have, primarily, used the guidelines of the American Academy of Pediatric Dentistry (AAPD) , which can be accessed online at: http://www.aapd.org/media/policies.asp.

The chapter topics have been selected to represent the essentials of pediatric dentistry. However, as with all books, there are some limitations. The cases were not meant to comprise an exhaustive survey of pediatric oral disorders. Rather, it was our intention that they represent the "bread and butter" of our discipline. Also, it was beyond the scope of this type of book to provide comprehensive citations; those are available in other reference texts, but we have listed a few key references for each case. We hope that students, educators, and clinicians will find this book a useful resource as we advance and broaden the scope of pediatric oral health care.

Clinical Cases in
Pediatric Dentistry

1

Medically Compromised Patients

Paddy Fleming

Clinical Cases in Pediatric Dentistry, First Edition. Edited by Amr M. Moursi.
© 2012 Blackwell Publishing Ltd. Pubished 2012 by Blackwell Publishing Ltd.

Case 1

Congenital Heart Disease

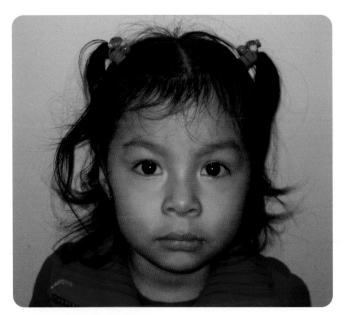

Figure 1.1.1 Facial photo

A. Presenting Patient
- 2-year-, 8-month-old Hispanic female
- New patient

B. Chief Complaint
- Referred from hospital pediatric cardiac unit for dental assessment and management of asymptomatic dental caries

C. Social History
- Single mother is primary caregiver and receives welfare
- No siblings

D. Medical History
Congenital Heart Defects
- Triscuspid atresia
- Hypoplastic right ventricle
- Restrictive ventricular septal defect (VSD)
- Sub-pulmonary narrowing

No Known Food or Drug Allergies
Current Medications
- Warfarin po 3 mg daily
- Furosemide po 20 mg daily

Several Past Surgeries and Hospitalizations

E. Medical Consult
For This Patient (see Fundamental Point 1):
- Baseline cardiac function
- Baseline INR range: 2.0 to 3.0
- Baseline hemoglobin: 11.7 g/dl
- Baseline pulmonary saturations: 97%
- Baseline blood pressure 80/40 mm Hg
- Baseline respiratory rate: 20/minute
- Baseline oxygen: 0.5 l/minute

F. Dental History
- No dental home
- Currently bottle feeding with sweetened liquids
- High caloric supplementation to increase weight
- Toothbrushing once a day with fluoridated toothpaste with little adult supervision
- No systemic fluoride exposure
- No history of dental trauma

G. Extra-oral Exam
- No significant findings

H. Intra-oral Exam
Soft Tissues
- Generalized erythematous mucosa
- Generalized edematous gingivae

Hard Tissues
- Proximal and smooth surface cavitations on maxillary incisors

BACKGROUND INFORMATION 1
Congenital Heart Disease (CHD)

- Incidence rate of approximately 8 to 10 cases/1,000 live births
- Most lesions occur individually; several form major components of syndromes or chromosomal disorders such as Down (trisomy 21) and Turner syndrome (XO chromosome)
- Known risk factors associated with CHD include maternal rubella; diabetes; alcoholism; irradiation; and drugs such as thalidomide, phenytoin sodium (Dilantin) and warfarin sodium (Coumadin)
- Turbulent blood flow is caused by structural abnormalities of the heart anatomy and presents clinically as an audible murmur
- CHD can be classified into acyanotic (shunt or stenotic) and cyanotic lesions depending on clinical presentation
- Acyanotic lesions are characterized by a connection between the systemic and pulmonary circulations or stenosis of either circulation (left to right shunts). The most common anomalies are:
  1. Atrial septal defect (ASD)
  2. Ventricular septal defect (VSD)
  3. Patent ductus arteriosus (PDA) caused by failure of closure of the ductus connecting the pulmonary artery with the aorta (normally closes soon after birth)
  4. Coarctation of the aorta
  5. Aortic stenosis
  6. Pulmonary stenosis
- All cyanotic conditions exhibit right to left shunting of desaturated blood. Infants with mild cyanosis may be pink at rest but become very blue during crying or physical exertion. Children with cyanotic defects are at significant risk for desaturation during general anesthesia
- The most common cyanotic lesions are:
  1. Tetralogy of Fallot which includes a VSD, pulmonary stenosis, overriding aorta and right ventricular hypertrophy
  2. Transposition of great vessels
  3. Tricuspid atresia
- If cardiac failure develops, the infant is digitalized and prescribed diuretics if necessary. Hospitalization, oxygen, nasogastric tube feeding, and antibiotic therapy for chest infection may also be required

FUNDAMENTAL POINT 1
Consult with Cardiologist and Hematologist to Obtain Baseline Information on:
Current Cardiac Status

- Blood pressure
- Respiratory rate
- Oxygen rate
- Pulmonary saturations
- Blood gases

Cardiac Medications
Current INR Range (Normal: Without Anticoagulant Therapy: –1; Target Range With Therapy: –2 to 3)

Previous Surgical Management
Future Surgical Management
Information is Then Used to:

- Assess risk of cardiac complications under general anesthesia (GA)
- Assess risk of infective endocarditis (IE) and need for antibiotic prophylaxis before invasive dental procedures
- Assess risk of hemorrhage during dental surgery
- Develop a perioperative anticoagulant management plan

- Fissure cavitations on molars
- Smooth surface demineralization on molars

Occlusal Evaluation of Primary Dentition
- Flush terminal plane
- Anterior open bite

Generalized Severe Plaque Accumulation

I. Diagnostic Tools
Bacteriology and Saliva Tests
- Not done

Radiographs
- Intra-oral periapical films (taken at time of dental treatment under general anesthesia)

Photographs
- Pre- and post-operative intra-oral photos (taken at time of dental surgery)

High Caries Risk Due to (Caries-risk Assessment Tool [CAT]) (see Fundamental Point 2):
- Special health needs child
- Visible cavitations
- Enamel demineralizations
- Low socioeconomic status
- Visible plaque score (4/6)
- Dietary chart (>3 sugar exposures/day)
- Medications that impair saliva flow

- Use of fluoridated toothpaste but no fluoridated water nor fluoride supplements
- Toothbrushing once a day

J. Differential Diagnosis
Developmental
- Enamel hypoplasia/hypomineralization

Infective
- Bacterial and/or fungal

Odontogenic
- Loss of tooth structure due to dental caries and/or attrition/abrasion/erosion

Inflammatory

Pulpal Pathology

K. Diagnosis and Problem List
Diagnosis
- Active early childhood caries
- Chronic hyperplastic gingivitis
- Periapical pathology
- Enamel hypoplasia

Problem List
- Untreated carious lesions
- Malocclusion
- Poor infant feeding practice

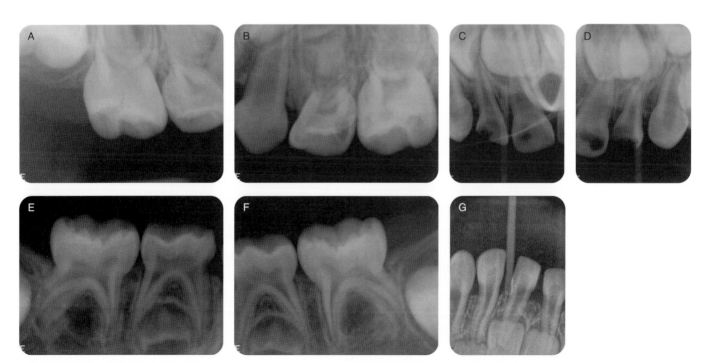

Figure 1.1.2a–g. Pre-op intra-oral radiographs

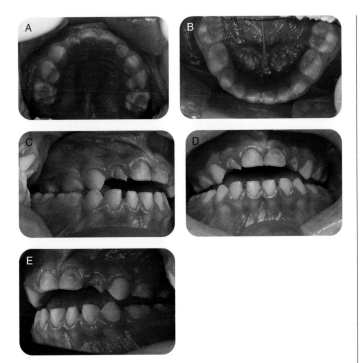

Figure 1.1.3a–e. Pre-op intra-oral photographs

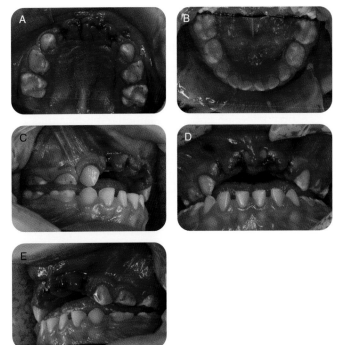

Figure 1.1.4a–e. Post-op intra-oral photographs

- Parent's limited understanding of potential medical complications
- High risk of infective endocarditis (IE)—see Background Information 2
- High risk of uncontrolled hemorrhage from invasive dental procedure
- Behavior assessment: uncooperative

L. Comprehensive Treatment Plan
Establishment of a Dental Home and Caries Prevention Plan

- Cease bottle feeding
- Improve and increase frequency of oral hygiene
- Limit sugar intake between meals
- Brush after oral medicine intake
- Commence 1 mg fluoride supplement daily

Caries Control Using 0.2% Chlorhexidine Gel or 0.12% Liquid: Apply With Cotton Tip Nightly Two Weeks Prior to Procedure

Remove Any Potentially/Pulpally Involved Teeth to Reduce Future Risk of Chronic Bacteremia

Comprehensive Treatment of Carious Lesions Under General Anesthesia Due to the Complex Medical History, Dental Needs, and Behavior Management Issues

BACKGROUND INFORMATION 2
Infective Endocarditis (IE)

- Both coronary heart disease (CHD) and rheumatic heart disease can predispose the scarred internal lining of the heart to bacterial or fungal infection known as infective endocarditis (IE)

- Bacteremia during or after an invasive dental procedure can lead to the formation of friable vegetations of blood cells and organisms on the scar tissue

- *Streptococcus viridans* is most frequently responsible for chronic IE, while *Staphylococcus aureus* is often implicated in the acute fulminating form (Hallett 2003)

- IE may be prevented by antibiotic prophylaxis but there is little or no evidence to support this practice

- In 2008, the National Institute for Health and Clinical Excellence in the UK recommended against IE prophylaxis for all patients undergoing any type of dental procedures. Despite a 78.6% reduction in the number of prescriptions in the two years after the guideline was introduced, there was no large increase in the incidence of cases of or deaths from IE

- Pre-operative antiseptic mouthwash can reduce oral bacterial load

- Focusing on good oral hygiene practices may be more important than antibiotic prophylaxis

IE Prevention With IV Antibiotic Prophylaxis.

Perioperative Anticoagulant Plan

Follow-up Care

Post-op and Home Care Instructions
- Discharge after recommencement of Warfarin
- Soft cold diet for two days
- Recommence tooth brushing after 24 hours
- Start prevention plan

Recall Plan
- Six weeks post-op, and four- to six-month recall thereafter

M. Prognosis and Discussion
- Prognosis for limiting caries progression and changing the diet is guarded in view of limited understanding of caries risk factors and medical complications by parent. Prognosis could be improved with additional home support.

N. Common Complications and Alternative Treatment Plans
- Noncompliance with dietary advice
- Post-operative bleeding or infection
- Continued caries progression

Alternative Treatment Plans May Include:
- Use of stainless steel crowns in all teeth presenting with decalcification or white spot lesions
- Alternative pulpal management, e.g., extraction vs. pulp therapy (must consider risks of chronic bacteremia)
- Alternative medications for anticoagulant management (e.g., Heparin)
- Alternative methods for behavior management

BACKGROUND INFORMATION 3
Anticoagulant Therapy

- Anticoagulants are usually prescribed for children with valvular heart disease and prosthetic valves to reduce the risk of embolization

- If dental extractions are required, it may be necessary to decrease the clotting times to facilitate adequate coagulation but not to such an extent so as to cause emboli or clotting around the heart valves

- Commonly used anticoagulant drugs are oral warfarin sodium (Coumadin), which is a vitamin K antagonist depleting factors II, VII, IX and X, or heparin sodium (Heparin), which inhibits factors IX, X, and XII

- Local hemostatic measures include application of topical thrombin, packing of the socket with microfibrillar collagen hemostat, oxidized regenerated cellulose, and suturing of attached gingivae. Splints or stomo-adhesive bandages may also be of benefit. There have been recent reports of the efficacy of a "fibrin sealant" (Tisseel Duo 500) in the management of coagulopathies, but its use on moist oral mucosa is limited

- It is recommended to consult the cardiologist regarding modification of the anticoagulant therapy before oral surgery. Some practitioners cease warfarin three to five days prior to the surgery date, commence enoxaparin sodium once daily via Insulfon, and admit the patient to the hospital on the day of the procedure. In this protocol, recommencement of warfarin and weaning of enoxaparin sodium 24 hours after surgery is required to re-establish correct international normalized ratio (INR), prothrombin time (PT), and activated partial thromboplastin time (APTT)

- However, recent studies on adults who had multiple dental extractions without modification of their anticoagulant therapy showed few or no post-operative complications. The American Dental Association stated in 2003 that the scientific literature does not support routine discontinuation of oral anti-coagulation therapy for dental patients because it can place them at unnecessary medical risk. Their coagulation status, based on the INR, must be evaluated before invasive dental procedures are performed and any changes in their anticoagulation therapy must be discussed with the patient's physician.

- The American College of Chest Physicians recommends that patients who are taking vitamin K antagonists and are about to undergo minor dental procedures continue with the therapy because it does not confer an increase in clinically important major bleeding. The 2008 College guidelines further state that it is reasonable to co-administer an oral pre-hemostatic agent at the time of the procedure until more adequately powered studies are done. In patients receiving aspirin, the College recommends continuing it around the time of the procedure.

- To date, there have been no studies on pediatric patients, only case reports.

Self-study Questions

1. *What important questions need to be asked when taking a medical history from a patient with congenital heart disease?*

2. *What are some common medications to improve cardiac function and reduce congestive heart failure in children?*

3. *Why are children with congenital heart disease more likely to develop dental caries in primary teeth?*

4. *How would non-compliance with preventive advice alter treatment planning?*

Answers are located at the end of the case.

Bibliography and Additional Reading

American Academy of Pediatric Dentistry. 2011–2012a. Guideline on Caries-risk Assessment and Management for Infants, Children, and Adolescents, Reference Manual. *Pediatr Dent* 33(6):110–17.

American Academy of Pediatric Dentistry. 2011–2012b. Guideline on Antibiotic Prophylaxis for Dental Patients at Risk for Infection, Reference Manual. *Pediatr Dent* 33(6):265–9.

Brennan MT, Wynn RL, Miller CS. 2007. Aspirin and bleeding in dentistry: an update and recommendations. *Oral Surg Oral Med Oral Pathol Oral Radiol Endod* 104:316–23. http://www.circulationaha.org, May 8, 2007.

Douketis JD, Berger PB, Dunn AS, et al. 2008. The perioperative management of antithrombotic therapy. American College of Chest Physicians evidence-based clinical practice guidelines. 8th ed. *Chest* 2008; 133:299–339S.

Dunn AS, Turpie AGG. 2003. Perioperative management of patients receiving oral anticoagulants—A systematic review. *Arch Intern Med* 163:901–8.

Grines CL, Bonow RO, Casey DE Jr, et al. 2007. Prevention of premature discontinuation of dual antiplatelet therapy in patients with coronary artery stents. *JADA* 138(5):652–5.

Hallett KB. 2003. Medically compromised children. In *Handbook of Pediatric Dentistry*, 2nd ed. AC Cameron, RP Widmer (eds). Mosby: London pp. 234–44.

Jeske AH, Suchko GD. 2003. Lack of a scientific basis for routine discontinuation of oral anticoagulation therapy before dental treatment. *JADA* 134:1492–7.

Lockhart PB, Loven B, Brennan MT, Fox PC. 2007. The evidence base for the efficacy of antibiotic prophylaxis in dental practice. *JADA* 138:458–74.

Napenas JJ, Hong CHL, Brennan MT, et al. 2009. The frequency of bleeding complications after invasive dental treatment in patients receiving single and dual antiplatelet therapy. *JADA* 140:690–5.

Perry DJ, Noakes TJC, Helliwell PS. 2007. Guidelines for the management of patients on oral anticoagulants requiring dental surgery. *Br Dent J* 203:389–93.

Thronhill MH, Dayer MJ, Forde JM, et al. 2011. Impact of the NICE guideline recommending cessation of antibiotic prophylaxis for prevention of infective endocarditis: before and after study. *BMJ* 342:d2392.

Wilson W, Taubert KA, Gewitz M, et al. Prevention of Infective Endocarditis—Guidelines from the American Heart Association.

SELF-STUDY ANSWERS

1. Nature of diagnosis (acyanotic or cyanotic), supportive medications, previous surgical corrections, future surgical corrections, current cardiac function, physical activity limitations, risk of IE

2. Oral elixirs including Digoxin and Furosemide, usually with sucrose or sorbitol base.

3. Enamel is often hypoplastic and susceptible to early childhood caries; high-caloric diet; use of sucrose-rich medications; medications may induce xerostomia; parental indulgence with sweets, juices, sodas, etc.

4. It may be necessary to extract all carious teeth, especially those with pulpal involvement, to reduce the risk of infection and IE.

Case 2

Cystic Fibrosis

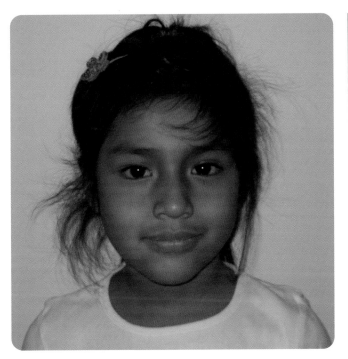

Figure 1.2.1a. Facial photograph

A. Presenting Patient
- 5-year-, 1-month-old female
- New patient

B. Chief Complaint
- Referral by general dentist for dental assessment and treatment of asymptomatic carious lesions

C. Social History
- Mother is primary care provider
- No siblings

D. Medical History
Cystic Fibrosis (CF) (see Background Information 1)
- Diagnosed at 3 years and 6 months of age
- Sees pediatrician every six weeks
- Has daily physiotherapy for removal of lung secretions
- Last acute chest infection: three weeks ago

No Known Drug or Food Allergies; Vaccinations Up-to-Date

Medications
- Flucloxacillin 250 mg qid: broad-spectrum antibiotic for prophylaxis against chest infections

- Pancreatin with each meal: pancreatic enzyme replacement
- Salbutamol inhaler bid: β-2 agonist
- Fluticasone Propionate inhaler bid: corticosteroid
- Vitamins A, D, and E supplements
- Ursodeoxycholic acid: dietary supplement to improve flow of bile

E. Medical Consult

If Parent is Not a Good Historian or if Child is Not Cooperative for Dental Care in Office, Contact Child's Pediatrician to:

- Review current medications and history of hospital admissions
- Establish respiratory status
- Discuss other means to treat this patient

F. Dental History

- Patient has dental home and has had restorations done in office
- Cariogenic diet
- Good oral hygiene habits with some parental supervision
- Uses toothpaste containing fluoride
- Has non-fluoridated water supply and no fluoride supplementation
- No history of trauma
- Behavior assessment: ± on the Frankl Palmer Scale

G. Extra-oral Exam

- No significant findings

H. Intra-oral Exam

Soft Tissues

- No significant findings

Hard Tissues

- No significant findings

Occlusal Evaluation of Primary Dentition

- Mesial step molars
- Right anterior crossbite
- Lower midline shift to the right (3 mm)
- Maxillary anterior crowding

Minimal Plaque Seen on Teeth

Dental Exam

- Severe enamel defects on maxillary left second primary molar and mandibular left second primary molar, which have been restored with amalgam. However, there is evidence of secondary caries at margins now

---

BACKGROUND INFORMATION 1
Cystic Fibrosis

- Autosomal recessive disorder
- Prevalence 1 in 2,500 live births in Caucasians
- Basic defect is a failure to code for cystic fibrosis transmembrane regulator (CFTR) protein which regulates electrolyte and water transport across cell membranes
- The optimal diagnostic test is the measurement of sweat electrolyte levels
- Complex, multisystem disease involving the upper and lower airways, pancreas, bowel, and reproductive tracts. The two main systems affected are respiratory and gastrointestinal.
- Respiratory issues: Viscous secretions accumulate in smaller airways which are prone to infection. Children are on long-term antibiotics to prevent chest infections, which must be treated aggressively. Healing occurs with scarring, further compromising the airway. Regular physiotherapy is required to encourage physical removal of secretions. Many children have reversible airway obstructions treated by salbutamol and steroid inhalers.
- Gastrointestinal issues: Damage to pancreas results in pancreatic enzyme insufficiency, thus oral pancreatic supplements are required with all meals. Fat-soluble vitamin supplements are taken due to the patients' reduced ability to absorb the vitamins. Incidence of celiac disease and Crohn's disease seems to be increased in CF patients.
- Long-term complications of CF include diabetes, liver disease, pneumothorax, sinusitis, nasal polyps, osteopenia, failure to thrive, and infertility
- The cornerstones of management include proactive treatment of airway infection and encouragement of good nutrition, as well as an active lifestyle
- For patients in late respiratory failure, heart-lung transplants are an option but are available in only a minority of cases

Oral Manifestations and Dental Treatment Considerations in Cystic Fibrosis Patients

- In spite of a high-carbohydrate diet the incidence of dental caries in cystic fibrosis (CF) patients has been found to be consistently lower than in healthy controls (Kinirons 1985, Narang, et al. 2003). This fact has been attributed to the long-term antibiotic therapy of these children (Kinirons 1992), high salivary pH (Kinirons 1985), and raised salivary calcium levels (Blomfield, et al. 1973)

- Patients with CF present increased levels of calculus and lower gingival health (Narang, et al. 2003). These patients have altered amounts of calcium and phosphate in their saliva, which affect calculus formation. However, pancreatin may have a role in decreasing calculus formation and reducing dental caries in these patients (Narang, et al. 2003)

- There is a higher prevalence of enamel defects, which can be attributed to severe systemic upset in infancy, especially in cases which patients are diagnosed late

- General anesthetic is strongly contra-indicated because of the compromised airway and increased incidence of post-operative chest infections

- Decisions on which antibiotic to give for acute dental conditions must be made in conjunction with the pediatrician. The choice of antibiotic should take into account the current regime and the types of antibiotics that may be required for future treatment

- Children with CF are high priority for dental prevention because the condition makes treatment of dental disease more difficult

- Liver disease may be a feature of older children with CF, resulting in complications involving bleeding, infection, and drug metabolism

- Nitrous oxide sedation may be contra-indicated in these children and should only be carried out after consultation with the pediatrician to establish respiratory capacity. The procedure should be carried out in a hospital environment. Careful monitoring of oxygen saturation levels is essential

- Mild enamel defects on mandibular right second primary molar and maxillary right second primary molar; the latter also has occlusal caries

- Evidence of moderate erosion on upper and lower incisors

I. Diagnostic Tools

- Right and left bitewings: no other radiographic lesions noted other than the ones mentioned above.

J. Differential Diagnosis

- N/A

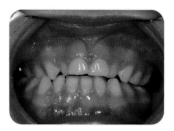

Figure 1.2.1b. Pre-op frontal intra-oral

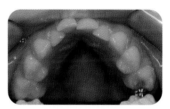

Figure 1.2.2. Pre-op maxillary intra-oral

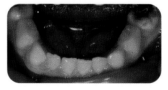

Figure 1.2.3. Pre-op mandibular intra-oral

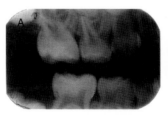
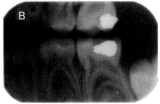

Figure 1.2.4a–b. Pre-op right and left bitewing radiographs

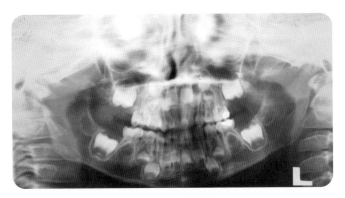

Figure 1.2.5. Pre-op panoramic radiograph

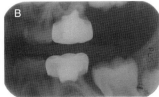

Figure 1.2.6a–b. Post-op right and left bitewing radiographs

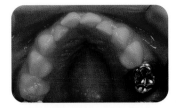

Figure 1.2.7. Post-op maxillary intra-oral

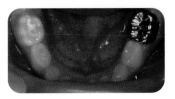

Figure 1.2.8. Post-op mandibular intra-oral

K. Diagnosis and Problem List

Diagnosis
- Early childhood caries with probable pulp involvement
- Occlusion problems
- Enamel hypoplasia
- Early tooth surface loss in incisors

Problem List
- Untreated carious lesions
- Poor dietary habits
- High caries risk (special health care needs, cariogenic diet, caries)
- Possible behavior management issues
- Correction of malocclusion

L. Comprehensive Treatment Plan
- Treatment of all carious lesions
- Establishment of a caries prevention plan

M. Prognosis and Discussion
- This patient was on a typical therapeutic regime. Involvement of the respiratory system meant that she was on ventolin and flixotide inhalers as well as flucloxacillin as prophylaxis against chest infections. Damage to the pancreas had resulted in the requirement of pancreatin, a combination of pancreatic enzymes. In addition, supplementation of fat-soluble vitamins was required as well as a diet high in refined carbohydrate and protein, and a full fat content.

In general, children with cystic fibrosis have low levels of dental caries. It is, therefore, surprising that three cavities were present. A number of factors may have contributed to this. All three teeth had enamel defects and two had been restored with amalgam which had developed secondary caries. Diet analysis revealed a high consumption of sweet drinks between meals, a finding further supported by the degree of erosion present.

The fact that there was some erosion present could be also considered unusual. No studies have specifically examined erosion in children with cystic fibrosis; however, salivary studies have demonstrated higher concentration of salivary bicarbonate and phosphates with consequent increased pH (Kinirons 1985). It would seem that, in this case, the high frequency of acidic drinks negated this protection.

The aims of prevention were to halt further development of oral lesions and to maintain the positive attitude that the patient displayed to dentistry. Ultimately, general anesthesia (GA) was strongly contra-indicated given her respiratory status and it was therefore extremely important not to reach a stage when this was necessary.

The patient was vulnerable to chest infections and her mother was naturally keen to protect her when these developed. This resulted in a number of cancelled appointments, especially during the winter and autumn.

The overall response to treatment was very positive. Compliance both with treatment and preventive messages was excellent and the overall prognosis could be considered very good.

N. Common Complications and Alternative Treatment Plans

- Extensively decayed maxillary left second primary molar and mandibular left second primary molar

- Pulpectomy or extraction if teeth are non-vital with infection. If extracted, space maintenance must be addressed

Self-study Questions

1. **Why do CF patients have a high rate of calculus?**
2. **What two main systems are affected in this condition?**
3. **Studies have shown that caries rates are low in this condition. What reasons have been given for this?**

4. **What precautions are required for treatment under general anesthesia in CF patients?**
5. **What are the long-term complications of CF?**

Answers are located at the end of the case.

Bibliography and Additional Reading

Aps JKM, Van Maele GOG, Martens LC. 2002. Caries experience and oral cleanliness in cystic fibrosis homozygotes and heterozygotes. *Oral Surg Oral Med Oral Pathol Oral Radiol Endod* 93:560–3.

Blomfield J, Warton KL, Brown JM. 1973. Flow rate and inorganic components of submandibular saliva in cystic fibrosis. *Arch of Dis Child* 48:267–74.

Davies JC, Alton EWFW, Bush A. 2007. Cystic fibrosis. *BMJ* 335:1255–9.

Haworth CS. 2010. Impact of cystic fibrosis on bone health. *Curr Opin Pulm Med* 616–22.

Kinirons MJ. 1985. Dental health of children with cystic fibrosis: An interim report. *J Paediatr Dent* 1:3–7.

Kinirons MJ. 1989. Dental health of patients suffering from cystic fibrosis in Northern Ireland. *Community Dent Health* 6:113–20.

Kinirons MJ. 1992. The effect of antibiotic therapy on the oral health of cystic fibrosis children. *Internat J Paediatr Dent* 2:139–43.

Mogayzel PJ Jr, Flume PA. 2011. Update in cystic fibrosis 2010. *Am J Respir Crit Care Med* 183:1620–4.

Narang A, Maguire A, Nunn JH, Bush A. 2003. Oral health and related factors in cystic fibrosis and other chronic respiratory disorders. *Arch Dis Child* 88:702–7.

Turcios NL. 2005. Cystic fibrosis—an overview. *J Clin Gastroenterol* 39:307–17.

SELF-STUDY ANSWERS

1. They have altered amounts of calcium and phosphate in their saliva, which affect calculus formation. However, pancreatin may have a role in decreasing calculus formation and reducing dental caries in these patients

2. Respiratory and gastro-intestinal

3. This fact has been attributed to the long-term antibiotic therapy of these children, high salivary pH, and raised salivary calcium levels

4. The precautions for treatment under general anesthesia are:
   - Avoid general anesthesia if possible
   - Make sure that there are no signs of pulmonary infection. May require sputum culture
   - Chest radiograph

   - Blood gases
   - Pulmonary function testing
   - Vigorous course of pre-op and post-op chest physiotherapy to clear as much of the secretions as possible
   - Check for diabetes (blood glucose) and liver disease (LFTs) pre-op
   - Check current antibiotic regimen
   - Peri-operative frequent suctioning and removal of secretions
   - Nasal polyps are a contra-indication to nasal intubation

5. Long-term complications of CF include diabetes, liver disease, pneumothorax, sinusitis, nasal polyps, osteopenia, failure to thrive, and infertility

Case 3

Hemophilia A

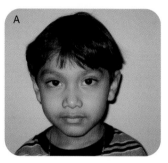 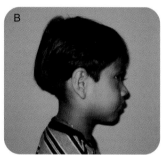

Figure 1.3.1a–b. Facial photographs

A. Presenting Patient
- 4-year-, 2-month-old Hispanic male
- New patient referred by his physician

B. Chief Complaint
- Child states, "My tooth hurts when I eat candy"
- Mother states, "Has only been a problem for one week"

C. Social History
- Patient attends preschool
- Middle class family, married parents, mother is primary caregiver, patient is the only child

D. Medical History
- Severe Hemophilia A
- Two emergency room visits in the past year for injury-associated bleeding (knee and elbow)
- Medications: IV Advate® (recombinant factor VIII) three times a week administered at home by mother
- The patient has no food or drug allergies and his vaccinations are up-to-date

E. Medical Consult
- Hemophilia Team

F. Dental History
- No dental home

- Fair oral hygiene; no adult supervision
- Three meals and two snacks daily. Special snack of candy bar or soda is given as reward after each IV infusion
- Brushes with fluoridated toothpaste once a day
- Lives in optimally fluoridated area
- No history of trauma

G. Extra-oral Examination
- No significant findings

H. Intra-oral Examination
Soft Tissues
- Marginal gingivitis around molars

Hard Tissues
- No significant findings

Occlusal Evaluation of Primary Dentition
- No significant findings

BACKGROUND INFORMATION 1
Hemophilia Management

- Hemophilia occurs in 1 out of every 5,000 males. Hemophilia A (factor VIII deficiency), the most common type (85% of the cases), and hemophilia B (factor IX deficiency) are X-linked recessive traits. Hemophilia C (factor XI deficiency) is an autosomal recessive trait most frequently presenting in Ashkenazi Jews

- Hemophilia presents as impaired secondary hemostasis (stabilization of the platelet plug with fibrin) while primary hemostasis (platelet plug formation) is normal. The disease is classified by level of factor activity (normal: 55% to 100%): severe(<1%), moderate (1% to 5%), and mild (>5%). The activated partial thromboplastin time (aPTT) is usually two to three times the upper limit of normal

- Patients with severe factor deficiencies may bleed spontaneously in muscles, skin, and joints, which may eventually develop arthropy, particularly in the ankles and knees. The incidence of joint pathology is decreased with prophylactic factor administration which is done multiple times a week in cases of moderate and severe hemophilia to increase factor levels to approximately 5%

- For breakthrough bleeds, additional factor replacement is needed together with administration of antifibrinolytic medications such as aminocaproic acid (AMICAR) or tranexamic acid (Cyklokapron). Desmopressin (DDAVP) increases plasma levels of factor VIII and may be useful in mild hemophilia A

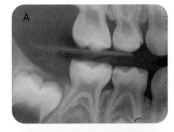
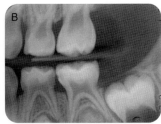
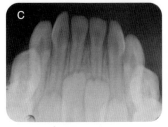
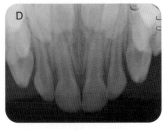

Figure 1.3.2a–d. Pre-op intra-oral radiographs. A. Right bitewing radiograph, B. Left bitewing radiograph, C. mandibular occlusal radiograph, D. Maxillary occlusal radiograph

J. Differential Diagnosis
- N/A

K. Diagnosis and Problem List
Diagnosis
- Severe hemophilia A
- Early childhood caries

Problem List
- High risk of bleeding with invasive dental procedures and nerve blocks
- Untreated caries on the interproximal surfaces of all primary molars and incipient lesions in the maxillary left molars
- High caries risk due to special health care needs, lack of dental home, presence of caries, cariogenic diet, oral hygiene without adult supervision, and visible plaque and radiographic findings

L. Comprehensive Treatment Plan
- Establishment of a dental home and a caries prevention plan
- Prevention of head and oral trauma (helmets and mouth guard)
- Contact hemophilia team for factor management before and after dental care. Plan oral intubation for general anesthesia (GA) to minimize risk of airway trauma, and an aggressive treatment such as restoring all primary molars with stainless steel crowns

Moderate Plaque Accumulation

Enamel Chipping on Incisal Edges of Mandibular Incisors

Intact Dentition on Visual Exam

I. Diagnostic Tools
- Two bitewing radiographs
- Maxillary and mandibular incisor occlusal radiographs
- Interproximal caries noted between molars

Dental Care for Patients with Hemophilia

- Most patients can receive outpatient dental treatment. Appointments should be planned to minimize the need for factor infusions. Treatment under GA in a hospital should be considered for patients with extensive treatment needs and those with moderate or severe hemophilia. Always consult the hemophilia team before any dental work

- Prevention of dental problems is essential

- Avoid iatrogenic trauma to the oral mucosa by careful use of saliva ejectors, rubber dam, Vaseline lubrication of soft tissues, proper impression technique, use of interproximal wedges, and gentle placement of radiograph film, particularly in the sublingual area

- For local anesthesia, careful technique and aspiration are essential

- In general, buccal, intrapapillary, and periodontal ligament infiltrations can be administered without factor replacement

- Due to the risk of dissecting hematoma formation and potential airway compromise, factor replacement should be raised to 30% to 40% before infiltration into a highly vascular area or loose connective tissue as well as before posterior superior alveolar or inferior alveolar nerve blocks

- Pulp treatment usually presents a low risk of bleeding and is generally preferable to extractions

- Factor replacement is needed for subgingival scaling. Periodontal surgery can be a great challenge to hemostasis

- Fixed or removable orthodontic appliances can be used. Minimize gingival trauma when fitting bands and cementing appliances

For Surgical Procedures

- Carry out treatment as atraumatically as possible

- Observe patients for a prolonged period of time post-surgery; consider hospitalization in moderate/severe cases

- Use local hemostatic agents: pressure, absorbable gelatin product, cellulose materials, thrombin, microfibrillar collagen, fibrin glue, cyanoacrylate, acrylic stents, bone wax, electrocautery, resorbable sutures, periodontal dressings, and epinephrine

- Bleeding can be aggravated by aspirin and other non-steroidal anti-inflammatory drugs. Codeine and acetaminophen are safe alternatives.

- Any swelling, rapid breathing, dysphagia, or hoarseness may be a sign of airway compromise caused by intubation and/or dental treatment. Patient should be sent to the hospital immediately for advanced airway management and the hematologist should be consulted.

- Schedule a follow-up dental appointment in two weeks to check for complications and to reinforce prevention plan
- Three month recall

M. Prognosis and Discussion

- Risk for future caries is high. Prognosis could be improved by establishing a dental home, improving dietary and hygiene habits, and frequent recall visits

N. Complications and Alternative Treatment Plan

- Hemophilia cases with inhibitors present a management challenge because bleeding episodes continue despite appropriate factor replacement. Inhibitors are factor-specific antibodies which develop in 25% to 35% of patients with hemophilia A and 3% to 5% of patients with hemophilia B. In such cases, dental care should be consolidated into one treatment session and may include use of a bypassing agent such as factor VIIa or activated prothrombin complex concentrate.

- The patient should be admitted post-operatively because complications may arise such as a compromised airway and bleeding from trauma to the maxillary midline frenum which may be managed by local and/or systemic measures.

Self-study Questions

1. Which laboratory screening test is affected by a reduced level of factor VIII or factor IX?

2. In addition to pre- and post-operative medications, what are special considerations for treatment under general anesthesia for patients with hemophilia?

3. Which analgesic medications are contra-indicated for a patient with a bleeding disorder and why?

4. What is the significance of inhibitors in hemophilia?

5. What local anesthesia techniques should be done only after factor replacement?

Answers are located at the end of the case.

Bibliography and Additional Reading

Brewer A, Correa ME. 2006. Treatment of hemophilia. *Guidelines for Dental Treatment of Patients with Inherited Bleeding Disorders*. Dental Committee, World Federation of Hemophilia. 40:1–9. Access at: www.wfh.org.

Sanders BJ, Shapiro AD, Hock RA, Weddell JA, Belcher CE. 2004. Management of the Medically Compromised Patient: Hematologic Disorders, Cancer, Hepatitis, and AIDS. In *Dentistry for the Child and Adolescent*, 8th ed. McDonald RE, Avery DR, Dean JA (eds), Mosby: St. Louis. pp.559–64.

Scott JP, Montgomery RR. 2007. Hereditary Clotting Factor Deficiencies (Bleeding Disorders). In *Nelson Textbook of Pediatrics*, 18th ed. Kliegman RM, Behrman RE, Jenson HB, Stanton BR. Saunders Elsevier: Philadelphia. Chapter 476. pp. 2066–9.

Scully C, Dios PD, Giangrande P, Lee C. 2002. Treatment of hemophilia. *Oral Care for People with Hemophilia or a Hereditary Bleeding Tendency*. World Federation of Hemophilia. 27:1–11. Access at: www.wfh.org.

Stubbs M, Lloyd J. 2001. A protocol for the dental management of Von Willebrand's disease, haemophilia A and haemophilia B. *Aust Dent J* 46:37–40.

SELF-STUDY ANSWERS

1. The activated partial thromboplastin time (aPTT) is usually two to three times the upper limit of normal

2. Nasotracheal intubation is contraindicated due to increased risk of airway trauma. Treatment venue is more appropriately in a hospital rather than in-office

3. Aspirin and nonsteroidal anti-inflammatory medications adversely impact hemostasis due to platelet inhibition

4. Bleeding episodes continue despite appropriate factor replacement levels. Care for these patients may include use of a bypassing agent such as factor VIIa or activated prothrombin complex concentrate

5. Infiltrations into a highly vascularized area or into loose connective tissue, and posterior superior alveolar and inferior alveolar nerve blocks.

Case 4

T Cell Lymphoblastic Leukemia/Chemotherapy

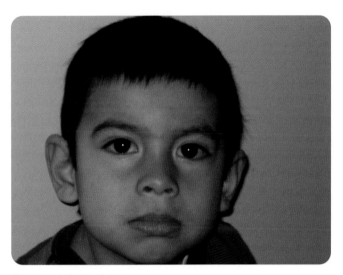

Figure 1.4.1. Facial photograph

A. Presenting Patient
- 3-year-, 4-month-old Caucasian male

B. Chief Complaint
- Referred by hospital oncology unit for dental assessment and management of oro-facial cellulitis

C. Social History
- Two-parent, middle class family unit, one sibling, mother is primary caregiver

D. Medical History
- Cell lymphoblastic leukemia
- Influenza A positive
- Norovirus positive
- No known food or drug allergies
- Vaccinations up to date

Current Medications
- Chemotherapy and supportive therapy (on Children's Oncology Group study): Five-week induction, five-week consolidation, eight-week

BACKGROUND INFORMATION 1
Acute Lymphoblastic Leukemia (ALL)
- Accounts for 80% to 85% of acute childhood leukemias with a peak incidence at four years of age
- Defined by the presence of more than 25% lymphoblasts in the bone marrow
- The most common signs and symptoms are anorexia, irritability, lethargy, anemia, bleeding (including oral), petechiae, fever, lymphadenopathy, splenomegaly, hepatomegaly, and bone pain
- The most common head, neck, and intraoral manifestations of leukemias are sore throat, lymphadenopathy, laryngeal pain, gingival bleeding, and oral ulceration
- Therapy is tailored to the risk of relapse dependent on cytogenetic markers, and includes a combination of induction chemotherapy, central nervous system prophylaxis, and maintenance chemotherapy for 2.5 to 3.5 years
- Intrathecal therapy (commonly methotrexate) has been used to replace cranial irradiation
- Cure rates for standard risk ALL are now over 90% on current protocols. If relapse occurs, 40% to 50% can be cured with chemotherapy and/or hematopoietic stem cell transplantation, which is reserved for very-high-risk or relapse patients
- Prognosis depends on age of onset, initial white cell count, cytogenetic abnormalities, and other features

interim maintenance, seven-week delayed intensification, reinduction if required, 12-week maintenance

- Multiple medications including Vincristine, Methotrexate, Prednisone

E. Medical Consult

Oncology Team

- Gather information about the underlying disease, time of diagnosis, modalities of treatment the patient has received since the diagnosis, planned treatment, surgeries, complications, prognosis, current hematological status, allergies, and medications
- Baseline complete blood count (CBC)
  - Platelets 81,000/mm3 (normal: 150,00 to 400,000)
  - White blood cells 4,100/mm3 (5,000 to 15,000)
  - Absolute neutrophil count (ANC) 2,600/mm3 (1,500 to 8,000)
  - Red blood cells 4.16×10^{12}/L (4 to 5.2)
  - Hematocrit 34% (34% to 40%)
  - Hemoglobin: 11.2 g/dL (11.5 to 13.5)

F. Dental History

- No dental home
- Good oral hygiene with supervision
- Cariogenic diet with high caloric supplementation to increase body weight
- Brushes once daily with fluoridated toothpaste
- Lives in an area without fluoridation
- No previous trauma history
- Behavior assessment: uncooperative for routine dental treatment

G. Extra-oral Exam

- No significant findings

H. Intra-oral Exam

Soft Tissues

- Localized marginal gingivitis with bleeding

Hard Tissues

- No significant findings

Occlusal Evaluation of the Primary Dentition

- Flush terminal plane
- Canines class I
- Anterior tooth contact on closure

Other

Multiple carious lesions on visual exam: Maxillary left first molar, maxillary right first molar, maxillary anterior teeth

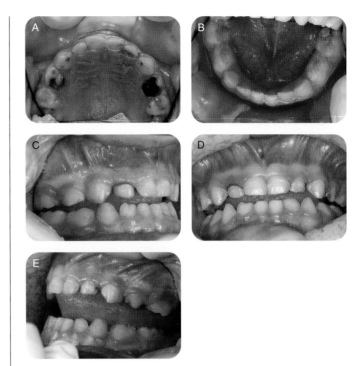

Figure 1.4.2a–e. Pre-op intra-oral photos

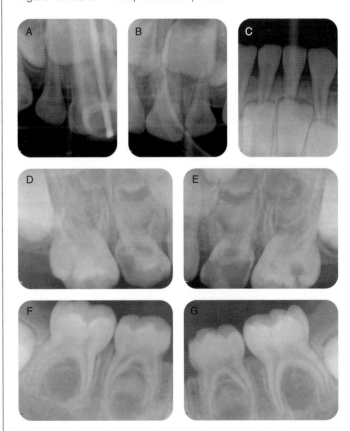

Figure 1.4.3a–g. Pre-op Intra-oral radiographs. A. Right maxillary occlusal radiograph, B. left maxillary occlusal radiograph, C. mandibular occlusal radiograph, D. right maxillary periapical radiograph, E. left maxillary periapical radiograph, F. right mandibular periapical radiograph, G. left mandibular periapical radiograph

- Fissure discolorations on molars
- Smooth surface demineralization on maxillary molars

I. Diagnostic Tools

- Intra-oral periapical films taken at time of dental care under general anesthesia

J. Differential Diagnosis

Developmental

- Enamel hypoplasia
- Enamel hypomineralization

Infective

- Bacterial
- Fungal

Odontogenic

- Loss of tooth structure
- Dental caries
- Attrition/abrasion/erosion

Inflammatory

- Pulpal pathology
- Oro-facial cellulitis

K. Diagnosis and Problem List

Diagnosis

- Active early childhood caries
- Acute apical periodontitis
- Facial cellulitis due to odontogenic infection

Problem List

- High caries risk due to:
  - Special health needs
  - Visible cavitations
  - Enamel demineralizations
  - Visible plaque
  - Cariogenic diet (>3 sugar exposures/day)
  - Usage of medications that impair salivary flow
  - Lack of fluoridated water and fluoride supplements
- Limited understanding of potential medical complications by parent
- High risk of oral sepsis and subsequent medical complications

L. Comprehensive Treatment Plan

- Explain importance of maintaining optimal oral health for children with acute lymphoblastic leukemia (ALL) being treated by chemotherapy (see Fundamental Point 1).

- Explain oral health care protocol (mucositis care), the risk of oral sepsis complicating medical management, and long-term oro-dental effects from therapy
- Caries control with antimicrobial therapy prior to surgical management
  - Prescribe 0.2% chlorhexidine gel application four times daily prior to procedure but avoid using alcohol-containing products when mucositis is present (it will sting and burn the mucosal tissues)
- Remove any potentially/pulpally involved teeth
- Remove any sources of tissue irritation
- Establish a caries prevention plan as well as a dental home
- Restore multi-surface caries lesions with stainless steel crowns due to their longevity and ability to prevent further caries progression
- Apply sealant on discolored molar fissures
- Apply fluoride varnish on demineralized areas
- Administer IV antibiotic prophylaxis at time of dental treatment to reduce risk of bacteremia if the patient is immunosuppressed and treatment cannot be delayed
- Address behavior management considerations
  - Provide comprehensive dental treatment under GA to facilitate all necessary procedures at the one time and to avoid delaying the cancer therapy. This can be done concurrently with other medical procedures such as lumbar puncture and bone marrow aspiration, if required

Post-op and Home Care Instructions

- Discharge after full recovery
- Soft, cold diet for 48 hours
- Recommence toothbrushing in 24 hours

Prevention Plan

- Recall plan
  - Six weeks post-op
  - Four-month review during chemotherapy
- Apply fluoride varnish to demineralized areas at both visits

M. Prognosis and Discussion

- Prognosis for limiting caries progression is fair in view of understanding of caries risk factors and potential medical complications by parent. However, the burden of a cancer diagnosis and all

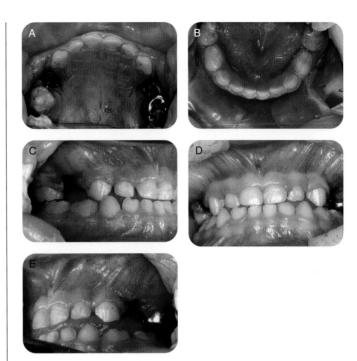

Figure 1.4.4a–e. Post-op intra-oral photos

of its complex treatment may push oral/dental care to a low priority status. Indulgence of the sick child with sweet candies and liquids can also be a problem.

- Prognosis for changing current dietary habits is uncertain in view of the difficulty in maintaining adequate nutrition during chemotherapy.

N. Common Complications and Alternative Treatment Plans

- Non-compliance with dietary advice
- Post-operative bleeding or infection
- Continued caries progression
- Acute and long-term oral complications related to chemotherapy (see Background Information 2)

Alternative Treatment Plans May Include:

- Alternative restorative materials, e.g., composite resin, amalgam, glass ionomers
- Alternative pulpal management, e.g., extraction vs. pulp therapy in posterior teeth (must consider risks of chronic bacteremia)
- Alternative methods for behavior management
- Nitrous oxide vs. outpatient sedation vs. GA vs. nothing

FUNDAMENTAL POINT 2
Dental Treatment During Cancer Treatment

- Ideally, all dental care should be completed before cancer therapy starts. When that is not possible, prioritize procedures and place temporary restorations until the patient is stable

- Infections, extractions, scaling, and sources of tissue irritation should be taken care of first, followed by carious teeth, root canal therapy, and replacement of faulty restorations. The risk of pulpal infection and pain determines which carious lesions should be treated first

- A complete blood count (CBC), including the absolute neutrophil count (ANC), is necessary before dental procedures

- Elective dental treatment should be delayed when the child is immunocompromised, i.e., the ANC is <1,000, although some oncology teams allow for invasive dental care to be done at ANC >500. In emergency cases, discuss antibiotic prophylaxis with the patient's physician before proceeding

- Because many acute lymphoblastic leukemia (ALL) patients have also been receiving systemic corticosteroids, the possibility of adrenocortical suppression should be considered and additional steroid cover provided as appropriate

- Primary teeth in need of pulpal therapy during the induction and consolidation phase of chemotherapy should be considered for extraction due to possibility of failure of the pulp treatment, which will lead to an odontogenic infection

- When pulpal therapy of permanent teeth is needed, the risk of bacteremia and potential septicemia must be weighed against the potential benefits of tooth conservation

- Braces should be removed if the patient has poor oral hygiene or is at risk for the development of moderate/severe mucositis. Smooth, well-fitting appliances (e.g., band and loops) can be kept if the patient has good oral hygiene

- Root tips, teeth with periodontal pockets >6mm, teeth with acute infection, significant bone loss, involvement of furcation, symptomatic impacted teeth, and non-restorable teeth should be removed at least seven to 10 days prior to initiation of therapy.

- A platelet count >75,000/mm^3 does not require additional support, but be prepared to treat prolonged bleeding with local measures after oral surgical procedures

- If the platelet count is <75,000/mm^3 and invasive procedures need to be carried out, consult with the physician before providing care

- Coagulation tests may be in order for individual patients, especially those with liver disease or coagulation problems

- Consult an experienced oral surgeon before oral surgical procedures in patients who have had or are currently on head and neck irradiation and/or bisphosphonates, given the risk of jaw necrosis

- Children in full remission can be treated routinely, although a CBC is prudent if an invasive procedure is planned

- There is no evidence to support the administration of antibiotic prophylaxis to prevent catheter-related infections associated with an invasive oral procedure in patients with chronic indwelling central venous catheters

BACKGROUND INFORMATION 2

Acute and Long-Term Effects of Chemotherapy on the Craniofacial Complex

- The cytotoxic drugs used during chemotherapy can cause damage to several body organs, including the craniofacial complex
- Neutropenia is defined as <1,500 neutrophils/mm^3 and can predispose the child to oral sepsis by commensal organisms
- Direct stomato-toxicity is caused by the cytotoxic action of the chemotherapeutic agents on oral mucosal cells leading to inflammation, thinning, and ulceration of the mucosa (mucositis)
- Recent case reports suggest that the incidence and severity of mucositis, the most common and painful side effect of chemotherapy, may be reduced with the concomitant administration of granulocyte colony stimulating factor (G-CSF) during chemotherapy
- Salivary function may also be diminished, although this response has not been reported as common in children
- Other acute oral side effects of chemotherapy include secondary infections, bleeding, and neurotoxicity
- These problems are commonly encountered in the induction and consolidation phases of chemotherapy when relative high doses of multi-agent therapy are employed
- Children younger than 10 years of age who receive chemotherapy and/or radiotherapy (total body irradiation or localized radiotherapy to the head and neck) may present dental developmental defects such as tooth agenesis; short, tapered roots; early apical closure; crown disturbances in size and shape; microdontia; enlarged pulp chambers; and dentin and enamel opacities and defects

Self-study Questions

1. What important questions need to be asked when taking a medical history from a patient with ALL?
2. What are some common side effects of chemotherapy?
3. Why are children with neutropenia at risk of oral sepsis?
4. How would non-compliance with preventive advice alter treatment planning?
5. How would management differ if the child had a poor medical prognosis?

Answers are located at the end of the case.

Bibliography and Additional Reading

Baddour LM, Bettmann MA, Bolger AF, et al. 2003. Nonvalvular cardiovascular device-related infections. *Circulation* 108:2015–31.

da Fonseca MA. 2004. Dental care of the pediatric cancer patient. *Pediatr Dent* 26:53–7.

da Fonseca MA. 1998. Pediatric bone marrow transplantation: oral complications and recommendations for care. *Pediatr Dent* 20:386–94.

da Fonseca MA. 2000. Long-term oral and craniofacial complications following pediatric bone marrow transplantation. *Pediatr Dent* 22:57–62.

Dahllof G. 1998. Craniofacial growth in children treated for malignant diseases. *Acta Odontol Scand* 56:378–82.

Goho C. 1993. Chemoradiation therapy: effect on dental development. *Pediatr Dent* 15:6–12.

Gotzche PC, Johansen HK. 2002. Nystatin prophylaxis and treatment in severely immunocompromised patients. *Cochrane Database Syst Rev* 2:CD002033.

Hallett KB. 2003. Medically compromised children. In *Handbook of Pediatric Dentistry*, 2nd ed. Cameron AC and Widmer RP (eds), Mosby: London.

Hong CHL, Allred R, Napenas JJ, et al. 2010. Antibiotic prophylaxis for dental procedures to prevent indwelling catheter-related infections. *Am J Medic* 123:1128–33.

Hong CH, Brennan MT, Lockhart PB. 2009. Incidence of acute oral sequelae in pediatric patients undergoing chemotherapy. *Pediatr Dent* 31:420–5.

Hong CH, da Fonseca M. 2008. Considerations in the pediatric population with cancer. *Dent Clin North Amer* 52:155–81.

Hou GL, Huang JS, Tsai CC. 1997. Analysis of oral manifestations of leukemia: A retrospective study. *Oral Dis* 3:31–8.

www.mascc.org

SELF-STUDY ANSWERS

1. Questions regarding the underlying disease, time of diagnosis, modalities of treatment the patient has received since the diagnosis, planned treatment, surgeries, complications, prognosis, current hematological status, allergies and medications

2. Mucositis, opportunistic infections, oral bleeding, salivary dysfunction, and neurotoxicity

3. They do not have enough neutrophils to defend them from an infection

4. Non-compliance with preventive measures such as daily oral hygiene would indicate a poor prognosis for minimizing adverse long-term oro-dental effects such as enamel demineralization and high caries rates

5. Management of children with a poor prognosis is generally palliative or symptomatic relief of pain and oral discomfort

Case 5

Liver Transplant

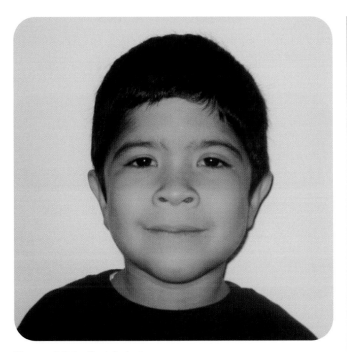

Figure. 1.5.1. Facial photo

A. Presenting Patient
- 4-year-, 11-month-old Caucasian male

B. Chief Complaint
- New patient referred by pediatric gastroenterology for dental assessment and treatment
- Mother noted decayed teeth but no symptoms
- Mother states that teeth have always been somewhat discolored but she is not concerned

C. Social History
- Lives at home with 6-year-old sibling and parents
- Middle class family

D. Medical History
- Biliary atresia, liver transplant at 13 months of age
- Medications: Tacrolimus 0.8 mg twice daily and Prednisolone 1 mg daily

- Frequent hospitalizations and hospital visits since birth for management of biliary atresia and liver transplant
- Allergic to eggs and nuts, no known drug allergies
- Vaccinations are up to date, including measles, mumps, and rubella, which is a live vaccine that was administered before the transplant when the patient was immunocompetent

E. Medical Consult
Pediatric Gastroenterologist
- All tests (liver function, urea and electrolytes, blood pressure) were within normal range for this patient

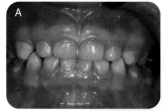
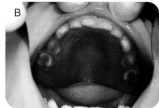
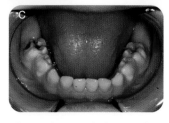

Figure 1.5.2a–c. Pre-op intra-oral photos. A. Anterior view, B. maxillary view, C. mandibular view

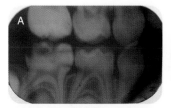
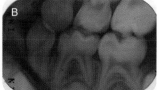
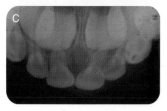

Figure 1.5.3a–c. Pre-op radiographs. A. Right bitewing radiograph, B. Left bitewing radiograph, C. Maxillary occlusal radiograph

BACKGROUND INFORMATION 1
Liver Function and Disorders
Some Important Functions of the Liver

- Metabolism of carbohydrates, lipids, and proteins
- Metabolism of drugs (detoxification) prior to excretion
- Synthesis of plasma protein (albumin) and clotting factors
- Storage organ for glycogen, vitamin B_{12}, and iron
- Breaks down hemoglobin; bilirubin and biliverdin are added to bile as pigment

Most Common Indications for Pediatric Liver Transplantation

- Chronic liver disease
  - Biliary atresia (most common reason for pediatric liver transplantation)
  - Alpha-1 antitrypsin deficiency
  - Autoimmune hepatitis
- Metabolic liver disease with extra-hepatic complications
  - Crigler-Najjar syndrome
  - Urea cycle defects
- Acute liver failure
- Hepatic tumors

F. Dental History

- No dental home
- Drank juices from a bottle until 4 years old
- Fair oral hygiene with parental supervision
- Uses toothpaste containing fluoride
- Optimal water fluoridation levels
- No history of dental trauma
- Asymptomatic dental decay

G. Extra-oral Exam

- No significant findings

H. Intra-oral Exam

- Soft and hard tissues: no significant findings
- Occlusal evaluation of primary dentition: class I canines and mesial step molars
- No visible plaque
- Carious lesions on primary molars

- Greenish discoloration of teeth consistent with history of biliary atresia
- Possible enamel hypomineralization and/or hypoplasia of mandibular right primary second molars with post-eruptive breakdown and caries
- Erosion of palatal surfaces of maxillary anterior teeth
- Cooperative for examination and radiographs

I. Diagnostic Tools

- Radiographs confirm extensive and deep decay involving mandibular right primary second molar

J. Differential Diagnosis

- Hemolytic disease of newborn
- Amelogenesis imperfecta
- Dentinogenesis imperfecta

- Coronal dentin dysplasia (Shields type II)
- Congenital porphyria

K. Diagnosis and Problem List

Diagnosis

- Early childhood caries
- Liver transplant
- Possible enamel hypomineralization and/or hypoplasia of mandibular right primary second molars with post-eruptive breakdown and caries
- Erosion of palatal surfaces of maxillary anterior teeth
- Intrinsic staining of teeth due to incorporation of unconjugated bile pigments in calcifying dental tissues

Problem List

- High caries risk due to:
  - Use of juice in a bottle until 4 years of age
  - Hospitalization as infant and young child due to biliary atresia

- Need for daily ingestion of medications
- Possible enamel hypomineralization/hypoplasia of mandibular primary second molars
- Special health care needs
- No dental home
- Untreated caries
- Immunosuppressant therapy to prevent rejection of liver transplant
- Significant dental treatment required in a 4-year-old with history of extensive medical intervention since birth

L. Comprehensive Treatment Plan

Establishment of a Caries Prevention Plan as well as a Dental Home
Comprehensive Dental Treatment Under General Anesthesia (GA)

- Intravenous administration of hydrocortisone 25 mg at time of induction because of long-term steroid use

---

FUNDAMENTAL POINT 2
Dental Treatment Considerations in a Child with Liver Disease

- Decreased metabolism (detoxification) of many drugs including lidocaine: administer less than maximum recommended dose of local anesthetic (lidocaine <4.4 mg/kg)

- Decreased metabolism (detoxification) of general anesthetic and sedative agents: except for nitrous oxide/oxygen analgesia/anxiolysis, the use of sedation or general anesthesia should be restricted to specialist hospital units

- Decreased production of vitamin-K-dependent blood clotting factors (II, VII, IX, X): Increased potential for post extraction bleeding

- Enlargement of spleen may cause platelet sequestration with associated low platelet count: Increased potential for post extraction bleeding

- Local measures to control post-extraction bleeding include the use of oxidized regenerated cellulose (Surgicel or Gelfoam) and the use of resorbable sutures

- Hematology consult if platelet count <75,000/mm^3: Consider platelet transfusion to prevent prolonged bleeding

- Varices (enlarged blood vessels) at base of esophagus due to obstruction of blood flow to diseased liver: Chronic gastrointestinal hemorrhage may result in anemia

- Greenish discoloration of teeth due to incorporation of unconjugated bile pigments, especially biliverdin, during period of calcification of teeth

- Yellow discoloration of skin and mucosa (jaundice) due to presence of unconjugated bilirubin in the tissues

- Do not use nonsteroidal anti-inflammatory drugs (NSAIDS) for analgesia because they increase the risk of gastrointestinal bleeding

- Use acetaminophen in reduced dosage for analgesia because high doses are hepatotoxic

---

- Stainless steel crown (SSC) restoration of mandibular right primary second molars following caries removal
- High-strength glass ionomer or composite resin restorations of occlusal lesions in both maxillary primary second molars and mandibular primary first molars
- Post-operative pain relief with acetaminophen 500 mg as a suppository and intra-oral buccal infiltration of 0.5 ml 2% lidocaine with epinephrine

Follow-up Care
- Post-operative and home care instructions
- Establishment of a frequent recall schedule

M. Prognosis and Discussion
Good Prognosis if Aggressive Preventive Plan is Established and Consistent Home and Professional Dental Care is Provided
- Three-month dental recall visits
- Fluoride varnish application biannually

- Fissure sealant application to the permanent first molars when erupted sufficiently to allow isolation for moisture control
- Promotion of twice daily toothbrushing with fluoride toothpaste and restriction in the frequency of ingestion of sugary drinks/juices and sugary snack foods

N. Common Complications and Alternative Treatment Plans
Extensively Decayed Mandibular Right Second Primary Molar
- Vital pulpotomy and SSC if pulp exposure
- Extraction of tooth if non-vital with infection and subsequent space management/maintenance when permanent first molar erupts

Distal Shoe Appliance Relatively Contraindicated in View of Immunosuppression

Long-term Complications of Steroid and Immunosuppression Agents with Dental Implications: Gingival Overgrowth, High Blood Pressure, Osteoporosis, etc.

FUNDAMENTAL POINT 3

Dental Management of Child Before Liver Transplantation

- Prevention: Educate child and caretakers on the importance of optimal oral care at time of transplantation and afterwards
- Treat/stabilize active dental decay so that the teeth will not be a potential source of infection at the time of transplantation and for the following three to six months
- Extract extensively decayed teeth and teeth with pulp or potential pulp pathology
- Consult the pediatric gastroenterology team: seek advice on coagulation status and ensure a platelet count of >75,000/ml³ before extracting teeth

Dental Management Following Liver Transplantation

- Regular dental visits for preventive and ongoing care from six months following transplant
- Immunosuppression issues
- Scrupulous cross-infection control measures
- Decreased immunosurveillance

- Increased risk of lymphomas (non-Hodgkins lymphomas or post-transplant lymphoproliferative disease)
- Increased risk of skin cancer: Reinforce safety in sun and the use of sunscreen with high sun protection factor
- Cyclosporine with/without the antihypertensive drug nifedipine may cause gingival hyperplasia and delayed eruption of teeth
- No gingival problems with tacrolimus, which is an alternative to cyclosporine
- Caution with use of NSAIDs for analgesia because these may increase the nephrotoxicity of cyclosporine and tacrolimus
- Glucocorticoids may be used in low dosage as immunosuppressant: Additional dosage not usually required tor dental treatment unless treatment provided under general anesthesia
- Azathioprine and mycophenolate mofetil are other immunosuppressant drugs that may be used following solid organ transplantation. They have no specific oral or dental side effects

Self-study Questions

1. *What is the most common liver disease in children that requires transplantation?*
2. *What is the most likely cause of greenish staining of teeth in children with liver disease?*
3. *What is the minimum platelet count that is recommended for dental extractions?*
4. *What analgesic should be prescribed with caution in children with liver disease and why?*
5. *What immunosuppressant medication may induce gingival hyperplasia?*

Answers are located at the end of the case.

Bibliography and Additional Reading

Golla K, Epstein JB, Cabay RJ. 2004. Liver disease: current perspectives on medical and dental treatment. *Oral Surg Oral Med Oral Pathol Oral Radiol Endod* 98:516–21.

Greenwood M, Meechan JG. 2003. General medicine and surgery for dental practitioners; Part 5: Liver disease. *Brit Dent J* 195:71–3.

Guggenheimer J, Eghtesad B, Stock DB. 2003. Dental management of the (solid) organ transplant patient. *Oral Surg Oral Med Oral Pathol Oral Radiol Endod* 95:383–9.

Schör K. 2007. Aspirin and Reye's syndrome—a review of the evidence. *Pediatr Drugs* 9:195–204.

Seow WK, Shepherd RW, Ong TH. 1991. Oral changes associated with end-stage liver disease and liver transplantation: implications for dental management. *J Dent Child* 58:474–80.

Sheehy EC, Heaton N, Smith P, Roberts GJ. 1999. Dental management of children undergoing liver transplantation. *Pediatr Dent* 21:273–81.

Wondimu B, Nemeth A, Modeer T. 2001. Oral health in liver transplant children administered Cyclosporine A or Tacrolimus. *Intern J of Paediatr Dent* 11:424–9.

SELF-STUDY ANSWERS

1. Biliary atresia
2. The incorporation of unconjugated bile pigments, especially biliverdin, during the period of calcification of teeth
3. 75,000/mm^3
4. Acetaminophen should be prescribed in reduced dosages for analgesia in children with liver disease because high doses may be hepatotoxic
5. Cyclosporin

Case 6

Chronic Benign Neutropenia

A. Presenting Patient
- 10-year-, 11-month-old Caucasian male

B. Chief Complaint
- New patient referred by pediatric hematologist with concerns about gingival inflammation.
- Mother states that "his gums are red and bleed during brushing."

C. Social History
- Lives at home with his parents
- Middle class family
- No siblings

D. Medical History
- Chronic benign neutropenia (absolute neutrophil count [ANC] of 300 cells/mm^3 at time of diagnosis)
- Chronic lower respiratory tract infection
- Medications: Azithromycin 250 mg oral prophylaxis on alternate days
- Granulocyte–colony stimulating factor (G-CSF) subcutaneous administration twice weekly
- Hospitalizations: Parenteral antibiotics and physiotherapy for management of recurrent pneumonia. Recent surgical resection of chronically infected lower lobe of left lung
- ANC today: 2,100 cells/mm^3 (see Fundamental Point 1)
- No known allergies to medications or foods
- Vaccinations up to date

E. Medical Consult
- Pediatric hematologist to confirm medical history and advise about any special precautions when providing dental treatment

F. Dental History
- Regular visits to a general dentist for routine care, including management of hypomineralized permanent first molars

BACKGROUND INFORMATION 1
Immunological Defects and Susceptibility to Infection
- An immunocompromised child has one or more defects of the immune system that are sufficiently severe to predispose him to life-threatening infection. A deficiency in the number or quality of phagocytic cells, humoral immunity (immunoglobulin and complement), or cell-mediated immunity is associated with an increased risk of infection by certain pathogens, depending on the type of defect. It is important to remember that immunological defects rarely exist in isolation and frequently there is more than one defect present

Infections in Children With Neutropenia or With Disorders of Neutrophil Function
- Patients are particularly susceptible to recurrent and severe bacterial or fungal infections of the lungs, paranasal sinuses, oropharynx and skin
- They are also susceptible to overwhelming infection, including those of dental origin
  See Table 1.6.1: Pathogens and immunological defects

- Brushes teeth twice each day with parental supervision
- Healthy low-cariogenic diet
- Uses toothpaste containing fluoride
- Optimal water fluoridation

G. Extra-oral Examination
- No significant findings

Table 1.6.1. Pathogens and immunological defects

Abnormality	Bacterial	Fungal	Viral	Protozoal
Neutropenia or qualitative defects of phagocytes	Gram-positive Staphylococci (coagulase positive and negative) Streptococci (enterococcus and *á*-hemolytic) Gram-negative *E.coli K.pneumoniae* *P. aeroginosa* Other Enterobacteriaceae	Candida spp Aspergillus spp		
Defective cell-mediated immunity	*Legionella* *Salmonella* Mycobacteria	Histoplasma capsulatum Cryptococcus neoformans Candida Aspergillus	Cytomegalovirus Varicella-zoster Herpes simplex Epstein-Barr Live viral vaccines (measles, mumps, rubella, polio)	*P. carinii* *T. gondii* Cryptosporidia
Immunoglobulin deficiency	*S. pneumoniae* *H. influenzae*		Enteroviruses	Giardia
Complement deficiency	*S. pneumoniae* *H. influenzae* Neisseria species			
Splenectomy	*S. pneumoniae* *H. influenzae* Neisseria species			Babesia

Reprinted from Reich, et al. 2003, with permission from Elsevier Publishing Ltd.

H. Intra-oral Examination

Soft Tissues

- Gingivitis, especially around mandibular and maxillary incisors

Bone Tissues

- No significant findings

Occlusal Evaluation of Mixed Dentition

- Class 1 molar relationship with crowding in the canine and premolar regions, more severe in the maxillary arch; overjet: 3 mm, overbite: 80%. There is a mandibular midline shift to the left associated with premature exfoliation of the mandibular left primary first molar (see Figure 1.6.1)

Dental Exam

- Minimal visible plaque with significant gingivitis
- Enamel hypomineralization affecting the permanent first molars with opacities on the labial surface of two permanent incisors
- Defective restoration of mandibular right permanent first molar and mandibular left primary second molar

I. Diagnostic Tools

Panoramic Radiograph (Exposed Six Months Before This Examination) (Figure 1.6.2)

- Unerupted premolars and permanent cuspids show insufficient space to erupt in good alignment. All permanent teeth, including permanent third molars, are present.
- The decayed and hypomineralized maxillary right permanent first molar has been restored since the radiograph was exposed. The restorations of the mandibular right permanent first molar and mandibular left primary second molar are defective and are scheduled for restoration by the local dentist

J. Differential Diagnosis

Gingivitis Due to:

- Poor plaque control
- Incompetent lips/mouth breathing causing drying of gingiva
- Crohn's disease (inflammatory bowel disease)

FUNDAMENTAL POINT 1
Neutropenia

- Neutrophils and monocytes are phagocytic cells that function within the body as the chief defense against infection by bacteria and fungi

- The neutrophil is the predominant phagocytic cell in the peripheral circulation

- Neutrophils have a major role in protecting those surfaces of the body that are in direct contact with the external environment

- The absolute neutrophil count (ANC) is a measure of the number of neutrophils in the blood.

- ANC values can determine what procedures can safely be performed
  - 1,500 to 8,000 cells/mm^3 is normal
  - 500 to 1,500 is safe (no restrictions)
  - 500 or less is low (restrictions apply)

- The normal lower limit for circulating neutrophils is 1,500 to 2,000 cells/mm^3. Severe neutropenia occurs with an ANC below 500 cells/mm^3, which puts the patient at risk of serious infection, including those of oral origin. With an ANC of 100 cells/mm^3 there is a dramatic increase in the incidence of severe infection.

Causes of Neutropenia
Different Diseases May Result in Low Numbers or Absence of Neutrophils. The Causes of Neutropenia In Children Include:

Neutropenias Present at Birth

- Severe congenital neutropenia (Kostmann syndrome) with associated severe periodontitis

- Cyclic neutropenia. Primary cyclic (every 21 days) decrease in maturation of precursor cells in bone marrow with recurring fever, skin infections, oropharyngeal disease, and periodontitis

- Neutropenia in association with a primary immunodeficiency

- Neutropenia in association with a metabolic disorder (Shwachmann-Diamond syndrome and Glycogen–storage disease type 1b)

- Neutropenia as part of certain syndromes (pancytopenia in Fanconi's anemia; dyskeratosis congenita with progressive marrow failure)

Neutropenias Acquired During Life

- Idiopathic neutropenia
- Autoimmune neutropenia
- Chronic benign neutropenia
- Hematological dysplasias and malignancies
- Solid tumor invasion of bone marrow
- Cancer chemotherapy and radiotherapy
- Drug toxicity
- Viral infections

Qualitative Defects of Phagocytes With a Normal Number of Neutrophils Occur in the Following Inherited Conditions:

- Chronic granulomatous disease (CGD)
- Leucocyte adhesion deficiency (LAD)

BACKGROUND INFORMATION 2
Medical Management of Neutropenia

Medical Management Depends on its Cause and Severity. The Primary Goal is to Prevent Infection With:

- Prophylactic antibiotics
- Granulocyte–Colony Stimulating Factor (G-CSF)
- Interferon gamma (IFN-γ) for management of chronic granulomatous disease (which presents a normal number of neutrophils but with a functional defect)

- Hematopoietic stem cell transplant (e.g., for Kostmann and Shwachmann-Diamond syndromes because of high risk of developing acute myeloid leukaemia; for chronic granulomatous disease, transplant is done to prevent life-threatening infection)

- Immunoglobulin and steroid therapy

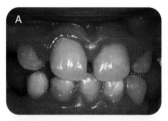
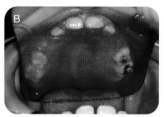
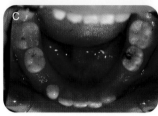

Figure 1.6.1a–c. Pre-op intra-oral photos. A. Anterior, B. maxillary, C. mandibular

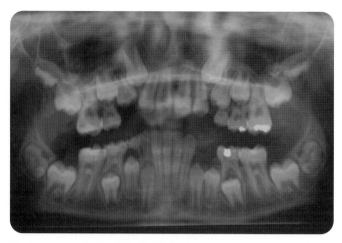

Figure 1.6.2. Panoramic radiograph

FUNDAMENTAL POINT 2
Oral Manifestations of Neutropenia or Disorders of Neutrophil Function

- Gingivitis
- Periodontitis
- Oral ulceration

- Prepubertal periodontitis
- Primary immunodeficiency disease
- HIV/AIDS
- Hematological dysplasia or malignancy
- Chemotherapy
- Poorly controlled diabetes mellitus

Hypomineralized Permanent First Molars
- Caries
- Chronological enamel hypoplasia
- Amelogenesis imperfecta
- Fluorosis (severe)

K. Diagnosis and Problem List
Diagnosis
- Gingivitis
- Hypomineralized permanent first molars
- Dental crowding and mandibular midline shift to the left

L. Comprehensive Treatment Plan
Treatment of Gingivitis
- Toothbrushing and flossing instruction

BACKGROUND INFORMATION 3
Molar-incisor-hypomineralization

- Molar-incisor–hypomineralization or idiopathic enamel hypomineralization usually manifests as hypomineralization or hypoplasia of one or more permanent first molars with opacities of one or more permanent incisors
- It may be associated with a history of illness during infancy or early childhood such as pneumonia, otitis media, and fever, or there may not be any relevant past medical history

---

- Chlorhexidine mouthwash (0.12%) or gel (0.2%) for initial period of two to three weeks to help resolve gingivitis
- Use of G-CSF leads to increase in ANC with a consequent reduction of the gingivitis

Treatment of Hypomineralized Permanent First Molars
- Interim restorations using resin or resin-modified glass ionomers
- Avoid use of stainless steel crown restorations because of anticipated exaggerated gingival response in association with medical history of neutropenia and associated gingivitis
- Prosthodontic referral when older for long-term restorations of permanent first molars

Caries Prevention

- Reinforce advice about balanced healthy diet
- Advise use of sugar-free preparations of liquid medications (antibiotics)
- Reinforce twice daily use of fluoride toothpaste
- Fissure sealant application on eruption of premolars and permanent second molars

Orthodontic Assessment

- Referral for orthodontic assessment of dental crowding and evaluation of hypomineralized permanent first molars

- Extraction of severely hypomineralized permanent first molars may be considered in some cases as part of the orthodontic treatment plan

M. Prognosis and Discussion

- Ongoing liaison and communication with hematologist who will continue to review and manage patient's neutropenia
- Regular review of gingival condition. Consult with periodontist for best time to refer for regular periodontal review into adulthood
- Referral for orthodontic management of crowding
- More definitive restorations of the hypomineralized permanent first molars may be provided in late teenage years or in young adulthood, preferably by a prosthodontist because of the history of neutropenia and gingivitis

N. Common Complications and Alternative Treatment Plans

- An exacerbation of gingivitis may be anticipated during fixed orthodontic appliance treatment and the orthodontist should be informed of this
- An alternative treatment is to monitor the development of occlusion, without orthodontic treatment, and accept some minor crowding and lower midline shift to the left
- Another option, following consultation with an orthodontist, is to extract the most severely hypomineralized permanent first molars to facilitate mesial movement of the unerupted and unaffected permanent second molars. Spontaneous space closure should occur in the majority of cases but there may be mesial inclination of the second permanent molars (Jalevik and Moller 2007).

Self-study Questions

1. **What is the absolute neutrophil count (ANC)?**
2. **What is the normal range of ANC values in a healthy child?**
3. **What is one of the primary aims of medical management of a child with neutropenia?**
4. **What are the predominant types of pathogens likely to cause infection in a child with neutropenia?**
5. **What oral conditions may be typically seen in a patient with neutropenia?**

Answers are located at the end of the case.

Bibliography

Deas DE, Mackey SA, McDonnell HT. 2003. Systemic disease and periodontitis: manifestations of neutrophil dysfunction. *Periodontol 2000* 32:82–104.

Fleming P, Palmer N. 2006. Pharmaceutical prescribing for children, part 6: Dental management and prescribing for the immunocompromised child. *Prim Dental Care* 13:135–9.

Jalevik B, Moller M. 2007. Evaluation of spontaneous space closure and development of permanent dentition after extraction of hypomineralized permanent first molars. *Int J Paediatr Dent* 17:328–35.

Parisi E, Glick M. 2003. Immune suppression and considerations for dental care. *Dent Clin N Am* 47:709–31.

Reich R, Fleisher TA, Shearer WT, Kotzin BL, Schroeder, Jr. HW. 2003. *Clinical Immunology: Principles and Practice*, Mosby: St. Louis.

Segel GB, Halterman S. 2008. Neutropenia in pediatric practice. *Pediatr Rev* 29:12–23.

William V, Messer LB, Burrow MF. 2006. Molar incisor hypomineralization: Review and recommendations for clinical management. *Pediatr Dent* 28:224–32.

SELF-STUDY ANSWERS

1. The absolute neutrophil count (ANC) is a measure of the number of neutrophils in the blood expressed as the number cells/mm^3 of blood

2. The normal range of ANC in healthy children is 1,500 to 8,000 cells/mm^3

3. Prevention of infections and their sequelae

4. Bacteria and fungi

5. Gingivitis, periodontitis, and/or oral ulceration

Case 7

Asthma

A. Presenting Patient
- 5-year-old Caucasian female
- New patient referral from community dental service

B. Chief Complaint and History of Present Illness
- Intermittent toothache over the past two weeks keeping child awake at night

C. Social History
- Lives at home with parents and two older siblings
- Low socio-economic status

D. Medical History
- Moderate persistent asthma: generally well-controlled with infrequent acute exacerbations
- Allergic rhinitis
- Allergies: dust mite, pollen
- Current medications: Beclomethasone twice daily, Albuterol as required, nasal corticosteroid spray
- Admitted with an acute asthmatic episode eight months ago
- No known food or drug allergies, vaccinations up to date

E. Medical Consult
- No need to contact pediatrician because asthma is generally well controlled

F. Dental History
- Has a dental home but despite numerous previous dental visits to manage early childhood caries (ECC), no treatment has been accomplished
- Diet: frequent consumption of fruit juices
- Poor oral hygiene
- Brushes once daily, unsupervised
- Only occasionally uses fluoridated toothpaste
- Lives in an area with water fluoridation of 0.8 ppm
- Very anxious concerning dental treatment

G. Extra-oral Exam
- Open mouth breathing

H. Intra-oral Exam
Soft Tissues
- White plaque-like lesions overlying hard palate
- Generalized gingivitis

Occlusal Evaluation of Primary Dentition
- Class I canines and molars

Dental Exam
- Heavy plaque
- Multiple teeth with carious lesions
- Surface wear consistent with bruxism is evident on some teeth

I. Diagnostic Tools
- Microbiology: swab of palatal mucosa
- Periapical radiographs (taken under general anesthesia)

J. Diagnosis and Problem List
Diagnosis
- Dental anxiety
- Severe ECC
- Oral candidiasis; pseudomembranous candidiasis of hard palate
- Tooth wear
- Pulpal pathology

Problem List
- Dental pain
- Risk of developing dental infection
- Very anxious child
- Impact of asthma medication on oral health

High Caries Risk Due to:
- Special health needs
- Use of medication that can impair salivary flow
- Presence of dental caries

BACKGROUND INFORMATION 1

Asthma

Definition

- Asthma is a common chronic disorder of the airways, characterized by variable and recurring symptoms, airflow obstruction, bronchial hyper responsiveness and an underlying inflammation.

Prevalence

- Estimated 300 million people suffer from asthma worldwide
- One of the most common chronic diseases among children

Etiology

- The etiology is not fully understood. Precipitating factors include pollens, mold spores, house dust, viral infections, cigarette smoke, cold air, extreme emotional arousal, exercise, and anti-inflammatory medication

Pathophysiology

- Airflow limitation is due to a number of changes influenced by airway inflammation
- Bronchoconstriction following irritant exposure
- Airway hyper responsiveness
- Airway edema and mucous hypersecretion

Signs

- Wheeze
- Tachypnea

Symptoms

- Wheeze
- Shortness of breath
- Chest tightness
- Cough

Classification

Based on Etiology

- Extrinsic: Allergic
- Intrinsic (specific triggers, e.g., exercise)

Based on severity

- Intermittent
- Persistent: Mild, moderate, severe

Management

Goals

- Reduce impairment and maintain (near) normal lung function and normal activity levels
- Reduce risk: Prevent exacerbations, minimize need for emergency care, prevent reduced lung growth, have no adverse effects of therapy

How

- Assessment and monitoring
- Patient education
- Control of environmental factors and co-morbid conditions
- Medications

FUNDAMENTAL POINT 1

Assessment of Asthma

History

- Type and severity of asthma
- Frequency of asthmatic attacks
- Precipitating factors
- Last acute episode and hospital admission
- Symptoms associated with sports/exercise
- Type of medication used regularly and during an acute episode

Consult With Pediatrician in Uncontrolled or Severe Cases. Consultation May Include Assessment of:

- Shortness of breath
- Coughing
- Wheezing
- Rate and depth of respiration
- Use of accessory muscles of respiration
- Auscultation of the lungs
- Oxygen saturation
- Pulmonary Function Test
- Peak Flow Test
- Spirometry

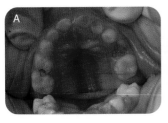
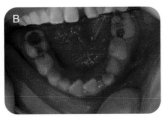

Figure1.7.1a–b. Pre-op intra-oral photos. A. Maxillary, B. Mandibular

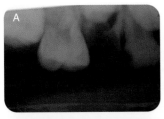
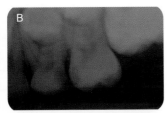
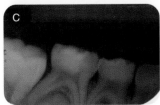
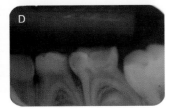
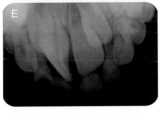

Figure 1.7.2a–e. Pre-op radiographs. A. maxillary right periapical radiograph, B. maxillary left periapical radiograph, C. mandibular right periapical radiograph, D. mandibular left periapical radiograph, E. Maxillary occlusal radiograph

- Low socio-economic status
- Frequent between-meal sugar exposure (fruit juice)
- Unsupervised toothbrushing only once a day
- Visible plaque

K. Comprehensive Treatment Plan
Preventive Plan
- Diet
  - Stop frequent juice intake
  - Limit between-meal snacks
- Oral hygiene
  - Brush twice daily (morning and night)

- Fluoride exposure
  - Consistently brush with fluoridated toothpaste
  - Continue to consume fluoridated water
- Visit dentist for regular review and biannual fluoride varnish application

Management of Oral Candidiasis
- Prevention
  - Consider use of aerosol holding chamber
  - Rinse with water following exposure to inhaled corticosteroids
- Treatment
  - Rinse with chlorhexidine mouthwash daily while candidiasis is present
  - Consider topical antifungal drug therapy in more persistent cases

Comprehensive Dental Treatment Under General Anesthesia (GA)
- Medical
  - Preventive asthma medication as normal
  - Many anesthetic gases are bronchodilators
- Dental
  - Removal of extremely carious, mobile (e.g., maxillary central incisors), and non-vital teeth
  - Restoration of remaining carious teeth: Stainless steel crown (SSC) restoration of two or more surface carious lesions, ferric sulphate vital pulpotomy and SSC if pulp exposed
  - Restoration of single surface carious lesions in molar teeth with high-viscosity glass ionomer cement
  - Space maintenance
- Behavioral management considerations
  - Comprehensive dental treatment under GA to facilitate all necessary procedures at one time
- Follow-up care
  - Post-op and home care instructions: Asthma medication as normal, resume toothbrushing
  - Recall plan: Two weeks post-op, establish regular recall schedule

L. Prognosis and Discussion
- Prognosis for limiting caries progression is guarded
- Prognosis for changing current dietary habits is guarded
- Prognosis for prevention of asthmatic attack is good because of regular use of asthma medication and bronchodilator effect of many anesthetic agents

BACKGROUND INFORMATION 2

Pharmacotheraputic Management of Asthma

- Therapy is initiated based on asthma severity and adjusted as necessary based on asthma control. Stepwise approach to asthma management
- Every patient with persistent asthma, regardless of disease severity, should use a daily controller medication, i.e., an inhaled corticosteroid (ICS)

Quick-relief Medication

- To treat acute symptoms and exacerbations
  - Inhaled short-acting beta agonists, e.g., Albuterol

Long-term Control Medication

- To maintain and achieve control of persistent asthma
  - First choice: ICS (e.g., Beclomethasone)
  - Inhaled long-acting beta$_2$-agonist
  - Leukotriene receptor antagonist
  - Systemic corticosteroids
  - Immunomodulators
- Long-term use of ICS within labeled doses is safe for children in terms of growth, bone mineral density, and adrenal function
- Low- to medium-dose ICS are not associated with the development of cataracts or glaucoma in children

Oral Implications of Asthma and/or its Management

Oral Mucosal Changes

- Gingivitis (associated with mouth breathing)
- Oral candidiasis (associated with use of inhaled corticosteroids)
- Dryness of mouth (associated with use of inhaled corticosteroids)

Dental Caries

- There is insufficient evidence to confirm the increased risk of dental caries and/or erosion in patients with asthma
- Lactose is the carrier for many devices; it gives taste so patient knows that a dose was dispensed
- Inhalers do not taste good; thus, patients increase consumption of flavored beverages

Asthma Medication

- Beta$_2$-agonist medications are associated with:
  - Decrease in salivary flow
  - Decrease in plaque pH
  - Muscle relaxation with subsequent gastroesophageal reflux and associated acid reflux

- Prognosis for prevention of further candidiasis is guarded because of regular use of inhaled corticosteroids and difficulty in rinsing mouth

M. Common Complications and Alternative Treatment Plans

- Non-compliance with dietary advice
- Continued caries progression
- Acute asthmatic episode (see management in Chapter 7)

- Alternative treatment plans may include:
  - Control behavior with conscious sedation
  - Alternative restorative materials, e.g., amalgam or composite for small single or two-surface restorations
  - Alternative pulpal management (e.g., pulpectomy) in non-vital teeth

BACKGROUND INFORMATION 3

Dental Management of Patients with Asthma

- Optimal asthma control is desired prior to dental treatment
- If wheezing, severe, or poorly controlled asthma: reappoint ± medical consult ± consider a hospital setting
- Asthma medication should be taken as normal on day of dental treatment. Bronchodilator should be brought along to the dental appointments
- Behavior management is essential to alleviate anxiety and reduce risk of an acute episode
- Non-steroidal anti-inflammatory drugs (NSAIDS) should be used with caution in all children with asthma: 4% of asthmatics are allergic to aspirin and other NSAIDS. Use acetaminophen instead
- Avoid use of opiates
- For patients taking long-term oral corticosteroids, steroid supplementation is necessary in anticipation of a stressful situation such as dental extractions or during general anesthesia
- Nitrous oxide is contraindicated in severe asthmatics: consult physician
- Unhumidified nitrous oxide may dry out secretions
- Use rubber dam whenever possible
- Certain materials used in the dental office can trigger attacks: sealants, enamel dust, cotton rolls, sulfites, dentrifices, methyl metacrylate
- Avoid long appointments

Conscious Sedation

- Oral: benzodiazepines (e.g., midazolam 0.5 mg/kg) in patients with mild/moderate asthma
- Inhalation sedation (e.g., nitrous oxide) in patients with mild/moderate asthma
- Intravenous: Use extreme caution in patients with asthma (consult pediatrician and anesthesiologist)

General Anesthesia

- Pre-anesthetic review for children with severe or uncontrolled asthma. Non-urgent dental treatment should be postponed until asthma is controlled

Self-study Questions

1. What important questions need to be asked when taking a medical history from a patient with asthma?
2. List some potential stimuli/triggers of an episode of asthma.
3. What are the four main areas of asthma management?
4. Name one inhaled medication used to prevent asthma and one inhaled medication used to provide quick relief from an acute episode of asthma.
5. Name a common oral manifestation of inhaled corticosteroid therapy.

Answers are located at the end of the case.

Bibliography

Cornell A, Shaker M, Woodmansee DP. 2008. Update on the pathogenesis and management of childhood asthma. *Curr Opin Pediatr* 20:597–604.

Ersin NK, Gülen F, Eronat N, et al. 2006. Oral and dental manifestations of young asthmatics related to medication, severity and duration of condition. *Pediatr Int* 48:549–54.

Guidelines for the diagnosis and management of asthma. National Heart, Lung and Blood Institute. http://www.nhlbi.nih.gov/guidelines/asthma/ Accessed on December 21, 2007.

Kil N, Zhu JF, VanWagnen C, Abdulhamid I. 2003. The effects of midazolam on pediatric patients with asthma. *Pediatr Dent* 25:137–42.

Redding GJ, Stoloff SW. 2004. Changes in recommended treatments for mild and moderate asthma. *J Fam Pract* 53:692–700.

Ryberg M, Möller C, Ericson T. 1991. Saliva composition and caries development in asthmatic patients treated with beta 2-adrenoceptor agonists: a 4-year follow-up study. *Scand J Dent Res* 99:212–8.

Steinbacher DM, Glick M. 2001. The dental patient with asthma—an update and oral health considerations. *JADA* 132:1229–39.

Tootla R, Toumba KJ, Duggal MS. 2004. An evaluation of the acidogenic potential of asthma inhalers. *Arch Oral Biol* 49:275–83.

SELF-STUDY ANSWERS

1. Type and severity of asthma, level of asthma control, precipitating factors, frequency of acute asthmatic episodes, last acute episode and whether admitted to the hospital, and type of medication used regularly and during an acute episode
2. Pollens, mold spores, house dust, viral infections, cigarette smoke, cold air, extreme emotional arousal, exercise, and certain anti-inflammatory medications
3. Assessment and monitoring, patient education, control of environmental factors and other asthma triggers, and pharmacotherapy
4. Beclomethasone and Albuterol
5. Oral candidiasis

Case 8

Crohn's Disease

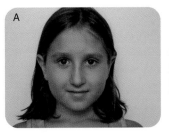 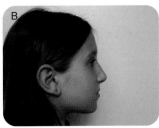

Figure 1.8.1a–b. Facial photographs at 6 month follow up visit

A. Presenting Patient

- 7-year-, 4-month-old Caucasian female

B. Chief Complaint and History

- New patient referred from pediatric gastroenterology for assessment of swollen lower lip and angular cheilitis as part of a diagnostic work-up of inflammatory bowel disease
- Mother noted progressive swelling of lower lip for the past three to four months concurrently with abdominal cramps and diarrhea

C. Social History

- Lives at home with both parents
- Sister (5 years old) and brother (2 years old)
- Middle class family
- Maternal aunt has Crohn's disease

D. Medical History

- Hospitalized because of weight loss, abdominal cramps, and diarrhea. Gastroenterologists undertaking investigations to determine if child has Crohn's disease (CD)
- Three-month history of abdominal cramps, diarrhea, anorexia, and weight loss
- No medications present during medical work-up
- No known allergies to foods or medications
- Vaccinations are up to date

Specific Examinations

- Weight: 21.5 kg (Below the 25th Percentile), Hemoglobin: 9.7 g/dl (Normal Range: 11 to 14), Platelets: 507 × 10⁹/l (Normal Range: 140 to 400), C Reactive Protein: 13 mg/l (Normal Range: <10), Albumin: 26 g/l (Normal Range: 35 to 50)
- Barium meal and follow-through showed irregular stricture involving the distal portion of the terminal ileum
- Upper endoscopy and colonoscopy reveal multiple regions with inflammation but mainly involvement of terminal ileum with large ulcers

Histopathology

- Biopsies from stomach, terminal ileum, and colon show focal areas of acute and chronic inflammation
- Gingival biopsy (mandibular incisor labial gingiva) shows marked chronic inflammation and non-necrotizing granulomas, which, in combination with acute and chronic inflammation in the other biopsies, supports the clinical diagnosis of CD with involvement of multiple regions of the GI tract

E. Medical Consult

- Pediatric gastroenterologist

F. Dental History

- One previous dental visit at 6 years of age and dentist noted decay-free primary dentition
- Poor oral hygiene during last two weeks due to illness; supervised by parents. Difficult to brush teeth because of swollen lower lip
- Reduced appetite during last three months but good diet before
- Uses toothpaste containing fluoride
- Lives in optimally fluoridated area
- No history of dental trauma

BACKGROUND INFORMATION 1

- Inflammatory bowel disease (IBD) can be sub-classified as ulcerative colitis (UC) or Crohn's disease (CD). Indeterminate colitis is the term used when unable to clearly discriminate between UC and CD.

Crohn's Disease

- Chronic granulomatous inflammatory disorder of unknown etiology, likely the result of an inappropriate inflammatory response in a genetically susceptible individual to an environmental stimulus

- May affect any part of the gastrointestinal (GI) tract from the mouth to the anus

- Typically involves the terminal segment of the small intestine (ileum) and first segment of the large intestine (colon)

- Peak incidence is in second and third decades of life with up to one-third of cases occurring before 20 years of age

- There is familial clustering with a history of IBD in approximately 15% of cases of CD

- There are probably several genes involved in conferring susceptibility to IBD and there may be genetic heterogeneity, with different genes having similar phenotypic expressions

- NOD2 is the best characterized susceptibility gene, mutations of which confer increased risk for CD. The gene encodes for a protein that is involved in recognizing pathogens and intracellular signaling of the innate immune response

Treatment of Crohn's Disease

- Medical induction and maintenance of remission of intestinal inflammation

- Nutritional support may require nasogastric infusion of formulated food in severe cases with malnourishment and growth retardation, to increase caloric intake

- Medical treatment of relapses/acute exacerbations

- Surgical intervention if there are intractable symptoms despite medical therapy or if there are intestinal complications such as obstruction, infection, fistula, perforation, or hemorrhage

BACKGROUND INFORMATION 2

Presentation of Crohn's Disease in Children

- Abdominal pain
- Diarrhea ± blood in stools
- Poor appetite
- Weight loss
- Impaired growth and pubertal delay
- Anemia due to malabsorbtion and blood loss
- Erythrocyte sedimentation rate (ESR) or C-reactive protein (CRP) and high platelet count are indicative of an inflammatory process
- Low albumin due to protein losing enteropathy oral soft tissue manifestations

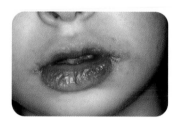

Figure 1.8.2. Swelling and angular cheilitis of lower lip

swelling of marginal and attached gingiva around mandibular incisors

- Early mixed dentition with class I relationship of permanent first molars. Mandibular permanent lateral incisors erupting lingual to permanent central incisors with retention of both mandibular primary lateral incisors and the mobile mandibular left primary central incisor

- Generalized plaque accumulation, particularly on labial aspect of incisors

- Caries-free dentition

G. Extra-oral Examination

- Bilateral angular cheilitis
- Gross swelling of lower lip with vertical fissures
- Dry lips

H. Intra-oral Examination

- Soft tissues: Swelling of lower labial mucosa, soft tissue tags and ulcers in lower labial sulcus, and

I. Diagnostic Tools

- Gingival biopsy when under general anesthesia for endoscopy and colonoscopy

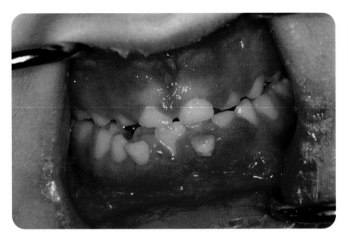

Figure 1.8.3. Intra-oral soft tissue inflammation and ulcerations

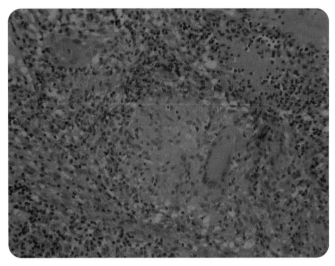

Figure 1.8.4. Histological image of gingival granuloma, formed by an aggregate of epithelioid macrophages. To the right of the center of the image is a multinucleated giant cell

J. Differential Diagnosis

- Orofacial granulomatosis (OFG) that may be associated with hypersensitivity to foodstuffs or additives
- Ulcerative colitis (UC): Inflammatory bowel disease affecting the colon in which there may be associated oral aphthous ulceration. Pyostomatitis vegetans with tiny yellow pustules in the oral mucosa has been reported in individuals with UC and CD
- Hereditary angioedema
- Allergic angioedema

K. Diagnosis and Problem List

- CD with oral lesions
- Retained primary incisors

L. Comprehensive Treatment Plan

- Gingival biopsy to obtain histological confirmation of granulomatous inflammation and diagnosis of CD

- Extraction of retained mandibular primary incisors
- Oral hygiene instruction
- Monitor developing occlusion

BACKGROUND INFORMATION 3
Orofacial Granulomatosis

- Orofacial granulomatosis (OFG) is a condition characterized by orofacial swelling with biopsy-positive non-necrotizing granulomas in a patient without Crohn's disease (CD) or other systemic disease

- May be associated with a hypersensitivity to certain food and drink additives such as benzoates, cinnamon, and tartrazine

- OFG that is associated with hypersensitivity to food additives may improve or resolve with an exclusion diet; however, compliance with such a diet may be very difficult

- Intra-lesional steroids may be required to treat lip swelling in OFG

- A child with OFG may not have overt symptoms or signs of CD but may subsequently develop intestinal CD

- A child with OFG should be referred to a specialist in oral medicine. Review by a pediatric gastroenterologist may also be required because OFG may precede the development of CD.

- Fissure sealant application to permanent first molars when erupted sufficiently to isolate for moisture control

M. Prognosis and Discussion

- Regression of oral lesions anticipated with treatment of CD
- Oral lesions may reappear if there is relapse of systemic CD

Initial Medical Treatment Following Diagnosis of CD

- 6 Mercaptopurine 25 mg daily
- Prednisolone 25 mg daily for four weeks. Then reduce dosage by 5 mg each week until tapered course is completed
- Iron supplements for treatment of anemia: 6 mg/kg daily of elemental iron

Dental Treatment

- Delay treatment in the dental office until medical improvement in CD
- Monitor retained mandibular primary incisors and anticipate spontaneous exfoliation
- Frequent preventive dental visits to encourage improved oral hygiene; professional application of fluoride varnish and fissure sealant application to permanent first molars
- If general anesthesia is planned, Prednisolone therapy may result in suppression of the normal adrenocortical response, with a risk of developing hypotension. Hydrocortisone should therefore be

---

BACKGROUND INFORMATION 4
Categories of Drugs Used in the Management of Crohn's Disease

Drug category	Drug	Comments
Anti-inflammatory	Glucocorticoids Prednisolone	Conventional corticosteroid, initial high dose to control disease
	Budesonide	Controlled ileal release corticosteroid
	Enteral nutrition	Typically exclusive use of elemental or semi-elemental diet for six to eight weeks (mechanism of action unknown)
	Aminosalicylates (ASA) Sulfasalazine Mesalamine	Active component, 5-ASA, acts locally in intestinal mucosa to inhibit inflammation
Antibiotic	Metronidazole Ciprofloxacillin	Antibacterial effect on intestinal flora
Immunomodulator	6-Mercaptopurine Azathioprine	Immunosuppressant Steroid-sparing
Biologic	Infliximab/Remicade	Monoclonal antibody that neutralizes bioactivity of the key inflammatory cytokine, tumor necrosis factor-alpha (TNF-α)

administered IV at induction of anesthesia by an anesthesiologist if general anesthesia is administered within three to six months of glucocorticoid therapy. There is no need for IV hydrocortisone or glucocorticoid medication prior to providing dental treatment under local analgesia in a dental office.

Self-study Questions

1. **What parts of the gastrointestinal tract may be affected in CD?**
2. **Name four possible orofacial manifestations of CD.**
3. **What is one of the key histopathological findings in CD?**
4. **What categories of drugs may be used in the management of CD in children?**
5. **Orofacial granulomatosis in some cases may be associated with a hypersensitivity to certain agents. What agents may be implicated?**

Answers are located at the end of the case.

Bibliography

Cameron AC, Widmer RP. 2003. *Handbook of Pediatric Dentistry. Chapter 6: Pediatric Oral Medicine and Pathology.* Mosby: Philadelphia.

Challacombe SJ. 1997. Oro-facial granulomatosis and oral Crohn's disease: Are they specific diseases and do They predict systemic Crohn's Disease? *Oral Dis* 3:127–9.

Harty S, Fleming P, Rowland M, et al. 2005. A prospective study of the oral manifestations of Crohn's disease. *Clin Gastroenter Hepatol* 3:886–91.

Scully C. 2004. *Oral and Maxillofacial Medicine. The Basis of Diagnosis and Treatment.* Wright, an imprint of Elsevier Science: London.

SELF-STUDY ANSWERS

1. Any part of the tract, including the mouth
2. Lip swelling and/or cheek swelling, angular cheilits, mucogingivitis, cobblestoning of buccal mucosa, mucosal tags, aphthous ulceration, and long, deep ulcers in the mandibular buccal sulcus are some of the possible orofacial manifestations of CD

3. Presence of non-necrotizing granuloma(s)
4. Anti-inflammatories (glucocorticoids, enteral nutrition, aminosalicylates), immunomodulators, biologics, and antibiotics may be used in management of CD in children
5. Certain food and drink additives such as benzoates, cinnamon and tartrazine

2

Oral Medicine and Oral-facial Pathology

Angus C. Cameron

Case 1

Acute Odontogenic Infection

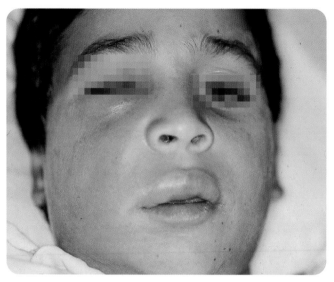

Figure 2.1.1. Facial photograph showing facial swelling

A. Presenting Patient
- 7-year-old Caucasian male
- New patient presenting as an emergency

B. Chief Complaint and History of Present Illness
- Child has woken in the morning with a large swelling in the upper jaw.
- Has not eaten or drunk any fluids since previous night (16 hours)
- The child has complained of a toothache for several days and was seen the day before by a dentist who prescribed oral penicillin. Two days later, patient returned to the dental office for extraction but because facial swelling had increased, he was referred to the children's hospital emergency department for treatment (see Fundamental Point 1).

FUNDAMENTAL POINT 1
Obtaining a History for a Facial Swelling
Major Questions to Consider
- **How long has the swelling been present?** This swelling has arisen quickly in relation to previous odontogenic pain. The speed of progression of the swelling indicates the acute nature of the pathology or perhaps an acute exacerbation of a previous chronic condition. The size and extent of the swelling is also important.
- **What is the fluid balance for this child?** Has the child been able to take oral fluids or food? Serious conditions in children may rapidly deteriorate when fluid balance is upset. Children may become dehydrated quickly. The ability to swallow may also indicate the extent to which the swelling involves the airway and the oral cavity.
- **Has the swelling arisen in spite of the prescription of antibiotics?** This swelling has arisen or increased in the presence of antibiotics. This may aid your diagnosis in that a highly virulent infection may be present, or it may indicate that the swelling is not a result of a bacterial organism. Furthermore, the antibiotics may not be addressing the cause of an infection or the dose and administration of these drugs may be inappropriate.
- **Is the pain waking the child at night?** The severity of any discomfort can be easily measured by assessing whether it is sufficient to wake the patient from sleep. Children (and most adults) are often unable to fall asleep with severe pain or discomfort and if they wake from sleep, then this is a good indicator of pain.

C. Social History
- Youngest of three children, both parents present
- Middle class family

D. Medical History
- Review of medical history reveals no significant findings, no known food or drug allergies, no medications; vaccinations are up to date

E. Medical Consult
- Infectious diseases

F. Dental History
- No dental home
- Episodic visits to several different local dentists for relief of pain only. No dental treatment provided due to uncooperative behavior.
- Other children in the family have been managed for extensive dental caries under general anesthesia.
- Poor oral hygiene habits, no adult supervision
- Cariogenic diet
- Uses toothpaste containing fluoride
- Lives in optimally fluoridated area
- No history of trauma

G. Extra-oral Exam (see Figure 2.1.1a)
- Examination is difficult because the child is extremely anxious and in pain.
- The child is febrile with a temperature of 38.5°C (101.3°F).
- Large swelling in the canine fossa on the right side of the face extending from the upper lip to the eye. The swelling is firm, red, warm and painful to touch. The eye is closed due to the swelling. The upper lip on the right is also swollen (Figure 2.1.1).

H. Intra-oral Exam
Soft Tissues
- Swelling is present and continuous with the extra-oral component, adjacent to the upper right second primary molar

Hard Tissues (Figures 2.1.2ab)
Mixed dentition
- Multiple carious lesions noted on the primary molars

Occlusal Evaluation of Mixed Dentition
- Class I primary canines, class II permanent molars

Other
- Generalized severe plaque accumulation and calculus deposits on lingual surfaces of mandibular incisors

- Multiple extensive carious lesions present. Large carious lesion is present on the mesial of the upper right second primary molar, which is mobile and sore to touch

I. Diagnostic Tools
- Bitewing radiographs (Figures 2.1.3a–b)
- Panoramic radiograph (Figures 2.1.4)
- It was not possible to obtain a maxillary right periapical radiograph given the patient's discomfort.

J. Differential Diagnosis
Infective
- Odontogenic infection
- Periorbital cellulitis

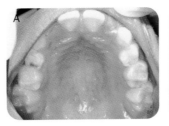
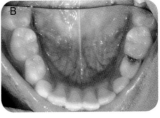

Figure 2.1.2a–b. Pre-op intra-oral photos. A. Occlusal maxillary, B. occlusal mandibular

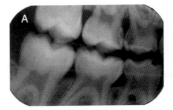
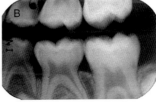

Figure 2.1.3a–b. Pre-op bitewing radiographs. A. Right bitewing radiograph, B. Left bitewing radiograph

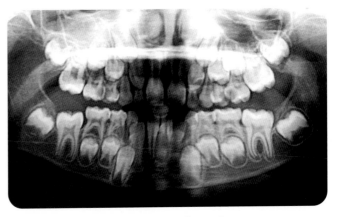

Figure 2.1.4. Pre-op panoramic radiograph

Immunological
- Insect bite

Neoplasia
- Sarcoma

Inflammatory
- Orofacial granulomatosis

K. Diagnosis and Problem List
Diagnosis
- Odontogenic infection

Problem List
- Acute odontogenic infection presenting with cellulitis
- Febrile illness
- Behavior management difficulties
- Untreated carious lesions in primary dentition
- Lack of dental home
- High caries risk (poor oral hygiene, cariogenic diet, extensive plaque accumulation, no dental home)

BACKGROUND INFORMATION 1
Management of Facial Infections
Antibiotics

- Serious infections should be treated quickly. While the removal of the cause of the infection may suffice in many circumstances, a large facial infection requires administration of antibiotics in appropriate dosage and route of administration.

- Antibiotics may be given in much higher dosages intravenously rather than orally, achieving higher plasma concentrations. An antibiotic of sufficiently broad spectrum should be used initially when the exact nature of an infective organism is unknown or has yet to be determined. Microbiological laboratory culture and sensitivity take at least several days to weeks (in the case of anaerobic infections) to yield results and so prescription of antibiotics is usually empirical.

- What antibiotic can the child tolerate in the oral form? Amoxicillin may be given three times a day with food, while penicillin VK may only be given on an empty stomach four times a day.

What to Do with the Tooth?

- Removal of the cause of the infection must be the mainstay of any treatment plan. The difficulties in treating children arise due to problems with behavior management. It is impossible to drain an infection through the apices of a primary molar tooth.

- Is there a collection of sub or supraperiosteal pus that needs to be drained? Most odontogenic infections in children of this age present as a cellulitis rather than an abscess, in which case there is little or no point in an incision and drainage. Fluctuant swellings usually indicate the presence of pus. Large submandibular swellings involving the first permanent molar may also require incision and drainage.

- If there is a large volume of pus to drain, is an extra-oral incision necessary? Pus will not drain up. Large swellings in the mandible require an extraoral approach.

- Consider what the child can cope with.

Should This Child Be Admitted?

- As noted above, any serious infection in the head and neck will probably require admission to a hospital. Hospital admission allows post-operative observation of the patient, allows for the administration of intravenous antibiotics and fluids, and allows monitoring of any complications. Children should only be discharged when fluid intake is adequate and the signs of infection are resolving. Following surgery to the mouth, it is important not to over-hydrate children because they will not feel like taking anything orally, delaying discharge. Maintenance fluids should be kept overnight but then reduced as the child improves to encourage oral intake.

Complications of Infections in the Head and Neck

- Always consider the risk of major complications when treating infections in the head and neck. While children improve quickly, they can also deteriorate equally fast when virulent organisms are involved or appropriate treatment is delayed. Such complications include the risk of posterior and/or inferior spread of infection along tissue planes, i.e., cavernous sinus thrombosis and possible brain abscess, spread into the tonsillar fossa, spread into the neck with respiratory obstruction, and/or mediastinal involvement.

L. Comprehensive Treatment Plan

- Admission to hospital for commencement of intravenous antibiotics and analgesics, and establishment of fluid balance (see Background Information 1).
- Emergency treatment in the operating room for extraction of teeth and drainage of abscess
- Comprehensive treatment of other carious lesions
- Establishment of a caries prevention plan

M. Prognosis and Discussion

Acute Phase Management

- The essential component of management of this case is the removal of the cause of the infection. Too often cases of acute infection are treated only with antibiotics. While in some cases the administration of antibiotics will resolve the acute phase of the infection, this swelling has increased in the face of antibiotics. The child is acutely febrile and the swelling has increased to close the eye due to collateral edema. Further spread of the infection posteriorly may involve the orbit with the risk of retrobulbar abscess or cavernous sinus thrombosis.

Choice of Management

- This child has had multiple attempts at treatment using routine behavior management techniques. In view of the severity of the infection, management under general anesthesia is the most preferable choice if available. It is recognized, however, that access to this modality of care may not be readily available and so other options such as conscious sedation should be considered.

Choice of Antibiotics

The swelling in this patient has arisen despite the administration of antibiotics, namely penicillin. It is therefore essential to change the antibiotic. Because the child is to be managed under general anesthesia, a first generation cephalosporin is an appropriate alternative. Depending on the severity of the infection, metronidazole could also be added because odontogenic infections are principally of mixed flora with a large Gram-negative component.

N. Complications (Dental)

- Failure of resolution of the infection
- Space loss associated with premature loss of the second primary molar
- Further restorative work required following the acute phase treatment

Self-study Questions

1. **What surgical approach would you consider in the management of this child?**

2. **What alternative antibiotics to penicillin are available in the management of this case?**

3. **What criteria would you consider for the use of pharmacological behavior management such as sedation or general anesthesia?**

4. **What long-term maintenance would you consider?**

Answers are located at the end of the case.

Bibliography and Additional Reading

Ellison SJ. 2009. The role of phenoxymethylpenicillin, amoxicillin, metronidazole and clindamycin in the management of acute dentoalveolar abscesses—a review. *Br Dent J* 206:357–62.

Khanna G, Sato Y, Smith RJ, Bauman NM, Nerad J. 2006. Causes of facial swelling in pediatric patients: correlation of clinical and radiologic findings. *Radiographics* 26:157–71.

Levi ME, Eusterman VD. 2011. Oral infections and antibiotic therapy. *Otolaryngol Clin North Am* 44:57–78.

López-Píriz R, Aguilar L, Giménez MJ. 2007. Management of odontogenic infection of pulpal and periodontal origin. *Med Oral Patol Oral Cir Bucal* 12:E154–9.

Robertson D, Smith AJ. 2009. The microbiology of the acute dental abscess. *J Med Microbiol* 58(Pt 2):155–62.

Seow WK. 2003. Diagnosis and management of unusual dental abscesses in children. *Aust Dent J* 48:156–68.

Swift JQ, Gulden WS. 2002. Antibiotic therapy—managing odontogenic infections. *Dent Clin North Am* 46:623–33.

SELF-STUDY ANSWERS

1. If there is a significant accumulation of pus subperiosteally, then the elevation of a buccal flap with copious irrigation should be considered. Unlike adults, children typically present initially with a cellulitis rather than a collection of pus. Most of the swelling is associated with collateral edema. Administration of antibiotics alone may localize and wall-off the infection, resulting in the formation of an abscess cavity and further tissue destruction.

2. First generation cephalosporin; Clindamycin, Metronidazole

3. Choice of any behavior management technique relies on the:
   - Ability of the child to cope with the treatment required
   - Medical contraindications
   - Future treatment needs of the patient
   - Potential complications
   - Presence of trismus
   - Local anesthesia issues

4. This child is at a high caries risk and requires a period of familiarization to the dental environment to improve behavior management.
   - Establishment of a dental home
   - Caries Control and Prevention: Familiarization, fluoridation, oral hygiene practices, diet analysis
   - Regular dental follow-up
   - Space maintenance as required
   - Behavior management

Case 2

Primary Herpetic Gingivostomatitis

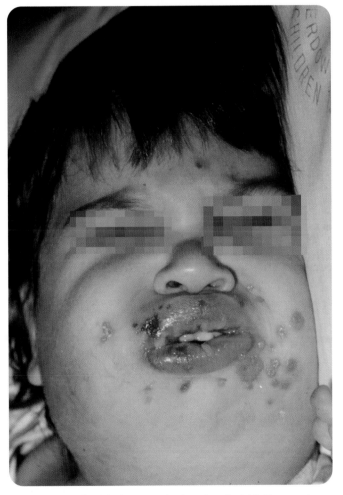

Figure 2.2.1. Facial photograph showing facial inflammation and ulcerations

A. Presenting Patient

- 20-month-old Arabic male
- New patient presenting as an emergency

B. Chief Complaint

- Child has been ill for two days with a very high fever.

- Child is unable to eat or drink because his mouth is extremely inflamed (see Fundamental Point 1).
- Child has been seen by his general medical practitioner who has prescribed antibiotics and referred to the dentist.

C. Social History

- Youngest of two children, older sister is four years of age and attends preschool
- Cared for by his grandmother during the day
- Low socio-economic status

D. Medical History

- Review of medical history showed no significant findings, no known food or drug allergies, no medications; vaccinations are up to date

E. Medical Consult

- Consultation with general pediatrics regarding fluid balance: The child has not had any fluid intake for more than 12 hours and hence admission to the hospital may be required.

F. Dental History

- No dental home
- First visit to the dentist
- Poor oral hygiene habits
- Cariogenic diet
- Brushes teeth infrequently with some adult supervision
- Lives in an optimally fluoridated area
- No history of trauma

G. Extra-oral Exam

- Examination is extremely difficult due to the state of the child's health.
- The child is generally unwell, lethargic, and irritable, with a temperature of 39°C (102.2°F).
- There is no extra-oral swelling, but there is marked inflammation and ulceration of the lips and the lateral commissures. Numerous ulcers and open lesions around the lips and face are present (Figure 2.2.1).

H. Intra-oral Exam

Soft Tissues (Figure 2.2.2)

- The gingival tissues are acutely inflamed with minor bleeding from the crevicular margin. There are multiple small ulcers, particularly on the dorsum of the tongue, and some areas of ulceration are noted on the attached gingiva. The hard palate, the fauces, and the pharynx are generally unaffected.

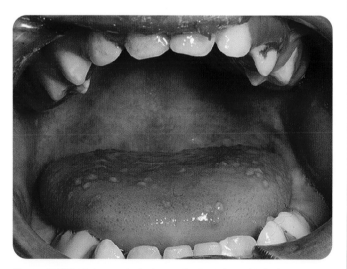

Figure 2.2.2. Intra-oral photograph showing gingival inflammation and mucosal ulcerations

Hard Tissue and Occlusal Evaluation

- Deferred at this appointment

Other

- Generalized heavy plaque accumulation

I. Diagnostic Tools

- A swab of the affected tissues could be considered for exfoliative cytology.
- Viral culture (may take many days to establish a result)
- Viral antibody detection

J. Differential Diagnosis

Infective: Viral Infection

- Primary herpetic gingivostomatis
- Coxsackie viral infection: herpangina, and hand, foot and mouth disease
- Other viral infections: infectious mononucleosis (Epstein Barr), varicella (chickenpox)

Immunological

- Autoimmune recurrent ulceration
- Erythema multiforme/Stevens Johnson syndrome
- Behcet's syndrome

Neoplasia

- Hematological malignancy

Inflammatory

- Orofacial granulomatosis

> **FUNDAMENTAL POINT 2**
> **Presentation of Herpetic Lesions**
>
> - The presentation of a young child with a prodrome of one to two days of febrile illness followed by the development of an acute stomatitis is characteristic of primary herpes infection. Typically, vesicles are not seen because they form rapidly and break down to form coalesced areas of ulceration; however, the primary signs are those of acute gingival inflammation. Commonly, the child will present to their local medical practitioner, and antibiotics are frequently prescribed, inappropriately, in the absence of a definitive diagnosis. It is not until the appearance of the ulcers that the true diagnosis is apparent.

FUNDAMENTAL POINT 3
Management of Herpetic Lesions

- The essential component of management of this case is symptomatic care. Maintenance of fluid balance is essential with a soft bland diet as tolerated. Pain should be controlled with analgesics and there is evidence that the use of topical antiseptics may be beneficial. Non-alcoholic chlorhexidine mouthwash may be used to swab the mouth to debride areas of slough that may be secondarily infected with oral bacteria causing more discomfort. It is advisable to use an aqueous solution of chlorhexidine because some formulations may contain up to 10% ethanol, which is particularly painful when applied to open ulcers.

K. Provisional Diagnosis annd Problem List

Provisional Diagnosis

- Primary herpetic gingivostomatitis (see Fundamental Point 2 and Background Information 1)

Problem List

- Acute viral infection
- Febrile illness
- Severe stomatitis
- Pain and discomfort resulting in decrease in fluid intake and possible dehydration.

L. Comprehensive Treatment Plan

- Admission to hospital for maintenance fluids, mouthwash and debridement, and pain control
- Soft diet as tolerated (see Fundamental Point 3)

M. Prognosis and Discussion

- The condition is self-limiting and should resolve within 10 to 14 days. If there is no resolution within this time, then a biopsy is indicated to exclude other conditions. The patient will be prone to recurrent episodes of herpes labialis in times of stress or immune compromise or when the lips are exposed to UV radiation.

- Topical anesthetics and coating agents help relieve pain and facilitate food intake. However, they should be used with extreme caution in children who cannot expectorate because of the potential for traumatic biting and numbness of the gag reflex, if swallowed, which may lead to aspiration.

BACKGROUND INFORMATION 1
Oral Herpes

- The causative agent in this condition is the *Herpes simplex* virus. This is usually the type I virus, although the presentation and course of a type II infection is identical.

- Initial infection comes from direct contact with another infected individual and the virus then infects the nerve and remains latent in the trigeminal ganglion.

- Reactivation of the virus results in herpes labialis.

- Because the disease is self-limiting, care should be symptomatic, except in severe cases or children with immune suppression. Acyclovir® has been shown to be effective in control of infection if administered within the first 72 hours of exposure. The usual dosage is 25 to 100 mg/kg/day given five times per day as an oral suspension. Intravenous administration is reserved for severe cases.

- Paracetamol is the most appropriate analgesic to prescribe, in the range of 15 mg/kg up to a maximum of 90 mg/kg/day.

- Eating ice cream or popsicles may help relieve oral discomfort and increase the fluid intake.

- Maintenance of oral hygiene is essential and it is important to warn the parents/caregivers to use separate utensils, change the child's toothbrush and pacifiers, etc., and avoid contact with other children.

- Parents should be warned that the child should not touch his eyes. The child must be hospitalized if ocular involvement occurs.

N. Complications

- Dehydration due to inadequate fluid intake
- Recurrent herpes labialis
- Contamination of other body parts (eyes, fingers, etc.)
- Transmission to other family members and children in school and daycare
- Disseminated herpes infection in children who are severely immunocompromised

Self-study Questions

1. **When should a child with primary herpes be admitted to hospital?**
2. **Should an antiviral medication be prescribed?**
3. **Should antibiotics be prescribed?**

4. **Will this child have another episode of this type of infection?**

Answers are located at the end of the case.

Bibliography and Additional Reading

Chung NY, Batra R, Itzkevitch M, Boruchov D, Baldauf M. 2010. Severe methemoglobinemia linked to gel-type topical benzocaine use: a case report. *J Emerg Med* 38:601–6.

Drugge JM, Allen PJ. 2008. A nurse practitioner's guide to the management of herpes simplex virus-1 in children. *Pediatr Nurs* 34:310–8.

Krol DM, Keels MA. 2007. Oral conditions. *Pediatr Rev* 28:15–21.

Nasser M, Fedorowicz Z, Khoshnevisan MH, Shahiri Tabarestani M. 2008. Acyclovir for treating primary herpetic gingivostomatitis. *Coch Database Syst Rev* 4:CD006700.

Usatine RP, Tinitigan R. 2010. Nongenital herpes simplex virus. *Am Fam Physician* 82:1075–82.

Wilson SS, Fakioglu E, Herold BC. 2009. Novel approaches in fighting herpes simplex virus infections. *Expert Rev Anti Infect Ther* 7:559–68.

Woo SB, Challacombe SJ. 2007. Management of recurrent oral herpes simplex infections. *Oral Surg Oral Med Oral Pathol Oral Radiol Endod* 103 (suppl 1):S12.e1–S12.e18.

SELF-STUDY ANSWERS

1. Hospital admission is only necessary if there is a risk of dehydration due to an inability to maintain an adequate intake of fluids. This is an uncommon event; however, the clinician must be aware of the dangers of inadequate fluid balance and should stress to the parents or caregivers that it is essential to encourage the child to drink as much as possible. Intake of solid food is not as important as fluids, but bland soft foods should also be encouraged. Young children will be hesitant to take anything orally in the acute phase.

2. The prescription of antivirals is contentious, and common practice dictates that acyclovir is only effective if administered within the first 72 hours of the appearance of the prodrome. In reality, few children will present to the dentist within this time period and have commonly visited their medical practitioner prior to the dentist. Acyclovir should always be used when managing children who are immunosuppressed.

3. There is really no indication for the prescription of antibiotics in cases of primary herpes because it is a viral infection.

4. Patients will not have another episode of this form of acute infection; however, they will be subject to recurrent cold sores appearing along the terminal distribution of the nerve pathways that have been involved (i.e., the particular division of the trigeminal nerve).

Case 3

Peripheral Giant Cell Granuloma

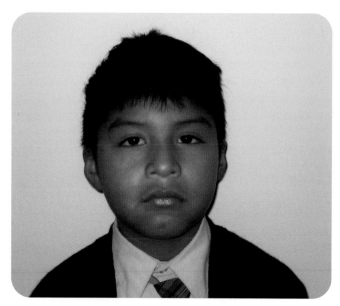

Figure 2.3.1. Facial photograph

A. Presenting Patient
- 7-year-old Hispanic male
- New patient presenting as an emergency

B. Chief Complaint and History of Present Injury
- The patient recently noticed a purple swelling between his mandibular permanent central incisors. The swelling is painless and occasionally bleeds when brushing the teeth, which is making him unwilling to brush so he will not damage the area (see Fundamental Point 1).

C. Social History
- Youngest of three children
- Attends primary school
- Middle class family

D. Medical History
- No significant findings, no known food or drug allergies, no medications, vaccinations are up to date

FUNDAMENTAL POINT 1
Obtaining a History for Intra-oral Lesions
Questions to Ask a Parent
- How long has the swelling been present? When did you first notice it?
- Has it changed in appearance (size, shape, color) recently?
- Has there been any spontaneous bleeding from this swelling or only on brushing?
- Is the lesion painful? Does it hurt spontaneously or only when stimulated?
- Is there anything that makes it better or worse?

E. Medical Consult
- N/A

F. Dental History
- Goes to dentist infrequently; last visit was more than 12 months ago
- Has had restorative work done in dental chair
- Poor oral hygiene with no adult supervision
- Normal diet
- Uses toothpaste containing fluoride
- Lives in an optimally fluoridated area
- Normal eruption of teeth with no difficulties in exfoliation of primary teeth
- No history of trauma

G. Extra-oral Exam
- No significant findings

H. Intra-oral Exam
Soft Tissues
- Mild gingivitis consistent with poor oral hygiene
- A well circumscribed 7 mm lesion and a large diastema are present between the mandibular

central incisors, which have been displaced laterally. The lesion is dark reddish to purple in color but does not blanch or hurt on pressure. The base appears to extend subgingivally and is not pedunculated. Bleeding is observed around the gingival margin upon probing (Figure 2.3.2).

Hard Tissues
- No significant findings

BACKGROUND INFORMATION 1
Oral Biopsy

- As in all areas of pathology, an accurate diagnosis is essential for determining appropriate management. Misdiagnosis can lead to serious complications such as infection, hemorrhage, spread of neoplastic tissue, or trauma to adjacent tissues or organs. Cases in which lesions are bilateral and symmetrical are almost never serious; they are usually developmental or are variations of normal tissues.

- As a general rule, if the diagnosis of a lesion cannot be determined and there is no resolution within two weeks, then further investigation is required.

- Biopsies may be incisional or excisional, usually depending on the size of the lesion. Smaller lesions should be completely excised with a border of normal tissue. Larger lesions may require a representative portion of tissue to be removed.

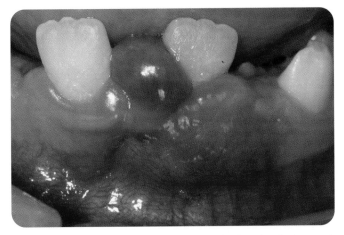

Figure 2.3.2. Pre-op intra-oral photograph showing lesion and diastema

---

Occlusal Evaluation of Mixed Dentition
- No significant findings

Other
- Caries-free dentition

I. Diagnostic Tools
- An excisional biopsy is required (see Background Information 1)

J. Differential Diagnosis
Inflammatory Hyperplasias
- Fibrous epulis/pyogenic granuloma
- Giant cell epulis/peripheral giant-cell granuloma

Neoplasias/Tumors
- Congenital epulis of the newborn
- Squamous papilloma/viral warts
- Condyloma acuminatum
- Melanotic neuro-ectodermal tumor of infancy

Developmental Anomalies
- Eruption cyst/hematoma
- Lymphangioma
- Hemangioma
- Vascular malformation
- Tuberous sclerosis

Traumatic
- Mucocoele

K. Provisional Diagnosis and Problem List
Provisional Diagnosis
- Peripheral giant-cell granuloma: In this case, there was no history of trauma and the provisional diagnosis is usually based on the clinical appearance.
- The relatively short standing duration of the lesion would exclude a developmental anomaly. An infective process such as a papilloma would not usually present unless the lesion is fungating or exophytic in appearance.
- The most common causes of an epulis are the pyogenic granuloma or the peripheral giant cell granuloma.
- The site and appearance is more suggestive of the latter but the presence of a tumour or neoplasm must not be excluded.

Problem List
- Red/purple swelling with unconfirmed diagnosis

L. Comprehensive Treatment Plan
- Excisional biopsy with border of normal tissue (Figure 2.3.3.)

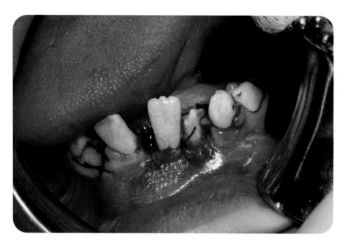

Figure 2.3.3. Post-op intra-oral photograph

BACKGROUND INFORMATION 2
Peripheral Giant Cell Granuloma

- The peripheral giant cell lesion is regarded as inflammatory in origin with an unknown etiology, although some authors have associated the overgrowth with mild irritation.
- The location is generally confined to the gingiva in the region of the primary dentition.
- The color is characteristic and may range from dark red to purple. It is generally darker than the pyogenic granuloma and it is not as vascular.
- Radiographically, there may be a characteristic cupping of the alveolar ridge with bone resorption.
- Histopathology is required to confirm the diagnosis in this case. The lesion is not thought to be related to the more aggressive central giant cell granuloma of bone, although the histology is similar.

- Regular follow-up to ensure that there is no regrowth
- Return to his dentist for recall exam and establishment of a prevention plan

M. Final Diagnosis

- Peripheral giant cell granuloma (see Background Information 2)

N. Prognosis and Discussion

- Hyperparathyroidism must be considered in the differential diagnosis when a giant cell lesion is found (see Fundamental Point 2). Central

FUNDAMENTAL POINT 2
Hyperparathyroidism

- Hyperparathyroidism must be considered in the differential diagnosis when a giant cell lesion is found. Central involvement necessitates further investigation. In the provisional diagnosis the presence of a vascular lesion must be excluded. Biopsy of such a lesion may result in profound hemorrhage and blood loss that may be life threatening, especially in the case of a vascular malformation. In this particular case, there was no blanching of the lesion when pressure was applied; nonetheless, in considering any invasive procedure, the surgeon must be aware of the possibility of profuse hemorrhage.
- There is an increased rate of regrowth if such giant cell lesions are not completely excised. However, this is not an indication for radical resection. Careful curettage of the bone ensures complete removal.

involvement would necessitate further investigation with blood tests for calcium and phosphate, and computerized tomography (CT) to assess the full extent of the lesion.

- The presence of a vascular lesion must be excluded in the provisional diagnosis. Biopsy of such a lesion may result in profound hemorrhage and blood loss that may be life threatening, especially in the case of a vascular malformation. In this particular case, there was no blanching of the lesion when pressure was applied; nonetheless, in considering any invasive procedure, the surgeon must be aware of the possibility of profuse hemorrhage.
- There is an increased rate of regrowth if such giant cell lesions are not completely excised. However, this is not an indication for radical resection. Careful curettage of the bone will ensure complete removal.

O. Complications

- Regrowth of lesion
- Misdiagnosis with the possibility of a vascular lesion and massive hemorrhage when performing a biopsy

Self-study Questions

1. **What investigations should be performed if hyperparathyroidism is suspected?**

2. **What is the difference between a pyogenic granuloma and the peripheral giant cell granuloma?**

3. **How much tissue should be removed in a biopsy?**

Answers are located at the end of the case.

Bibliography and Additional Reading

Flaitz CM. 2000. Peripheral giant cell granuloma: a potentially aggressive lesion in children. *Pediatr Dent* 22:232–3.

Grand E, Burgener E, Samson J, Lombardi T. 2008. Post-traumatic development of a peripheral giant cell granuloma in a child. *Dent Traumatol* 24:124–6.

Motamedi MH, Eshghyar N, Jafari SM, et al. 2007. Peripheral and central giant cell granulomas of the jaws: a demographic study. *Oral Surg Oral Med Oral Pathol Oral Radiol Endod* 103:e39–43.

Padbury AD, Tozum TF, Taba M, et al. 2006. The impact of primary hyperparathyroidism on the oral cavity. *J Clin Endocrinol Metab* 91:3439–45.

Pinto LP, Cherubinim K, Salum FG, Yurgel LS, de Figueiredo MA. 2006. Highly aggressive brown tumor in the jaw associated with tertiary hyperparathyroidism. *Pediatr Dent* 28:543–6.

Suliburk JW, Perrier ND. 2007. Primary hyperparathyroidism. *Oncologist* 12:644–53.

SELF-STUDY ANSWERS

1. Blood tests to determine levels of parathyroid hormone, calcium, phosphate, and alkaline phosphatase. CT is indicated to assess the full bony extent of any central lesion.

2. The pyogenic granuloma arises from mild irritation from plaque, calculus, or other foreign bodies, and may occur anywhere in the oral cavity. Some regard this lesion as a variant of the fibrous epulis with an increased vascular component. They are usually found interproximally and are commonly pedunculated with no osseous involvement.

3. Biopsies must always include a border of normal tissue so that the pathologist can observe the interface between the lesion and the healthy tissue. As a general rule, the clinician who will manage the case to conclusion should perform the biopsy (i.e., the surgeon who will ultimately manage a condition should be responsible for the biopsy). The size of the lesion determines the extent of the biopsy. Small lesions should be excised completely. If a large tissue deficit or functional disability may result following an excisional biopsy, then an incisional biopsy may be required. There must be adequate tissue to allow for histopathological examination and any tissue taken for an incisional biopsy must be representative of the lesion in its entirety.

Case 4

Eruption Cysts in a Newborn, Natal/Neonatal Teeth

A. Presenting Patient
- 2-day-old Caucasian male
- Newborn infant presenting as an emergency

B. Chief Complaint
- The mother and obstetrician have noticed two purplish swellings on the mandibular anterior alveolar ridge following delivery. There are no feeding difficulties at the moment. The pediatrician requested a dental consult.

C. Social History
- Only child to non-consanguineous parents
- Middle class family

D. Medical History
- Review of medical history reveals no significant findings, no known drug allergies, no medications. Child was born at term with a birth weight of 4,200 g (9.25 lbs). Delivery by forceps with a prolonged labor but good APGAR scores (8 and 10).

E. Medical Consult
- N/A

F. Dental History
- N/A

G. Extra-oral Examination
- Minor bruising on the face and scalp due to the delivery by forceps, but the mouth is not involved.

H. Intra-oral Examination
Soft Tissues
- There are two well circumscribed lesions on the lower alveolus on either side of the midline. They are symmetrically placed and identical in size, measuring approximately 4 mm in diameter (Figure 2.4.1).
- The lesions are dark purple but do not blanch on pressure. They are soft and fluctuant, and the base

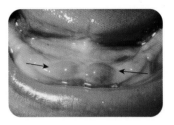

Figure 2.4.1. Intra-oral photograph showing two well circumscribed lesions (arrows)

appears to extend into the bone and is not pedunculated.

Hard Tissues
- No significant findings

I. Diagnostic Tools
- No other investigations are required in this case

J. Differential Diagnosis
Inflammatory Hyperplasias
- Fibrous epulis/pyogenic granuloma

Neoplasias/Tumors
- Congenital epulis/granular cell tumor of infancy
- Melanotic neuro-ectodermal tumor of infancy
- Congenital epithelial tumor

Developmental Anomalies/Harmatomas
- Eruption cyst/hematoma
- Bohn's nodules/dental laminar cysts
- Dentigerous cyst/odontogenic keratocyst
- Lymphangioma
- Hemangioma
- Vascular malformation
- Natal/neonatal teeth

K. Provisional Diagnosis and Problem List
Provisional Diagnosis
- Eruption cysts (see Fundamental Point 1)
- Natal/neonatal teeth (see Background Information 1)

BACKGROUND INFORMATION 1
Natal and Neonatal Teeth

- A natal tooth is present at birth (Figure 2.4.2), whereas the neonatal tooth erupts within a month of delivery. In almost every case, it is the normal primary tooth that has appeared early and not a supernumerary tooth. Therefore, the loss of a natal or neonatal tooth represents the loss of the primary tooth, but that will not affect the development of the permanent successor.

- The incidence of natal teeth is between 1:2,000 and 1:3,500 live births. There are no accurate figures on the incidence of neonatal teeth.

- Treatment options depend on the degree of mobility of the tooth and the risk that the tooth will exfoliate. It is important to remember that only five-sixths of the crown of a primary incisor has formed at birth; hence, the mobility of the tooth. Despite the theoretical risk, there has never been a reported case of aspiration of natal or neonatal teeth.

- If the tooth is excessively mobile or there are feeding difficulties, then it may be extracted.

- When extracting natal or neonatal teeth, it is essential to remove the dental papilla (pulp). If this is left behind, hard tissue or even a root may form.

- Local anesthesia is usually not required and the airway must always be protected.

- See Chapter 5, Case 1 for more on natal teeth.

Problem List
- Bilateral swellings on the alveolar ridge in a newborn

L. Comprehensive Treatment Plan
- Reassurance and monitoring
- If teeth erupt, extraction or monitoring

M. Prognosis and Discussion
- The cyst will resolve with the eruption of the new tooth and there is usually little need to surgically drain these lesions unless it is infected. If this is the case, the patient will be systemically ill because this represents an acute infection. Chronically infected eruption cysts cannot exist

FUNDAMENTAL POINT 1
Diagnosis of Eruption Cysts

- The eruption cyst or hematoma is an extremely common variation of normal eruption and not considered to be pathological unless the lesion is infected. The cyst represents an enlargement of the follicle around a newly erupting tooth. Because natal and neonatal teeth are common, it is not unusual to see an eruption cyst in a newborn infant. An eruption cyst must not be confused with a vascular lesion. To test this, apply pressure to the lesion to determine whether the area changes in color due to any blood emptying. Lesions that are bilateral and symmetrical are almost invariably benign and histopathology is not required.

- The most common lesions that may mimic eruption cysts in a newborn include vascular anomalies (hemangiomas or lymphangiomas), neuroectodermal tumors of infancy, or other odontogenic cystic lesions. A case has been reported of an odontogenic keratocyst mimicking an eruption cyst in a 19-month-old infant. (Chiang and Huang 2004)

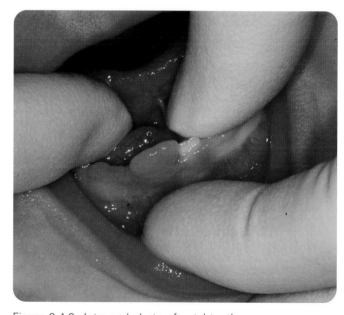

Figure 2.4.2. Intra-oral photo of natal tooth

because drainage would allow for eruption of the tooth and resolution of any infection. Parents are usually more worried about the appearance of the condition and are best reassured that the condition will resolve spontaneously.

- The premature emergence of a primary tooth is of little cause for concern except that root development will not be accelerated and so the tooth is likely to show increased mobility. The major concern is to ensure that the mother can adequately feed the infant without pain or trauma to the nipples. This is usually not a problem if the tooth is in the lower arch as the tongue will protect the nipple during feeding. However, if there is ulceration of the ventral surface of the tongue or the tooth is excessively mobile, then consideration should be given to its removal.

N. Complications

- Infection of the cyst
- Misdiagnosis with the possibility of a vascular lesion and massive hemorrhage when the primary tooth erupts or if there is surgical intervention.
- Aspiration/swallowing of loose teeth
- Riga-Fede disease: An ulceration affecting the ventral surface of the tongue in infants, caused by continual protrusive and retrusive movement of tongue over the lower incisors or natal/neonatal teeth. It typically presents between 1 month and 1 year of age. Treatment options include monitoring the ulcer only, smoothing of the incisal edge of the offending tooth, or extraction. See Chapter 5, Case 1 for more on Riga-Fede disease.

Self-study Questions

1. **What is the difference between a natal tooth and a neonatal one?**
2. **What happens if a neonatal tooth is lost soon after birth?**

3. **How is a natal tooth extracted?**
4. **What is Riga-Fede disease? How is treated?**

Answers are located at the end of the case.

Bibliography and Additional Reading

Chiang ML, Huang WH. 2004. Odontogenic keratocyst clinically mimicking an eruption cyst: report of a case. *Journal of Oral Pathology & Medicine* 33:373–5.

Chung NY, Batra R, Itzkevitch M, Boruchov D, Baldauf M. 2010. Severe methemoglobinemia linked to gel-type topical benzocaine use: a case report. *J Emerg Med* 38:601–6.

Cunha RF, Boer FA, Torriani DD, Frossard WT. 2001. Natal and neonatal teeth: review of the literature. *Pediatr Dent* 23:158–62.

Leung AK, Robson WL. 2006. Natal teeth: a review. *J Natl Med Assoc* 98:226–8.

Padmanabhan MY, Pandey RK, Aparna R, Radhakrishnan V. 2010. Neonatal sublingual traumatic ulceration—case report and review of the literature. *Dent Traumatol* 26:490–5.

Stamfelj I, Jan J, Cvetko E, Gaspersic. 2010. Size, ultrastructure, and microhardness of natal teeth with agenesis of permanent successors. *Ann Anat* 192:220–6.

Vucicevic Boras V, Mohamad Zaini Z, Savage NW. 2007. Supernumerary tooth with associated dentigerous cyst in an infant. A case report and review of differential diagnosis. *Aust Dent J* 52:150–3.

Ziai MN, Bock DJ, Da Silveira A, Daw JL. 2005. Natal teeth: a potential impediment to nasoalveolar molding in infants with cleft lip and palate. *J Craniofac Surg* 16:262–6.

SELF-STUDY ANSWERS

1. A natal tooth is present at birth, whereas a neonatal tooth erupts within a month of delivery.

2. There are few complications associated with the early loss of a primary incisor soon after birth. There is always a theoretical risk that a natal or neonatal tooth may be inhaled or swallowed. Invariably, the permanent tooth erupts normally and space loss does not present a problem because the inter-canine width is preserved. If the hard tissue of a natal tooth is removed, leaving some of the pulpal remnants behind, then a root may form from the dental papilla. If such a tooth is extracted, it is important to remove (curette) all associated tissue.

3. It is essential that the airway is protected when performing any invasive procedure on an infant. Place a piece of gauze behind the teeth at the back of the mouth to avoid accidental swallowing or aspiration of the tooth. It is usually convenient to use the knee to knee position with the child's head in the operator's lap. Young babies are best managed by wrapping them with a blanket to keep them secure, which also minimizes movement. Local anesthesia is usually not required because the tooth is only indicated for extraction in cases where there is extreme mobility. Commonly, the hard tissue of the crown is removed, leaving the dental papilla (pulp) behind. The tissue must be removed with a curette to ensure that there is no subsequent formation of hard tissue. Bleeding is controlled with local measures and feeding can start immediately.

4. It is an ulceration affecting the ventral surface of the tongue in infants, caused by continual protrusive and retrusive movement of the tongue over the lower incisors or natal/neonatal teeth. Treatment options include monitoring the ulcer only, smoothing of the incisal edge of the offending tooth, or extraction.

Case 5

Gingival Enlargement/Heart Transplant

A. Presenting Patient
- 10-year-old Causasian male
- Child referred by cardiologist regarding gingival enlargement following cardiac transplantation.

B. Chief Complaint
- Gingival overgrowth following heart transplant is causing gaps between the teeth, especially in the anterior region.

C. Social History
- Youngest of three children
- Attends primary school
- Middle-class family

D. Medical History
- Heart transplantation following cardiomyopathy five months ago
- Medications: cyclosporine and nifedipine (see Backgroung Information 1)
- No known food or drug allergies, vaccinations up to date

E. Medical Consult
- Cardiology

F. Dental History
- Has had regular dental care
- Fair oral hygiene habits which are further compromised by the gingival enlargement. No adult supervision.
- Strict diet, low in fat and simple carbohydrates
- Uses fluoridated toothpaste twice daily
- Lives in an optimally fluoridated area
- No history of dental trauma

G. Extra-oral Exam
- Slightly cushingoid appearance to face due to long-term corticosteroid therapy.

BACKGROUND INFORMATION 1
Gingival Enlargement

- Gingival enlargement, independent of gingivitis, is invariably related to medications or several hereditary conditions of which gingival fibromatosis is the most important. Clearly, if a child is on an immunosuppressive medication such as cyclosporine or a calcium channel blocker such as nifedipine, then the diagnosis is straightforward. Phenytoin-induced gingival enlargement depends on oral hygiene, whereas cyclosporine enlargement appears to have a particular threshold dose for some individuals. In all cases, the maintenance of meticulous oral hygiene is essential, although it must be realized that it is often extremely difficult for children to maintain their oral health in the presence of such enlarged tissues.

- A number of treatment options exist, such as changing the medication. This is obviously done in consultation with the physician, and general medical requirements always take precedence over oral considerations. In the case of cyclosporine, tacrolimus is often used as a substitute and there are drugs such as sodium valproate (Epilim) or carbamazepine (Tegretol) can be used as alternatives to phenytoin without the complications of gingival enlargement. The differential diagnosis in cases of enlargement should also include isolated gingival lesions such as epulides, of which the most common is the pyogenic granuloma.

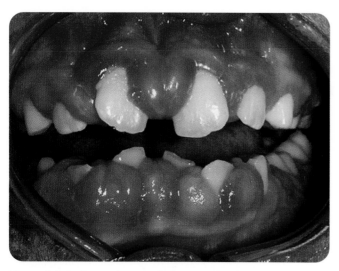

Figure 2.5.1. Pre-op intra-oral photograph of gingival enlargement

H. Intra-oral Exam

Soft Tissues (Figure 2.5.1)

- The keratinized gingiva is grossly enlarged with expansion of the interdental papilla and cervical tissues.
- Presence of gingivitis is consistent with poor oral hygiene.
- The tissues are firm and fibrous but not inflamed.

Hard Tissues

- No significant findings

Occlusal Evaluation of Mixed Dentition

- Class I canine and molar relationship with protuberant maxillary incisors spacing in both arches secondary to the gingival overgrowth.

Other

- Normal exfoliation of primary teeth but slightly delayed eruption and ectopic displacement of the permanent dentition.
- Caries-free

I. Diagnostic Tools

- Visual clinical exam only; no other investigations are required to determine the diagnosis

J. Differential Diagnosis

- Drug-induced gingival enlargement: cyclosporine, nifedipine, phenytoin (Dilantin)
- Hereditary gingival fibromatosis
- Other localized gingival enlargements such as epulides

K. Provisional Diagnosis and Problem List

- Gingival enlargement induced by cyclosporine and nifedipine (see Background Information 2)

BACKGROUND INFORMATION 2
Mechanisms of Gingival Overgrowth

- The precise mechanisms by which cyclosporine causes overgrowth of gingival tissues has yet to be fully determined. Nonetheless, there is increasing risk in younger children, those who express HLA-A24 antigen, and those with poor oral hygiene. The question of dose relationship is contentious, although it appears that a threshold may exist above which enlargement may occur.

- Cyclosporine causes an increase in fibroblast proliferation, possibly in response to elevated IL-6 and TGF-β1. There is an increase in the volume of extracellular collagen and decreased collagen loss. There is little doubt that oral hygiene is very important in reducing overgrowth and in some studies the use of antibiotics such as metronidazole was beneficial in controlling the gingival growth.

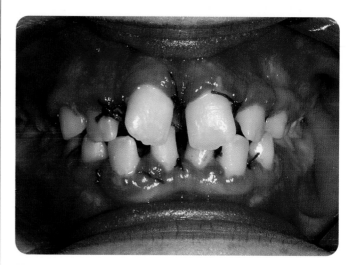

Figure 2.5.2. Post-op intra-oral photo following gingivectomy

Problem List

- Severe gingival enlargement with ectopic tooth eruption

L. Comprehensive Treatment Plan

- Consultation with treating physician
- Full mouth gingivectomy with infective endocarditis prophylaxis (see Figure 2.5.2 and Fundamental Point 1)
- Institution of preventive program with hygienist

FUNDAMENTAL POINT 1

Management of Gingival Enlargement

Surgical Resection of Gingival Overgrowths

- The choice of surgical procedure depends on the degree of overgrowth in each patient. No one procedure is better than another.

- The use of a diathermy or soft tissue lasers (diode, Nd:YAG, or CO_2) are useful when only minor work is required.

- The classical gingivectomy may be indicated when a major resection of the all of the gingiva is required. The disadvantage of this technique (using a bevel incision) is the large amount of open tissue that is left, making the post-operative period extremely uncomfortable for the patient and increasing the risk of infection.

- Flap surgery with apically repositioned flaps ensures primary closure of the wounds, less bleeding, and a better post-operative recovery period.

Orthodontic Treatment in Children Following Organ Transplantation

- There is no contraindication to orthodontic treatment in the post-transplant patient. Indeed, in these cases, orthodontics is impossible without removal of the excessive soft tissue which will also allow for better oral hygiene practices.

- It is important to observe the displacement of the teeth secondary to the growth of the gingival tissues and intervene where there is tooth movement.

Importance of Dental Care for the Transplant Recipient

- Dental care for transplant recipients is an essential part of their medical well being.

Immunosuppressed children are susceptible to infections from even minor wounds. It should be noted that pulp therapy in primary teeth is contraindicated in these children.

- Pre-transplant care
  - Excellent oral hygiene and preventive protocols (fluoride, fissure sealants, etc.)
  - Aggressive removal of any present and/or potential pathology that may compromise the child during immunosuppression.

- Post-transplant care
  - Continuation of excellent oral hygiene practices, including regular reviews and preventive monitoring.
  - Avoid elective dental treatment during immunosuppression periods. In consultation with the patient's cardiologist, use antibiotic prophylaxis if the patient is immunosuppressed and the dental treatment cannot be postponed. Although similar dosages may be used as in prophylaxis against endocarditis, the antibiotics are targeting secondary infections principally in the surgical site (not distant sites). Organ transplantation does not put the child at a greater risk of developing endocarditis, except if valvulopathy develops.
  - Protocols for the use of antibiotics for prophylaxis against endocarditis are constantly changing and the reader is advised to consult the most up-to-date protocols for their jurisdiction, such as those published by the American Heart Association and the National Institute for Health and Clinical Excellence (NICE) in the United Kingdom.

- Orthodontic treatment
- Maintenance and recalls

M. Prognosis and Discussion

- The long-term prognosis in this case is unknown due to our lack of knowledge regarding the precise mechanisms of action of cyclosporine. However, oral hygiene has been much improved and surgical

resection should allow the patient easier access for cleaning.

N. Complications

- Regrowth of gingival tissues
- Other oral growths
- Oral squamous cell carcinomas in long-term transplant survivors

Self-study Questions

1. *What type of surgical excision is preferable in cases in which all of the gingival tissues are involved?*
2. *When should orthodontic treatment be commenced in children with drug-induced gingival enlargement?*
3. *What is the role of the dentist in determining drug regimens in the management of complex medical conditions?*

4. *What is the antibiotic of choice when performing any gingival surgery on a child with a heart transplant?*

Answers are located at the end of the case.

Bibliography and Additional Reading

Burch M, Aurora P. 2004. Current status of paediatric heart, lung, and heart-lung transplantation. *Arch Dis Child* 89:386–9.

Chabria D, Weintraub RG, Kilpatrick NM. 2003. Mechanisms and management of gingival overgrowth in paediatric transplant recipients: a review. *Internat J Paediatr Dent* 13:220–9.

Doufexi A, Mina M, Ioannidou E. 2005. Gingival overgrowth in children: epidemiology, pathogenesis, and complications. A literature review. *J Periodontol* 76:3–10.

Euvrard S, Kanitakis J, Claudy A. 2003. Skin cancers after organ transplantation. *N Engl J Med* 348:1681–91.

Gould FK, Elliot TSJ, Foweraker J, et al. 2006. Guidelines for the prevention of endocarditis: report of the Working Party of the British Society for Antimicrobial Chemotherapy. *J Antimicr Chemother* 57:1035–42.

Kaur G, Verhamme KMC, Dieleman JP, et al. 2010. Association between calcium channel blockers and gingival hyperplasia. *J Clin Periodontol* 37:625–30.

Lockhart PB, Loven B, Brennan MT, et al. 2007. The evidence base for the efficacy of antibiotic prophylaxis in dental practice. *J Am Dent Assoc* 138(4):458–74.

Mavrogiannis M, Ellsi JS, Seymour RA, Thomason JM. 2006. The efficacy of three different surgical techniques in the management of drug-induced gingival overgrowth. *J Clin Periodontol* 33:677–82.

Nishimura RA, Carabello BA, Faxon DP, et al. 2008. ACC/AHA 2008 Guideline Update on Valvular Heart Disease: focused update on infective endocarditis. *Circulation* 2008; 188:887–96.

Schowengerdt KO. 2006. Advances in pediatric heart transplantation. *Curr Opin Pediatr* 18:512–7.

Seymour RA. 2006. Effects of medications on the periodontal tissue in health and disease. *Periodontol 2000*; 40:120–9.

Wilson W, Taubert KA, Gewitz M, et al. 2007. Prevention of infective endocarditis: Guidelines from the American Heart Association. *Circulation* 2007; 116:1736–54.

SELF-STUDY ANSWERS

1. There is no hard and fast rule as to which type of surgical excision is used in these cases. Where small amounts of tissue need to be removed, then the classical gingivectomy technique may be used. Where large amounts of tissue require removal, it is often better to use a flap procedure so that primary closure may be achieved. This is usually tolerated better by the patient and a better gingival contour may be achieved.

2. It is essential to seek an early orthodontic opinion in such cases. Selective gingivoplasty ranging to a full-mouth gingivectomy may be required to allow tooth eruption. Orthodontics should not be attempted unless the child and caretaker can maintain an adequate level of oral hygiene. While tooth alignment will not prevent gingival overgrowth, it may facilitate better oral hygiene that complicates such cases.

3. It is important for the dentist to be able to give appropriate advice to the treating physicians/oncologists/pediatricians in regard to the medications that are prescribed. Esthetics are of great concern to these children who have often undergone long hospitalization and many invasive medical procedures. To acquire oral health problems in addition to a heart transplant, for example, is burdensome and must be avoided. It is essential, therefore, for the dentist to be an integral part of the management team and to give good feedback to the treating doctors concerning oral health.

4. The transplant recipient who is on anti-rejection medication requires only the routine antibiotic medication to prevent post-operative infections. Children who have received a new heart are not at risk of developing endocarditis, except if they develop valvulopathy. However, perioperative and post-operative antibiotics are required to cover the immunosuppressed child from potential infection of tissues involved in the surgery. In the absence of any allergies, a broad-spectrum antibiotic such as amoxicillin, which is active against Gram-positive facultative oral organisms, is appropriate.

Case 6

Premature Loss of Primary Teeth—Hypophostasia

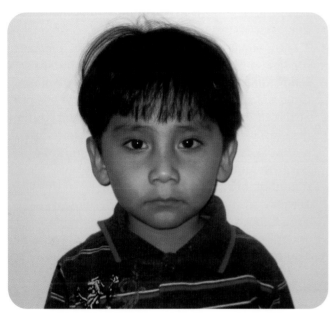

Figure 2.6.1. Facial photo

A. Presenting Patient
- 3-year-, 6-month-old Hispanic male
- New patient referred by his general dentist regarding exfoliation of mandibular primary central incisors.

B. Chief Complaint
- The mandibular central incisors have spontaneously fallen out.

C. Social History
- Youngest of three siblings
- High socio-economic status
- Lives with both parents

D. Medical History
- Review of medical history revealed no significant findings, no known drug or food allergies, no medications, vaccinations are up to date
- No family history of metabolic or genetic problems

E. Medical Consult
- Referral to pediatrics for lab tests and evaluation

F. Dental History
- Has a dental home
- Well-controlled normal diet
- Has good oral hygiene, brushes teeth every night with supervision
- Lives in optimally fluoridated area
- No history of dental trauma
- Normal eruption chronology and sequence of primary teeth, with the mandibular central incisors emerging around 7 months of age

G. Extra-oral Exam (Figure 2.6.1)
- No significant findings

H. Intra-oral Exam (Figure 2.6.2)
Soft Tissues
- The sites where the lower primary teeth have been lost have healed with no sign of infection or inflammation and the remaining gingival tissues are uninflamed.

Bone Tissues
- No significant findings

Occlusal Evaluation of Primary Dentition
- Mesial step molars, lateral incisors palatally positioned, maxillary anterior diastema

Dental Exam (Figure 2.6.2)
- No visible plaque
- Teeth appear morphologically normal with no enamel or dentin anomaly
- The maxillary central incisors and the mandibular lateral incisors are very mobile
- Caries-free

I. Diagnostic Tools
Panoramic Radiograph (Figure 2.6.3)
- No significant findings other than the premature loss of the mandibular primary central incisors

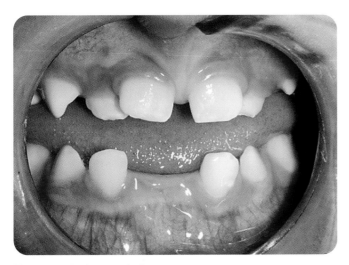

Figure 2.6.2. Intra-oral photo

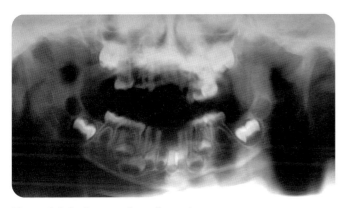

Figure 2.6.3. Panoramic radiograph

Tests With Normal Values
- Full blood count with differential white cell count
- Electolytes, urea, creatinine
- Calcium/phosphate
- Erythrocyte sedimentation rate (ESR)

Alkaline Phosphatase
- 70 U/L (normal: >100)

Urinary Phosphoethanolamine
- 87 μmol/mmol creatinine (normal: 10 to 25)

Pyridoxyl-5-phosphate
- 366 mmol/L (normal: 11–295)

J. Differential Diagnosis (see Fundamental Point 1)

Neutropenias
- Cyclic neutropenia
- Congenital agranulocytosis

Qualitative Neutrophil Defects
- Prepubertal periodontitis
- Juvenile periodontitis
- Leucocyte adhesion defect
- Papillon–Lefèvre syndrome
- Chèdiak–Higashi disease
- Acatalasia

Metabolic Disorders
- Hypophosphatasia

Connective Tissue Disorders
- Ehlers–Danlos syndrome (types IV and VIII)
- Erythromelalgia
- Acrodynia
- Scurvy

Neoplasia
- Langerhans' cell histiocytosis
- Acute myeloid leukemia

Self-injury
- Hereditary sensory neuropathies
- Lesch–Nyhan syndrome
- Psychotic disorders

K. Provisional Diagnosis and Problem List
Diagnosis
- Hypophosphatasia (see Background Information 1)

Problem List
- Premature exfoliation of primary teeth

L. Comprehensive Treatment Plan
- Confirmation of diagnosis by blood chemistry.
- Hard tissue pathology of exfoliated teeth examined under polarized light microscopy to determine amount of cellular cementum.
- Radiographic skeletal survey to assess for any rachitic changes in the long bones.
- Genetic counseling and screening of other family members.
- There is no specific treatment for hypophosphatasia other than maintenance of excellent oral hygiene to ensure that teeth are preserved as long as possible to remain caries-free.
- Future prosthetic rehabilitation

M. Prognosis and Discussion
- The fact that this patient has no other clinical manifestations is positive and it is likely that only the primary teeth will be affected.

FUNDAMENTAL POINT 1
Differential Diagnosis with Gingival Inflammation

- While uncommon, early loss of teeth is one of the most important diagnostic signs in oral medicine. All conditions that present with early loss of teeth are serious and potentially life threatening; thus, early recognition and diagnosis are essential. Any unexplained tooth loss needs immediate investigation. Teeth may exfoliate due to metabolic disturbances, periodontal disease, connective tissue disorders, neoplasia, loss of alveolar bone support, or self-inflicted trauma. The major diagnostic criterion is the state of the gingival tissues.

- The formulation of a differential diagnosis is essential, and serious conditions such as immune disorders must be excluded first.

- In this patient's case, the gingiva is entirely normal and the teeth exfoliated due to a deficiency in cellular cementum. This condition is quite distinct from all of the other diseases mentioned above in this regard.

- The appearance of the gingiva is also not consistent with trauma or self-injurious behavior.

- The majority of teeth are lost from periodontal disease. Gingivitis is common in children, but periodontal disease is extremely rare and indicates an underlying immune disorder based on quantitative or qualitative white cell disorders.

- The main organisms involved in periodontal disease are *Actinobacillus actinomycetemcomitans*, *Prevotella intermedia*, *Eikenella corrodens*, and *Capnocytophaga sputigena*. All are present in response to altered immune status but only some, particularly the *Actinobacilli*, secrete leukotoxins.

- Specific white cell function tests are required to assess chemotaxic disorders to altered degranulation of neutrophils. In cases of cyclic neutropenia, sequential differential white cell counts are required to confirm a diagnosis.

- The presence of gingival inflammation is an important indicator as to the status of the immune system and may be used to determine whether therapy with agents such as human granulocyte-colony stimulating factor (h-GCSF) may be discontinued or recommenced.

BACKGROUND INFORMATION 1
Hypophosphatasia

- Hypophosphatasia is an uncommon inherited metabolic disorder in which there is a deficiency in the activity of tissue non-specific alkaline phosphatase. It is characterized by a defective bone mineralization with highly variable clinical features, ranging from the premature loss of primary teeth to neonatal death. Importantly, the milder cases in which there is no long-bone involvement are diagnosed due to their dental manifestations.

- Frequency is 1:100,000 live births, transmitted as an autosomal recessive disorder or maybe a spontaneous mutation.

- In children with only dental involvement the prognosis is very good. Permanent teeth rarely exfoliate.

- The root surface shows an absence of cellular cementum that may account for the exfoliation of these teeth. Ground, hard tissue sections of exfoliated teeth should be performed.

- Screening of long bones with densitometry is important to assess for rachitic changes that may affect growth.

- Genetic counseling should be offered to families because this condition may be extremely variable in its expressivity.

- Severe cases have been treated with hematopoietic stem cell transplantation and enzyme replacement therapy with mixed success.

- Hypophostasia has extreme variability in expression and an uncertain mode of inheritance; thus, the parents and eventually the child must understand the risk of transmission to future offspring. Any genetic counseling should be undertaken by someone trained in this area.

- Bone healing appears to be normal but there have been no cases yet reported of the use of osseointegrated implants to rehabilitate such patients.

N. Complications

- Continuing loss of teeth and prosthetic rehabilitation

Self-study Questions

1. **What are the main white cell disorders associated with premature loss of primary teeth?**

2. **What changes might you expect to observe in the roots of exfoliated teeth with hypophosphatasia?**

3. **What biochemical and blood tests would you order if you suspect a child has hypophosphatasia?**

4. **When should a family be referred to a geneticist?**

Answers are located at the end of the case.

Bibliography and Additional Reading

Hartsfield JK Jr. 1994. Premature exfoliation of teeth in childhood and adolescence. *Adv Pediatr* 41:453–70.

Meyle J, Gonzéles JR. 2001. Influences of systemic diseases on periodontitis in children and adolescents. *Periodontol 2000*; 26:92–112.

Mornet E. 2008. Hypophosphatasia. *Best Pract Res Clin Rheumatol* 22:113–27.

Reibel A, Manière MC, Clauss F, Droz D, Alembik Y, Mornet E, Bloch-Zupan A. 2009. Orodental phenotype and genotype findings in all subtypes of hypophosphatasia. *Orphanet J Rare Dis* 4:6.

van den Bos T, Handoko G, Niehof A, et al. 2005. Cementum and dentin in hypophosphatasia. *J Dent Res* 84:1021–5.

SELF-STUDY ANSWERS

1. Periodontal disease in children indicates a serious underlying immune disorder. The microorganisms associated with prepubertal periodontitis are *Actinobacillus actinomycetemcomitans, Prevotella intermedia, Eikenella corrodens,* and *Capnocytophaga sputigena.* While these organisms may directly affect host immune responses, it is now believed that it is the underlying immune deficiency that results in an overgrowth of these organisms. Diagnosis of these conditions is often difficult and specialized tests of neutrophils are needed to assess function, chemotaxis, and integrity of these cells.

2. An exfoliated tooth may be sent for histopathological examination. Teeth should be prepared for hard tissue ground sections and not decalcified. It is possible to observe an absence of cellular cementum that is characteristic of hypophosphatasia under polarized light microscopy.

3. A child that is suspected of hypophosphatasia should have the following tests:

- Blood tests: Full blood test with differential white cell count; erythrocyte sedimentation rate (ESR); electrolytes, urea, and creatinine; Calcium, phosphate, and alkaline phosphatase
- Urine tests: Vitamin B_6 (pyridoxyl-5-phosphate); phosphoethanolamine (requires specialized metabolic assays that are only available to certain laboratories)
- Bone densitometry should be considered to assess the calcification of the long bones and for any rachitic changes that might be present

4. The question of genetic testing must be handled in a sensitive and professional way. Genetic counseling must be performed by clinicians or psychologists or counselors with appropriate training and knowledge about the particular problem. In most cases, both the parents and the child should be involved and often other siblings as well. This is naturally an emotional experience but it is important for families to have appropriate knowledge from a professional rather than looking up information on the Internet.

Case 7

Amelogenesis Imperfecta

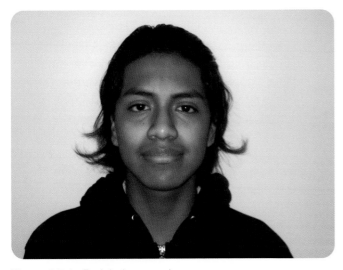

Figure 2.7.1. Facial photograph

A. Presenting Patient
- 13-year-old male
- New patient referred for assessment and management of enamel defects

B. Chief Complaint
- Patient was concerned with the appearance of his teeth as well as the sensitivity experienced.

C. Social History
- Patient has just started high school
- Oldest of five children
- Middle-class family
- His father, paternal grandmother, younger brother, paternal aunt, and first cousins have teeth with a similar appearance
- No diagnosis of any dental anomaly has been previously made

D. Medical History
- Review of medical history revealed no significant findings, no known drug or food allergies, no medications, vaccinations are up to date

E. Medical Consult
- Department of Genetics

F. Dental History
- Regular visits to local school dental clinic
- Regular diet
- Fair oral hygiene, brushes twice daily
- Uses fluoridated toothpaste
- Lives in optimally fluoridated area
- No history of trauma
- Cooperative for dental treatment

G. Extra-oral Exam (Figure 2.7.1)
- No significant findings

H. Intra-oral Exam
Soft Tissues
- Minor gingivitis

Hard Tissues
- No significant findings

Occlusal Evaluation of Permanent Dentition
- Class I molar and class I canine, overbite: 40%, overjet: 2 mm, on a class I skeletal base. There appeared to be loss of occlusal vertical dimension.

Other (Figures 2.7.2a–c)
- Minimal plaque and calculus deposits
- Teeth exhibited classical features of small, discrete pinpoint-to-pinhead sized pits, which were arranged in horizontal and vertical rows.
- All teeth exhibited yellow discoloration and were sensitive to cold, which had progressively worsened.
- Localized areas of loss of enamel in occlusal region subject to occlusal stresses. These defects were most prominent on the first permanent molars.
- Open contacts present between most teeth

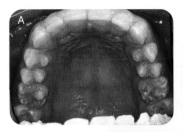
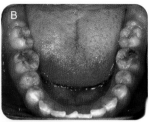
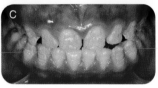

Figure 2.7.2a–c. Pre-operative intraoral photos. A. Pre-op maxillary photo, B. pre-op mandibular photo, C. pre-op anterior photo

- Occlusal caries detected in the mandibular first permanent molars.

I. Diagnostic Tools
- Panoramic radiograph showed reduced enamel thickness and normal contrast between enamel and dentin.

J. Differential Diagnosis
- Amelogenesis imperfecta (AI)
- Fluorosis
- Generalized chronological enamel hypoplasia
- Generalized chronological hypoplasia in association with other syndromes

K. Diagnosis and Problem List
Diagnosis
- Hypoplastic pitted autosomal dominant amelogenesis imperfecta (type IA Witkop classification, 1989) (see Background Information 1)

Problem List
- Poor esthetics
- Tooth sensitivity
- Loss of occlusal vertical dimension
- Dental caries

L. Comprehensive Treatment Plan (see Fundamental Point 1)
- Full dental records, including study models, facebow for articulator, radiographs, and intra-oral photographs
- Detailed interdisciplinary discussion of treatment plan, involving prosthodontist, orthodontist, and dental technician
- Detailed discussion with patient and parents regarding treatment plan

BACKGROUND INFORMATION 1
Amelogenesis Imperfecta
- Amelogenesis imperfecta (AI) is a diverse group of hereditary conditions that primarily affect the quality and/or the quantity of dental enamel, resulting in poor development or complete absence of the enamel of the teeth. It is caused by improper differentiation of ameloblasts in the absence of systemic involvement with the phenotypic manifestations of mutant genes influencing different levels of enamel development. There are four proven candidate genes for AI: amelogenin (AMELX), enamelin (ENAM), enamelysin (MMP20), and kallikrein 4 (KLK4). Various population studies of AI indicate a prevalence of between 1:718 and 1:14,000.

- The clinical appearance can be remarkably varied and both dentitions are affected. The eruption process of permanent teeth is affected by AI, with follicular cysts, delayed eruption, and retention or impaction of teeth being reported. The most frequent dental anomaly associated with AI is taurodontism. The radiologic appearance of AI varies with the type. In the smooth hypoplastic type, the enamel layer is conspicuously thin and its radiodensity is greater than the adjacent dentin, whereas in the hypocalcified type the enamel layer appears absent. In the hypomaturation type, the radiodensity of the enamel is almost equal to that of normal dentin.

- AI carries a high morbidity, including tooth sensitivity, poor esthetics, dental caries, anterior open bite, advanced dental age and/or failure of dental eruption, pre-eruptive tooth resorption, gingival inflammation, and loss of occlusal vertical dimension. The treatment and prognosis are highly variable and relate to the severity of the enamel involvement.

- Management of carious lesions on mandibular first permanent molars.
- Crowns with complete axial coverage on first and second permanent molars and esthetic crowns for all premolars with partial mesial and distal coverage.

FUNDAMENTAL POINT 1

Planning and Treatment for Amelogenesis Imperfecta

- The restoration of esthetics and function of the dentition in patients with amelogenesis imperfecta (AI) often presents the dentist with a major challenge. For a young child or adolescent, the long-term aim of treatment is to maintain the maximum amount of dental hard tissue possible until the patient reaches an age at which advanced restorative techniques can be employed to rehabilitate the dentition. In the short-term, it is frequently necessary to intervene to improve esthetics, maintain tooth structure, maintain or increase occlusal vertical dimension, and relieve the symptoms of tooth sensitivity. Treatment varies according to the age of the patient, stage of dental development, and existing condition of the dentition on presentation.

- The aim of the treatment of this patient was to provide well-fitting and retentive cast and indirect Artglass restorations with minimal to no tooth preparation such that tooth structure was protected, function was maintained, symptoms were controlled, and esthetics were improved.

The ultimate objectives were to ensure that the development of the dentition and the form of the dental arches were not compromised.

- The use of adhesive cast gold crowns on the first and second permanent molars served to increase the occlusal vertical dimension by approximately 4 to 5mm. The gold crowns would also support the occlusal vertical dimension and reduce the occlusal load on the Artglass crowns. All other posterior teeth were restored with Artglass crowns. The anterior teeth were restored with Artglass veneers.

- The design of the castings and crowns for the posterior teeth was based on occlusal and axial coverage. No reduction of occlusal and only minor axial surface reduction was performed. Artglass veneers were constructed for anterior teeth and based on full labial, palatal, and lingual coverage and partial mesial and distal coverage. Tooth preparation was restricted to maxillary permanent central and lateral incisors. Minimal tooth preparation prior to prosthodontic treatment has been well documented, minimizing unnecessary tooth surface loss.

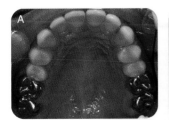
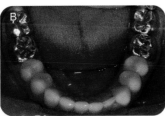
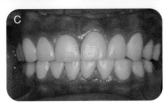

Figure 2.7.3a–c. Post-operative intra-oral photos. A. Post-op maxillary photo, B. post-op mandibular photo, C. post-op anterior photo

- Esthetic veneers with partial mesial and distal coverage for all permanent anterior teeth
- Review, prevention, and long-term maintenance

M. Post-operative Intra-oral Photographs
(Figures 2.7.3 a–c)

N. Prognosis and Discussion

- The use of Artglass as an indirect restorative material has been shown to be successful in the short and medium term, with superior marginal integrity and fracture resistance in comparison to other indirect materials. Additionally, composite resin can be added to the material, and axial surfaces can be thin and tapered. The use of cast restorations has been well documented for the management of AI. In this case, cast gold crowns have been used to restore both the first and second permanent molars in preference to cast NiCr crowns. Research indicates that properly fabricated cast gold restorations provide extremely predictable and long-term restorations. All treatment proved uneventful, with excellent esthetic results. Sensitivity was eliminated and the teeth protected from further wear. The occlusal vertical dimension was re-established without complications. The ultimate objective at this stage is to ensure that the development of the dentition and the form of the dental arches are not compromised.

O. Common Complications and Alternative Treatment Plans

Failure of Restorations Due to:
- Debonding
- Fracture
- Caries

Alternative Treatments for Permanent Molars
- Preformed stainless steel crowns
- Nickel chromium cast crowns or onlays
- Porcelain fused to metal crowns
- Direct composite resin crowns or onlays
- Indirect composite resin crown or onlays

Alternative Treatments for Anterior Teeth
- Direct composite resin veneers or crowns
- Porcelain veneers or crowns

Self-study Questions

1. **What alternative materials may be used for the restoration of the permanent molars?**
2. **What alternative materials may be used for the restoration of the anterior teeth?**
3. **What is the radiographic appearance of AI?**
4. **What are the major challenges the dentist faces with the restoration of esthetics and function of the dentition in patients with AI?**

5. **What are the most commonly reported problems in the eruption of permanent teeth with AI?**
6. **What is the most common dental anomaly associated with AI?**

Answers are located at the end of the case.

Bibliography and Additional Reading

Bailleul-Forestier I, Berdal A, Vinckier F, de Ravel T, Fryns JP, Verloes A. 2008. The genetic basis of inherited anomalies of the teeth. Part 2: syndromes with significant dental involvement. *Eur J Med Genet* 51:383–408.

Bailleul-Forestier I, Molla M, Verloes A, Berdal A. 2008. The genetic basis of inherited anomalies of the teeth. Part 1: clinical and molecular aspects of non-syndromic dental disorders. *Eur J Med Genet* 51:273–91.

Hu JC, Chun YH, Al Hazzazzi T, Simmer JP. 2007. Enamel formation and amelogenesis imperfecta. *Cells Tissues Organs* 186:78–85.

Hu JC-C, Simmer JP. 2007. Developmental biology and genetics of dental malformations. *Orthod Craniofacial Res* 10:45–52.

Ng FK, Messer LB. 2009. Dental management of amelogenesis imperfecta patients: a primer on genotype-phenotype correlations. *Pediatr Dent* 31:20–30.

Poulsen S, Gjorup H, Haubek D, et al. 2008. Amelogenesis imperfecta—a systematic literature review of associated dental and orofacial abnormalities and their impact on patients. *Acta Odontol Scand* 66:193–9.

Witkop Jr CJ. 1988. Amelogenesis imperfecta, dentinogenesis imperfecta and dentin dysplasia revisited: problems in classification. *J Oral Pathol* 17:547–53.

SELF-STUDY ANSWERS

1. Alternatives for permanent molars:
   - Preformed stainless steel crowns
   - Nickel chromium cast crowns or onlays
   - Porcelain fused to metal crowns
   - Direct composite resin crowns or onlays
   - Indirect composite resin crown or onlays

2. Alternatives for anterior teeth:
   - Direct composite resin veneers or crowns
   - Porcelain veneers or crowns

3. The radiologic appearance of AI varies with the type. In the smooth, hypoplastic type, the enamel layer is conspicuously thin and its radiodensity is greater than the adjacent dentin, whereas in the hypocalcified type the enamel layer appears absent. In the hypomaturation type, the radiodensity of the enamel is almost equal to that of normal dentin.

4. For a young child or adolescent, the long-term aim of treatment is to maintain the maximum possible amount of dental hard tissue until the patient reaches an age at which advanced restorative techniques can be employed to rehabilitate the dentition. In the short-term, it is frequently necessary to intervene to improve esthetics, maintain tooth structure, maintain or increase occlusal vertical dimension, and relieve the symptoms of tooth sensitivity. Treatment varies according to the age of the patient, stage of dental development, and existing condition of the dentition on presentation.

5. Follicular cysts, delayed eruption, and retention or impaction of teeth have been reported with the eruption of permanent teeth with AI.

6. The most frequent dental anomaly associated with AI is taurodontism.

3

Complex Pulp Therapy

Anna B. Fuks

Clinical Cases in Pediatric Dentistry, First Edition. Edited by Amr M. Moursi.
© 2012 Blackwell Publishing Ltd. Published 2012 by Blackwell Publishing Ltd.

Case 1

Indirect Pulp Treatment

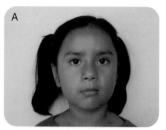 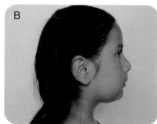

Figure 3.1.1a–b. Facial photographs

A. Presenting Patient
- 6-year-, 6-month-old Hispanic female
- Recall visit two years after last appointment

B. Chief Complaint and History of Present Injury
- Patient's father stated that his daughter "complained of toothache the last few days in the lower back right side, and I can see she has several cavities. She has not been to the dentist for a long time."

FUNDAMENTAL POINT 1

Questions to Ask When Obtaining a History Regarding Pain

- Describe the pain. Does it linger or subside after stimulus is removed? Is the pain spontaneous?
- What are the frequency, severity, duration, triggering agents of the pain (thermal, food, sleeping)?
- What are the symptoms (fever, swelling)?
- What has been the analgesic use?

C. Social History
- Middle class
- Patient is in 1st grade

D. Medical History
- No significant findings, no known drug or food allergies, no medications, vaccinations are up to date

E. Medical Consult
- N/A

F. Dental History
- Dental home was established at the age 16 months when initial signs of early childhood caries were observed on the maxillary primary incisors. Fluoride varnish applications were recommended every three months at that time
- Despite recommendation for routine six-month recalls, two years have passed since last visit
- Cariogenic diet
- Poor oral hygiene, brushes once daily, unsupervised
- Uses toothpaste containing fluoride
- Lives in an optimally fluoridated area
- No history of dental/oral trauma
- Cooperative behavior for all past dental care

G. Extra-oral Exam
- No significant findings

H. Intra-oral Exam
Soft Tissues
- No significant findings

Hard Tissues
- No significant findings

Occlusal Evaluation of Primary Dentition
- Mesial step molars, class III right canines, class I left canines

Other
- Moderate plaque accumulation
- Several teeth with moderate to extensive carious lesions
- Mandibular right primary second molar with an extensive carious lesion

I. Diagnostic Tools
- Periapical radiograph of the mandibular right primary second molar at the time of the initial appointment (Figure 3.1.2) shows a large occlusal carious lesion. It was treated with a pulpectomy as an emergency
- Right and left bitewing radiographs were taken after the initial visit, which focused on emergency treatment of the mandibular right primary second molar (Figures 3.1.3 a, b)
- The bitewing radiographs showed deep carious lesions on the maxillary right primary second molar and on the mandibular left primary second molar (Figure 3.1.3.)

J. Differential Diagnosis
For the Maxillary Right and the Mandibular Left Primary Second Molars:
- Deep carious lesions with possible pulp involvement

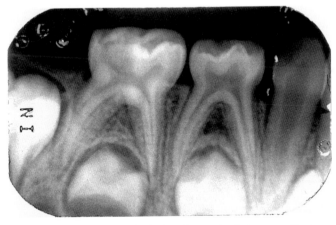

Figure 3.1.2. Pre-op periapical radiograph of the mandibular right primary second molar

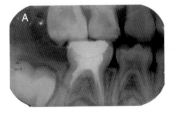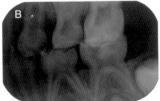

Figure 3.1.3a–b. Bitewing radiographs after pulpectomy and prior to IPT treatments. A. Right bitewing radiograph, B. left bitewing radiograph

- Deep carious lesions with partial necrosis
- Deep carious lesions with total necrosis

K. Diagnosis and Problem List
Diagnosis
- Extensive carious lesions in several primary molars
- Deep carious lesion on the right mandibular second primary molar (treated with a pulpectomy in the initial appointment as an emergency)
- Maxillary right and mandibular left primary second molars with deep carious lesions without signs or symptoms of irreversible pulpits and no soft tissue pathology
- No radiographic signs of pulpal nor peri-radicular pathology

Problem List
- High caries risk due to several factors: cariogenic diet, poor oral hygiene, moderate plaque accumulation, unsupervised brushing, no regular dental visits
- Several untreated carious lesions with possible reversible and/or irreversible pulp involvement

L. Comprehensive Treatment Plan
- Emergency treatment of the right mandibular primary second molar
- Explanation to the father of the importance of maintaining a primary second molar, particularly prior to the eruption of the first permanent molar
- Indirect pulp treatment (IPT) technique was chosen for the deep lesions of the maxillary right and mandibular left primary second molars, considering that they were asymptomatic and amenable to be properly sealed with leakage-free restorations
- Comprehensive treatment of other carious lesions: Consider using nitrous oxide analgesia given the length of the procedures
- Follow up care including:
  - Immediate post-op and home care instructions
  - Prevention plan
  - Recall visits every three months, including fluoride varnish application and caries risk re-evaluation
  - Follow up radiographs after six months

IPT Technique
- Local anesthesia and rubber dam
- Caries removal leaving affected dentin over the pulpal floor
- Coverage of the affected dentin with glass ionomer cement. This material was chosen due to its

BACKGROUND INFORMATION 1
Indirect Pulp Treatment

- Indirect pulp treatment (IPT) is recommended for teeth that have deep, carious lesions approximating the pulp but without signs or symptoms of pulp degeneration.

- In this procedure, the deepest layer of the remaining carious dentin is covered with a biocompatible material to prevent pulp exposure and additional trauma to the tooth. This results in the deposition of tertiary dentin, which increases the distance between the affected dentin and the pulp, and in the deposition of peritubular (sclerotic) dentin, decreasing dentin permeability. It is important to remove the carious tissue completely from the dentino-enamel junction (DEJ) and from the lateral walls of the cavity to achieve optimal interfacial seal between the tooth and the restorative material, thus preventing microleakage.

- The dilemma that clinicians face lies in the assessment of how much caries to leave on the pulpal or axial floor. The carious tissue that should remain on the floor of the cavity preparation is a quantity that, if removed, would result in overt exposure. It is difficult to determine whether an area is an infected carious lesion or a bacteria-free demineralized zone. The best clinical marker is the quality of the dentin: soft, mushy dentin should be removed, and hard, discolored dentin can be indirectly capped.

- The ultimate objective of this treatment is to maintain pulp vitality by:
  - Arresting the carious process
  - Promoting dentin sclerosis (reducing permeability)
  - Stimulating the formation of tertiary dentin
  - Remineralizing the carious dentin.

- Two materials have been most commonly used in IPT: $Ca(OH)_2$ and zinc oxide–eugenol paste. Lately, glass ionomer cements have also been successfully used in this procedure. Massara, Alves, and Brandao (2002) demonstrated that glass ionomer creates conditions that lead to remineralization and recommended it as a good base for IPT.

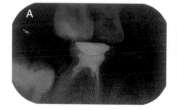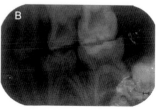

Figure 3.1.4a–b. Post-IPT bitewing radiographs. A. Post-op right bitewing radiograph, B. Post-op left bitewing radiograph

biocompatible properties, ability to promote remineralization of the demineralized dentin, and fluoride release capacity
- Both teeth received a Class I restoration using a composite resin material followed by a fissure sealant

M. Clinical and Radiographic Follow-up
- Ten months after IPT on the maxillary right primary second molar (Figure 3.1.4a) and on the mandibular left primary second molar (Figure 3.1.4b). Notice the retraction of the distal pulp horn due to the formation of reactionary dentin on both teeth

N. Prognosis and Discussion
- Prognosis for caries: The recommended protocol for decreasing caries risk depends on the parents' understanding and compliance in reducing the identified risk factors and in attending regular recall exams. In the present case, the parent brought the child for a recall visit 10 months after the completion of the initial comprehensive dental treatment, instead of the recommended six months. At that time, new lesions were identified

- Prognosis for IPT: The prognosis for IPT is usually good. Partial caries removal in asymptomatic primary or permanent teeth reduces the risk of pulp exposure. Success rates of IPT have been reported to be higher than 90% in primary teeth; thus, its use is recommended in patients in whom a pre-operative diagnosis suggests no signs of pulp degeneration. The value of taking a good history complemented by a careful clinical and radiographic examination cannot be overestimated. Studies investigating the long-term outcome of partial caries removal have used either composite resins or stainless steel crowns as the restorative material. A recent systematic review of the literature (Ricketts et al. 2006) reported no difference in the incidence of pulp exposure, in the progression of the decay and on the longevity of restorations, irrespective of whether the removal of decay had been minimal (ultraconservative) or complete. In the present case, the longevity of the composite restoration also depends on a periodic clinical follow-up to check the integrity of the margins of the restoration to rule out microleakage. In addition, the presence of a new proximal lesion might jeopardize the success of the IPT by contamination of bacteria and/or their toxins. Therefore, in children with high caries risk,

using a stainless steel crown over an IPT is suggested. The most relevant factor noted in the present case that can contribute to a poor prognosis is the patient's lack of compliance with dental appointments

O. Common Complications and Alternative Treatment Plans

- The most common complications of a failing IPT are pulp necrosis and/or a periapical lesion. These may be the result of an initial misdiagnosis of an irreversibly inflamed or necrotic pulp or due to a poor restoration leading to microleakage.
- Alternative treatments include pulpotomy or pulpectomy

Self-study Questions

1. **What could have prevented the amount and severity of the carious lesions in the present case?**
2. **Could a sealant have prevented these lesions?**
3. **Has the adopted approach to prevent pulp exposure (IPT) been evaluated and supported by the literature?**

4. **When is an IPT contraindicated for primary molars?**
5. **Should poor compliance and high caries risk influence the choice of treatment?**

Answers are located at the end of the case.

Bibliography and Additional Reading

Fuks AB. 2005. Pulp therapy for the primary dentition. In: *Pediatric Dentistry, Infancy through Adolescence* 4th Edition. Pinkham JR, Casamassimo PS, Fields HW Jr., McTigue DJ, Nowak AJ (eds). Elsevier Saunders: St. Louis. pp. 375–93.

Massara MLA, Alves JB, Brandão PRG. 2002. Atraumatic restorative treatment: Clinical, ultrastructural and chemical analysis. *Caries Res* 36:430.

Ricketts DNJ, Kidd EAM, Innes N, Clarkson J. 2006. Complete or ultraconservative removal of decayed tissue in unfilled teeth. Cochrane Database of Systematic Reviews. Jul 19; 3:CD003808.

SELF-STUDY ANSWERS

1. If the child's parents would have had a better compliance and followed the six-month recall protocol, at least the severity of the lesions could be controlled and new lesions prevented

2. Probably yes. Sealants are indicated for primary and permanent teeth with pits and fissures that are predisposed to plaque retention. If the sealant covering the susceptible fissure is intact, it can definitely prevent the development of caries

3. Yes. A systematic review of the literature (Ricketts et al. 2006) reported no difference in the incidence of pulp exposure, in the progression of the decay and on the longevity of restorations, irrespective of whether the removal of decay had been minimal (ultraconservative) or complete

4. IPT is contraindicated for primary molars when there is a history of spontaneous pain or any clinical and/or radiographic pathological signs. The tooth must be vital to be treated with IPT

5. Yes. In patients with high caries risk and poor compliance, it is preferable to use radical treatment approaches, such as stainless steel crowns, instead of multi-surface restorations

Case 2

Partial Pulpotomy in Traumatized Primary Incisors

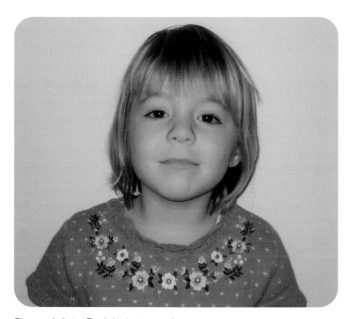

Figure 3.2.1. Facial photograph

A. Presenting Patient
- 4-year-, 2-month-old Caucasian female
- New patient presenting as an emergency

B. Chief Complaint
- Mother stated, "My daughter fell while playing with other children in the kindergarten yard and fractured her two upper front teeth"

C. Social History
- Second of three children
- Both parents are well educated
- Middle class, mother works part time

D. Medical History
- No significant findings, no known food or drug allergies, no medications, vaccinations are up to date

E. Medical Consult
- N/A

F. Dental History
- Has dental home
- Eating habits include a balanced diet rich in proteins and low in carbohydrates. The child eats regular meals and the parents demand that their children limit the ingestion of sweets to after meals
- Fair oral hygiene habits, brushes twice daily with parental supervision
- Uses toothpaste containing fluoride
- Optimal water fluoridation levels
- No history of previous trauma

G. Extra-oral Exam
- Mild swelling of the upper lip

H. Intra-oral Exam
Soft Tissues
- Bruises on labial mucosa, gingival laceration on maxillary anterior area, and laceration of the labial frenum

Hard Tissues
- No significant findings

Occlusion Evaluation of Primary Dentition
- Mesial step molars, class I canines

Other
- Moderate plaque accumulation over the fractured teeth
- Caries-free primary dentition
- Maxillary central incisors with complicated crown fractures
- Mild sensitivity to percussion on both maxillary central incisors
- Physiologic mobility on both traumatized incisors
- Extremely apprehensive

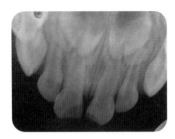

Figure 3.2.2. Anterior maxillary periapical radiograph showing crown fractures with pulp involvement

I. Diagnostic Tools

- Anterior maxillary periapical radiograph (Figure 3.2.2). Bitewing radiographs were not taken because the patient has periodical examinations at her family dentist

J. Differential Diagnosis

- Complicated crown fractures of maxillary primary central incisors
- Complicated crown–root fractures
- Complicated crown fractures associated with subluxation

K. Diagnosis and Problem List

Diagnosis

- Based on the history of pain, clinical examination, and radiographic findings, the most probable diagnosis is complicated crown fractures of maxillary primary central incisors

Problem List

- Maxillary primary central incisors with exposed pulps and pulp polyps needing emergency treatment
- Child has never had a local anesthetic

L. Comprehensive Treatment Plan

- Emergency treatment of the exposed pulps
- Explanation to the mother of the importance of maintaining the vitality of both teeth
- Behavioral management considerations (consider using nitrous oxide analgesia)
- Follow-up care including:
  - Post-op and home care instructions
  - Recall plan
- Radiographs should be taken after 3, 6, 12, 18, and 24 months and thereafter at yearly intervals until physiologic exfoliation of the teeth

M. Prognosis and Discussion

- Long-term studies have shown very high success rates of pulp capping and partial pulpotomy with

---

FUNDAMENTAL POINT 1
Complicated Crown Fracture

- Definition: Enamel-dentin fracture with pulp exposure
- Diagnosis: Clinical and radiographic findings reveal a loss of tooth structure with pulp exposure
- Treatment objectives: Maintain pulp vitality and restore normal esthetics and function. Injured lips, tongue, and gingiva should be examined for tooth fragments.
- Pulpal treatment alternatives are pulpotomy, pulpectomy, and extraction

Primary Teeth

- Keep treatment as simple as possible, taking into consideration the child's behavior and the life span of the tooth. Decisions often are based on life expectancy of the traumatized primary tooth and vitality of the pulpal tissue
- Risk of treatment and possible sequelae to the permanent tooth should be assessed versus the functional benefit resulting from treatment to the primary tooth

---

FUNDAMENTAL POINT 2
Advantages of Partial Pulpotomy

- Preserves cell-rich coronal pulp
- Increases healing potential due to preserved pulp
- Physiologic apposition of cervical dentin
- Obviates need for root canal therapy
- Preserves natural color and translucency
- Maintains pulp test responses

---

respect to pulp survival. Radiographic evidence of hard tissue closure of the perforation can be seen three months after pulp capping. Most of the studies were done in permanent teeth

- The primary factor to pulp survival after crown fracture is compromised pulp circulation due to luxation injuries. Crown fracture with concomitant luxation injury has been shown to have an

BACKGROUND INFORMATION 1

Partial Pulpotomy (Cvek Pulpotomy) Indications and Technique

Indications: Traumatic Pulp Exposures

- Initially performed only in permanent teeth. Presently, there is enough evidence that this procedure can also be applied in primary teeth

Technique

- After the diagnosis is completed, the tooth is anesthetized.

- If possible, pulpal procedures should always be performed under rubber dam isolation and aseptic conditions to prevent further introduction of microorganisms into the pulp tissues (Figure 3.2.3). Care must be taken when placing the rubber dam on a traumatized tooth. If any loosening of the tooth has occurred, the rubber dam clamps must be applied to adjacent uninjured teeth

- In traumatically exposed pulps, only tissue judged to be inflamed is removed. Cvek (1994) showed that with pulp exposures resulting from traumatic injuries, regardless of the size of the exposure or the amount of lapsed time, pulpal changes are characterized by a proliferative response with inflammation extending only a few millimeters into the pulp. When this hyperplastic, inflamed tissue is removed (about 2 mm), healthy pulp tissue is encountered. In teeth with carious exposure of the pulp, it may be necessary to remove pulp tissue to a greater depth to reach uninflamed tissue.

- The instrument of choice for tissue removal in the pulpotomy procedure is an abrasive diamond bur, using high speed with adequate water cooling. This technique has been shown to create the least damage to the underlying tissue.

- Care must be exercised to ensure removal of all filaments of the pulp tissue coronal to the amputation site; otherwise, hemorrhage will be impossible to control.

- After pulpal amputation, the preparation is thoroughly washed with physiologic saline or sterile water to remove all debris; the water is removed by vacuum and cotton pellets (Figure 3.2.4). Air should not be blown on the exposed pulp, because it will cause desiccation and tissue damage.

- Hemorrhage is controlled by cotton pellets slightly moistened with saline (i.e., wetted and blotted almost dry) placed against the stumps of the pulp. Completely dry cotton pellets should not be used because fibers of the dry cotton will be incorporated into the clot and, when removed, will cause hemorrhage. Dry cotton pellets are placed over the moist pellets, and slight pressure is exerted on the mass to control the hemorrhage.

- Hemorrhage should be controlled in this manner within several minutes. It may be necessary to change the pellets to control all hemorrhage. If hemorrhage continues, the clinician must carefully check to be sure that all filaments of the pulp coronal to the amputation site were removed and that the site is clean.

- Sodium hypochlorite (2.5% NaOCl) can be placed on the exposure site to cause hemostasis before pulp capping. It also has the beneficial effect of killing bacteria. It was reported that when used as a hemostatic agent there was no damage to pulpal cells and it did not inhibit pulpal healing, odontoblastic cell formation, or dentinal bridging.

- If hemorrhage cannot be controlled, pulpal amputation should be performed at a more apical level. Once the hemorrhage is controlled, Ca(OH)$_2$ or mineral trioxide aggregate (MTA) is placed in the canal against the pulp stump. A thin layer of intermediate restorative material or flowable composite resin is placed over the Ca(OH)$_2$ or MTA and light cured (Figure 3.2.5); otherwise, the material would be washed out during the acid etching procedure. The tooth is then sealed with an etched bonded composite strip crown restoration (Figure 3.2.6).

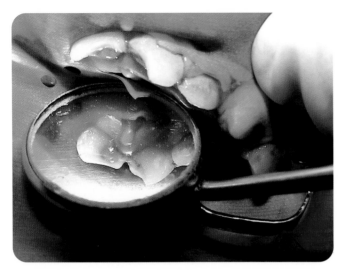

Figure 3.2.3. Placement of rubber dam after administration of a local anesthetic

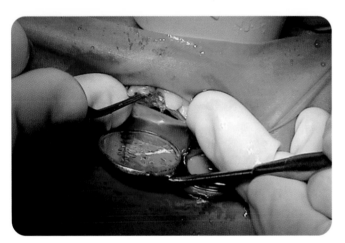

Figure 3.2.4. After pulp amputation, the area is rinsed with saline, and hemostasis is achieved with cotton pellet pressure

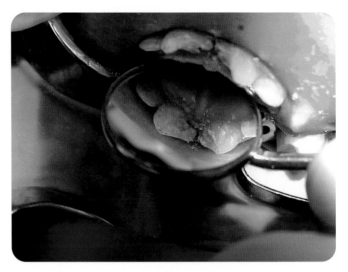

Figure 3.2.5. After hemostasis, the amputated areas are covered with calcium hydroxide or mineral trioxide aggregate, followed by intermediate restorative material

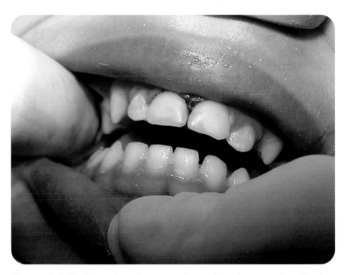

Figure 3.2.6. Completed restorations showing good esthetic results. The pulps remained vital

increased incidence of pulpal necrosis. Cvek (1994) reported 96% success with partial pulpotomy using Ca(OH)$_2$ on traumatically exposed permanent pulps. Size of the exposure or time between injury and treatment was not critical as long as the superficially inflamed pulp tissue was removed before capping. These studies included both mature teeth and teeth with immature roots. Subsequent investigations have verified these findings. In a long-term follow-up study of partial pulpotomy in permanent teeth, those judged to be healed at three years remained healed 10 to 15 years later.

• Only in the last few years did partial pulpotomy with Ca(OH)$_2$ or mineral trioxide aggregate (MTA)

start to be used as treatment modalities for traumatized primary incisors with pulp exposure. This was probably due to the traditional belief that pulpotomy with Ca(OH)2 results in internal root resorption. Today we know that most pulp dressing agents can lead to this pathologic complication, and may be due to the condition of the exposed pulp. Because the pulp is normal in traumatized exposures (except for the exposure area), removing the affected tissue brings about a good prognosis.

• The recommended treatment for traumatized primary teeth with pulp exposure is pulpectomy and full coverage, stainless steel crown [SSC] or composite strip crown (see Chapter 4, Flowchart C). Most root canal filling pastes cause discoloration of the tooth that can be seen through the composite crown. In addition, the tooth becomes brittle and more prone to fracture.

N. Complications and Alternative Treatment Plans

- Unsuccessful partial pulpotomy can result in pulp necrosis and/or a periapical abscess with or

without a fistula. These complications can be the result of chronic irritation due to microleakage from an improperly adapted SSC or defective strip crown. Another reason for failure can be related to recurrent trauma, a relatively common finding in young children. These complications can also occur if the initial treatment was a pulpectomy and SSC.

- Extraction is an alternative, but less desirable in a young child

Self-study Questions

1. **What are the treatment objectives for a complicated crown fracture?**
2. **What is the treatment recommended by the American Academy of Pediatric Dentistry for a complicated crown fracture in a traumatized primary incisor?**
3. **According to Cvek, what are the pulpal changes resulting from a traumatic pulp exposure?**
4. **What are the advantages of using sodium hydrochloride (NaOCl) to control pulpal**

hemorrhage during a pulpotomy procedure?
5. **What are the advantages of a partial pulpotomy over a pulpectomy for treatment of a complicated crown fracture?**
6. **What are the most commonly used pulp dressing materials in partial pulpotomy, and what are their properties?**

Answers are located at the end of the case.

Bibliography and Additional Reading

Casas M, Fuk AB. 2011. Pulp therapy in primary and young permanent teeth. In: *The Handbook of Pediatric Dentistry*, 4th Edition. Nowak AJ, Casamassimo PS (eds). *American Academy of Pediatric Dentistry*, pp. 91–8.

Camp JH, Fuks AB. 2006. Pediatric endodontics: Endodontic treatment for the primary and young permanent dentition. In: *Pathways of the Pulp*, 9th Edition. Cohen S, Hargreaves KM (eds). Mosby Elsevier: St. Louis. Chapter 22.

Cvek M. 1994. Endodontic management of traumatized teeth. *Textbook and Color Atlas of Traumatic Injuries to the Teeth*, 3rd Edition. In: Andreasen JO, Andreasen FM (eds). Munksgaard: Copenhagen.

Kupietzky A, Holan G. 2003. Treatment of crown fractures with pulp exposure in primary incisors. *Pediatr Dent* 25:241–48.

Fuks AB, Heling I. Pulp therapy for the young permanent dentition. In: *Pediatric Dentistry Infancy through Adolescence*, 4th Edition. Pinkham JR, Casamassimo PS, Fields HW Jr., McTigue DJ, Nowak AJ (eds). Elsevier Saunders: St. Louis. Chapter 33.

SELF-STUDY ANSWERS

1. To maintain pulp vitality and restore normal esthetics and function
2. Pulpectomy followed by a SSC or a composite strip crown
3. Cvek has shown that with pulp exposures resulting from traumatic injuries, regardless of the size of the exposure or the amount of lapsed time, pulpal changes are characterized by a proliferative response with inflammation extending only a few millimeters into the pulp (Cvek, 1994)
4. NaOCl, when placed on the exposure site, causes hemostasis, has a beneficial effect of killing bacteria, and does not damage the pulpal cells
5. Partial pulpotomy allows for the preservation of cell-rich coronal pulp, increases the healing potential due to preservation of the pulp, allows the physiologic apposition of cervical dentin, obviates the need for root canal therapy, and preserves the natural color and translucency
6. Calcium hydroxide and MTA. Both stimulate the healing of the pulp and the formation of a dentin bridge

Case 3

Cervical Pulpotomy in Cariously Exposed Primary Molars

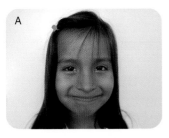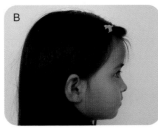

Figure 3.3.1a–b. Facial photographs

A. Presenting Patient

- 5-year-, 6-month-old Hispanic female
- New patient presenting as an emergency

B. Chief Complaint

- Mother confirmed the patient's complaint of pain in the lower left quadrant while eating; it subsides after a few minutes without taking analgesics

C. Social History

- Fourth of nine children
- Lower socio-economic status

D. Medical History

- Review of medical history revealed no significant findings, no known drug or food allergies, no medications, vaccinations are up to date

E. Medical Consult

- N/A

F. Dental History

- No dental home
- Eating habits include a low-protein, high-carbohydrate diet
- Poor oral hygiene, brushes without supervision
- Uses toothpaste containing fluoride
- Optimal water fluoridation levels
- No history of trauma
- Seven-day history of pain without history of swelling or fever

G. Extra-oral Exam

- No significant findings

H. Intra-oral Exam

Soft Tissues

- Generalized gingivitis

Hard Tissues

- No significant findings

Occlusal Evaluation of Primary Dentition

- Mesial step molars and class I canines

Other

- Extensive plaque accumulation
- Several teeth with extensive carious lesions: maxillary first primary molars, mandibular left first primary molars, maxillary lateral and central incisors

I. Diagnostic Tools

- Periapical radiograph of the maxillary incisors (Figure 3.3.2.)
- Two bitewings (Figure 3.3.3.)
- Unable to obtain posterior periapical radiographs (uncooperative behavior for the periapical radiographs)
- Radiographic lesions on maxillary first and second primary molars, maxillary lateral and central incisors, left mandibular first primary molar, mandibular primary canines, and mandibular right first and second primary molars

J. Differential Diagnosis

- Deep carious lesions
  - Reversible pulp inflammation
  - Irrreversible pulp inflammation
  - Partial pulp necrosis
  - Total pulp necrosis

K. Diagnosis and Problem List

Diagnosis

- Based on the history of pain, clinical examination, and radiographic findings, the most probable

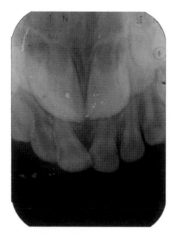

Figure 3.3.2. Periapical radiograph of the maxillary incisor

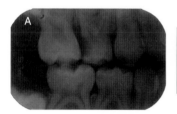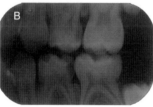

Figure 3.3.3a–b. Bitewing radiographs. A. Right bitewing radiograph, B. Left bitewing radiograph

diagnosis for the left mandibular first primary molar is a deep carious lesions with reversible pulp inflammation

Problem List
- Several untreated carious lesions
- High caries risk due to several factors (cariogenic diet, poor oral hygiene with extensive plaque accumulation)
- Lack of dental home

L. Comprehensive Treatment Plan
- Urgent treatment of the left first primary molar with formocresol pulpotomy and stainless steel crown (SSC)
- Explanation to the mother of the importance of maintaining the primary molars for proper occlusion
- Comprehensive treatment of other carious lesions
- Follow-up care including:
  - Post-op and home care instructions
  - Caries prevention plan
  - Appropriate prevention and recall plan

M. Radiographic Follow-up
- Post-operative bite-wing radiographs (Figure 3.3.4.)

FUNDAMENTAL POINT 1
Pulpotomy In Primary Teeth
Treatment Objectives
- Eradicate potential for infection
- Maintain tooth in a quiescent state
- Preserve space for underlying permanent tooth
- Retain primary tooth if permanent tooth is congenitally absent

Indications for a Pulpotomy
- Tooth with deep caries without pulp exposure
- Carious or traumatic pulp exposure with transitory thermal and/or chemical stimulated pain
- Physiologic mobility
- Normal soft tissues
- No percussion sensitivity (except in cases of food impaction)
- Intact continuous ligament space
- Intact periapical and/or furcation bone

Confounding Factors in Diagnosis of Pulp Status
- Color of pulpal hemorrhage not a reliable indicator of pulp histological status
- Excessive bleeding is strongly correlated with degenerative changes
- One-third of teeth with carious pulp exposures have "normal" pulps
- One-third of teeth with deep caries with no pulp exposures have "abnormal" pulps

---

N. Prognosis and Discussion
- The pulpotomy procedure is based on the rationale that the radicular pulp tissue is healthy or is capable of healing after surgical amputation of the affected or infected coronal pulp. The presence of any signs or symptoms of inflammation extending beyond the coronal pulp is a contraindication for a pulpotomy. In the present case, removing the soft and mushy dentin in the three first primary molars resulted in pulp exposure, and the teeth were treated with a formocresol pulpotomy and restored with SSCs
- The ideal dressing material for the radicular pulp should:

BACKGROUND INFORMATION 1
Pulpotomy Technique for Primary Teeth
Technique

- Excavate caries, amputate coronal pulp, achieve hemostasis, treat radicular pulp with medicament, restore with permanent restoration

Formocresol (FC) Pulpotomy

- Dilute FC using one part FC to four parts vehicle (three parts glycerine: one part water) and apply for five minutes
- Dilution mixture settles out; re-mixing indicated
- Method of action: tissue fixation
- Histological zones in FC-treated radicular pulp
  - Acidophilic zone: Fixation (coronal)
  - Pale staining zone: Atrophy (middle)
  - Broad zone of inflammatory cells (apical)
- Bactericidal
- 62% to 97% acceptable outcome
- No dentinal bridging, but calcific changes evident
- Persistent chronic inflammation
- Small risk of succedaneous tooth damage
- Exfoliation accelerated
- Cellular toxicity
- Immune sensitization risk
- Humoral and cell–mediated responses: Controversial
- Mutagenic and carcinogenic potential: Controversial

Ferric Sulfate (FS)

- 15.5% in aqueous base, pH = 1
- Method of action: Hemostatic, denatures protein, and forms ferric ion complex that occludes cut blood vessels
- Shorter application time than FC (10 to 15 seconds)
- Equivalent outcome to FC
- Self-limiting internal resorption reported

Mineral Trioxide Aggregate (MTA)

- Method of action: Mineralization, dental cement with discrete crystals and amorphous structure, pH = 12.5
- Pulp canal obliteration common
- Equivalent outcome to FC
- Promising clinical results

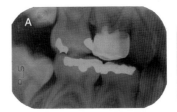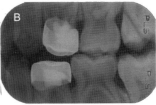

Figure 3.3.4a–b. Post-op bitewing radiographs. A. Post-op right bitewing radiograph, B. post-op left bitewing radiograph

- Be bactericidal
- Be harmless to the pulp and surrounding structures
- Promote healing of the radicular pulp
- Not interfere with the physiologic process of root resorption
- A good deal of controversy surrounds the issue of pulpotomy agents, and, unfortunately, the "ideal" pulp dressing material has not yet been identified. The most commonly used pulp dressing material is formocresol (Buckley's solution: formaldehyde, cresol, glycerol, and water). Clinical and radiographic studies have demonstrated that formocresol pulpotomies have success rates up to 97%. Although many studies have reported the clinical success of formocresol pulpotomies, an increasing body of literature has questioned the use of formocresol. (Fuks 2005)

O. Common Complications and Alternative Treatment Plans
Unsuccessful pulpotomy in a primary molar might result in internal resorption progressing into the bone, an inter-radicular pathological lesion, and/or a periapical abscess, with or without a parulis. In most of these situations, the teeth must be extracted.

Self-study Questions

1. *Which teeth are good candidates for pulpotomy?*

2. *What are the contra-indications for a pulpotomy?*

3. *What are the objectives of a pulpotomy?*

4. *What are the complications of a pulpotomy failure in a primary molar?*

5. *What are the desirable characteristics of an ideal pulp dressing?*

Answers are located at the end of the case.

Bibliography and Additional Reading

Casas M, Fuks A, 2007, Pulp therapy in primary and young permanent teeth, In: *The Handbook of Pediatric Dentistry, American Academy of Pediatric Dentistry*, 3rd Edition. Nowak, AJ, Casamassimo, PS (eds), American Academy of Pediatric Dentistry, Chicago, pg. 77–85.

American Academy of Pediatric Dentistry. 2011–2012. Guideline on pulp therapy for primary and young permanent teeth. *Reference Manual*. pp.212–19.

Fuks AB. 2005. Pulp therapy for the primary dentition. In: *Pediatric Dentistry*, Infancy Through Adolescence, 4th Edition Pinkham JR, Casamassimo PS, McTigue DJ, Fields HW Jr., Nowak AJ (eds). Elsevier Saunders: St. Louis. pp. 375–93.

SELF-STUDY ANSWERS

1. Teeth with carious or traumatic pulp exposure with transitory thermal and/or chemical stimulated pain, with physiologic mobility, normal soft tissues, no percussion sensitivity (except in cases of food impaction), intact continuous ligament space, and intact periapical and/or furcation bone

2. Teeth with carious or traumatic pulp exposure with spontaneous pain, persistent thermal and/or chemical stimulated pain, pathologic mobility, inflamed soft tissues, parulis, percussion sensitivity, widened and/or discontinuous ligament space, furcation and/or periapical radiolucencies, external and/or progressive internal resorption, dystrophic intrapulpal calcifications, less than one-third physiologic root resorption

3. To maintain tooth vitality and to cause no harm to the succedaneous tooth

4. Unsuccessful pulpotomy in a primary molar might result in internal resorption progressing into the bone, in an inter-radicular pathological lesion, and/or a periapical abscess, with or without a parulis

5. The ideal dressing material for the radicular pulp should be bactericidal, harmless to the pulp and surrounding structures, promote healing of the radicular pulp, and not interfere with the physiologic process of root resorption

Case 4

Root Canal Treatment in a Primary Molar

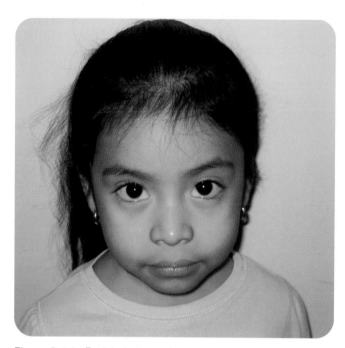

Figure 3.4.1. Facial photograph

A. Presenting Patient
- 5-year-, 2-month-old Hispanic female
- New patient presenting as an emergency

B. Chief Complaint
- Mother stated that the child "had excruciating pain awaking her from sleep last night, and the gums close to the right lower back tooth were swollen and red."

C. Social History
- Seventh of 10 children
- Lower socio-economical status

D. Medical History
- Review of medical history revealed congenital deafness, no known drug or food allergies, no medications, vaccinations up to date

E. Medical Consult
- N/A

F. Dental History
- No dental home
- Was taken for the first time to a dental office for an emergency visit the day before and antibiotics were prescribed
- Poor oral hygiene habits
- Low-protein, high-carbohydrate diet
- Uses toothpaste containing fluoride
- Optimal water fluoridation levels
- No history of trauma

G. Extra-oral Exam
- No significant findings

H. Intra-oral Exam
Soft Tissues
- Swelling and redness around lower right primary second molar

Hard Tissues
- No significant findings

Occlusal Evaluation of Primary Occlusion
- Vertical terminal plane (P) flush occlusal pattern

Other
- Moderate plaque accumulation
- Several teeth with extensive carious lesions

I. Diagnostic Tools
- Two bitewing radiographs
- Anterior periapical (maxillary) radiograph
- Periapical radiograph of lower right second primary molar
- Parent brought radiographs taken at another dentist's office the day before; radiographs show extensive pathological radiolucency in the inter-radicular area of the lower right second primary molar

J. Differential Diagnosis

- Acute dento-alveolar abscess
- Periodontal abscess
- Periapical granuloma
- Dentigerous cyst
- Radicular cyst

K. Diagnosis and Problem List

Diagnosis

- Deafness
- Based on the history of pain, the clinical examination, and the radiographic findings, the most probable dental diagnosis is acute dento-alveolar abscess in the lower right second primary molar
- Extensive caries lesions in other primary teeth

Problem List

- High caries risk due to several factors (cariogenic diet, poor oral hygiene with moderate to extensive plaque accumulation, special health care needs)
- Several untreated carious lesions
- Lack of a dental home
- Extremely apprehensive

L. Comprehensive Treatment Plan

- Emergency treatment of abscessed tooth (extraction or root canal treatment [RCT])
- Explanation to the mother of the importance of maintaining a second primary molar, particularly prior to the eruption of the first permanent molar, focusing on the difficulty of placing and maintaining a distal shoe
- Behavioral management considerations (consider using nitrous oxide)
- Comprehensive treatment of other carious lesions
- Follow up care including:
  - Post-op and home care instructions
  - Prevention plan
  - Recall plan, including any necessary consultations (orthodontic, endodontic, oral surgery, etc.)

M. Radiographic Follow-up

- See Figures 3.4.2 to 3.4.5

N. Prognosis and Discussion

Taken from Fuks (2005)

- The goal of pulpectomy is to maintain primary teeth that would otherwise be lost. The pulpectomy procedure is indicated in teeth that show evidence of chronic inflammation or necrosis

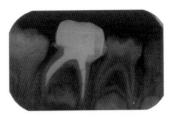

Figure 3.4.2. Radiograph, immediate post root canal treatment (RCT). Notice extensive pathologic radiolucent inter-radicular area

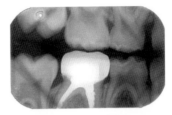

Figure 3.4.3. 15 months post-op radiograph. Notice inter-radicular area has healed with bone apposition

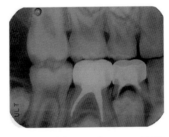

Figure 3.4.4. 4 years and 8 months post-RCT showing treatment success

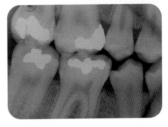

Figure 3.4.5. Radiograph showing fully erupted premolar in appropriate occlusion

in the radicular pulp, in teeth with carious exposure in which the radicular pulp exhibits clinical signs of hyperemia following coronal pulp amputation, or in teeth with evidence of necrosis of the radicular pulp, with or without caries involvement

- Conversely, pulpectomy is contraindicated in cases of infection involving the crypt of the succedaneous tooth, in teeth with non-restorable crowns, with perforation of the pulpal floor, with internal

BACKGROUND INFORMATION 1
Root Canal Treatment in Primary Molars

- Root canal treatment (RCT) can be performed in primary molars with irreversible pulpitis, determined as continuous bleeding exceeding five minutes, dark to purple blood color, or pulp necrosis. Although color of the pulpal hemorrhage alone is not a reliable indicator of pulp status. Radiographic periapical or inter-radicular radiolucencies, without involvement of the follicle of the permanent tooth, are not considered contraindication for RCT. The same is true for teeth with internal resorption without perforation and for those with external resorption not involving the permanent tooth follicle, as long as more than two-thirds of the root is intact

Technique

- RCT is usually completed in one visit. Under local anesthesia and rubber dam isolation, caries is removed and access to the pulp chamber is gained. The inflamed or necrotic pulp is then removed and mechanical preparation of the canal is performed using a series of 21-mm K-type endodontic files (Unitek Corp., Monrovia, CA) up to file no. 30. The working length is estimated from the preoperative radiograph. The root canals are then irrigated with alternating chlorhexidine or sodium hypochloride and saline, and dried with paper points. Because the morphology of the root canal system in primary teeth is extremely complex and difficult to clean mechanically, chemical disinfection is more effective.

- A root canal filling material containing iodoform is introduced into the root canal using a lentulo spiral mounted on a slow speed hand-piece, and the teeth are sealed with reinforced zinc oxide eugenol (ZOE)

- A postoperative radiograph is taken after each treatment to determine the extent of the filling material in the canals.

- "Flush" is determined when the filling material reaches the apex of the roots without excess beyond the apex, "underfilling" when the filling material is short of the apex, and "overfilling" when the filling material is extruded beyond the apex. Overfilling canals tend to result in more failures of the RCT.

- The patient is asked to return up to one month later for coronal restoration. In the absence of clinical pathologic signs of inflammation, the root-treated primary molars are restored with an amalgam or composite restoration if sufficient tooth structure remains to allow retention of the restoration. Otherwise, a stainless-steel crown is used. The estimated time left till natural shedding, determined by the extent of physiologic root resorption, also may influence the type of restoration to be placed. This factor, however, has less influence on the selection of the type of restoration.

Evaluation of RCT

- Patients should return every six months for recall examinations, in which the root-treated molars are evaluated clinically and radiographically. RCT is considered successful if the tooth is painless and presents healthy surrounding soft tissues and normal mobility, and if radiographs show decrease or no change in the pre-existing pathologic radiolucent defects. The treatment is considered a failure when pre-existing radiolucent defects grow in size or new defects appear. Moskovitz, Sammara, and Holan (2005) showed that although not statistically significant, overfilling resulted in more failures than underfilling.

resorption perforating into the underlying bone, and with external resorption of more than one-third of the root

- However, there is disagreement among clinicians about the utility of pulpectomy procedures in primary teeth. Difficulty in the preparation of primary root canals that have complex and variable morphologic features and the uncertainty about

teeth with gross loss of root structure; advanced internal or external or periapical resorption; and the effect of instrumentation, medication, and filling materials on developing succedaneous teeth dissuade some clinicians from using the technique. The behavior management problems that sometimes occur in pediatric patients have surely added to the reluctance among some dentists to perform RCT in primary teeth. These problems notwithstanding, the success of pulpectomies in primary teeth has led most pediatric dentists to prefer them to the alternative of extractions and space maintenance.

- Certain clinical situations may justify pulpectomy even with the knowledge that the prognosis may not be ideal. An example of such a case is pulp destruction of a primary second molar that occurs before the first permanent molar erupts. A premature extraction of the primary second molar without placement of a space maintainer usually results in mesial eruption of the first permanent molar with subsequent loss of space for the second premolar. Although a distal shoe space maintainer could be used, maintaining the natural tooth is definitely the treatment of choice. Therefore, a pulpectomy in a primary second molar is preferable, even if that tooth is maintained only until the first permanent molar has adequately erupted and is followed eventually by extraction of the primary second molar and placement of a space maintainer.

O. Common Complications and Alternative Treatment Plans

- Enlargement of a previously existing periapical or inter-radicular radiolucency and the development of a new lesion in a tooth without a pre-operative pathologic radiolucency are real failures and should eventually be extracted. However, in cases in which the pre-operative radiolucency remains unchanged, the patient should be recalled in six months for re-evaluation. Unsuccessful root canal treatment in a primary tooth may result in its premature exfoliation due to pathologic root resorption that can be followed by premature eruption of the permanent successor. Cystic lesions have been described less frequently as complications of primary root canal treatments

- The dentigerous cyst is an uncommon complication of root canal treatment in primary molars. The cystic lesion in Figure 3.4.6 was observed six and a half years after the successful endodontic treatment presented above. Extraction of the exfoliating primary molar and marsupialization of the cyst resulted in normal eruption and occlusion of the permanent premolar

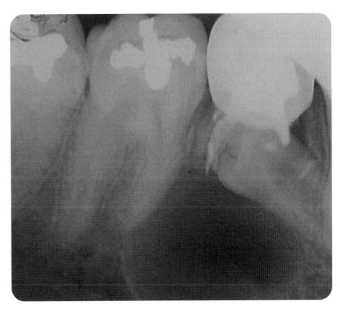

Figure 3.4.6. Radiograph showing dentigerous cyst as a complication of root canal treatment in a primary molar

Self-study Questions

1. **What are the indications for a pulpectomy according to the Guidelines of the American Academy of Pediatric Dentistry?**

2. **When is a root canal treatment contra-indicated for primary molars?**

3. **What are the radiographic signs of root canal treatment failure, and how should they be handled?**

4. **According to Moskovitz, Sammara, and Holan (2005), which root-treated teeth are more prone to failure: the underfilled, flush, or overfilled?**

5. **What is more effective for disinfection of the root canal system in primary teeth: mechanical or chemical debridement?**

Answers are located at the end of the case.

Bibliography

Fuks AB. 2005. Pulp therapy for the primary dentition. In: Pediatric Dentistry, Infancy through Adolescence, 4th Edition. Pinkham JR, Casamassimo PS, McTigue DJ, Fields HW Jr., Nowak AJ (eds). Elsevier Saunders: St. Louis, pp. 375–93.

Moskovitz M, Sammara E, Holan G. 2005. Success rate of root canal treatment in primary molars. *J Dent* 33:41–7.

SELF-STUDY ANSWERS

1. In teeth with carious exposure in which the radicular pulp exhibits clinical signs of hyperemia or evidence of necrosis of the radicular pulp, with or without caries involvement, following coronal pulp amputation

2. In teeth with non-restorable crowns, with perforation of the pulpal floor, with internal resorption perforating into the underlying bone, with external resorption of more than one-third of the root, or involving the follicle of the permanent tooth

3. Enlargement of a previously existing periapical or inter-radicular radiolucency and the development of a new lesion in a tooth without a pre-operative pathologic radiolucency are real failures and should eventually be extracted. However, in cases in which the pre-operative radiolucency remains unchanged, the patient should be recalled in another six months for re-evaluation

4. Although the differences were not statistically significant, overfilling resulted in more failures than underfilling or flush

5. Because the morphology of the root canal system in primary teeth is extremely complex and difficult to clean mechanically, chemical disinfection is more effective

Case 5

Partial Pulpotomy in a Cariously Exposed Young Permanent Molar

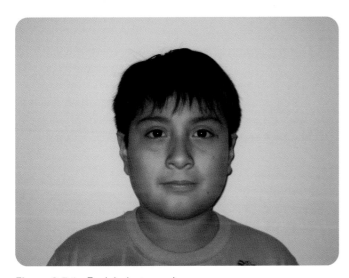

Figure 3.5.1. Facial photograph

A. Presenting Patient
- 8-year-, 6-month-old Hispanic male
- Patient of record presenting for an emergency

B. Chief Complaint
- Mother confirmed the patient's complaint of pain in the lower right quadrant for five days while eating sweets or drinking cold. The pain subsides after a few minutes, without taking analgesics.

C. Social History
- Oldest of five children
- Single mother
- Low socio-economic class

D. Medical History
- No significant findings, no known drug or food allergies, no medications, vaccinations up to date

E. Medical Consult
- N/A

F. Dental History
- History of pain for five days, with no swelling or fever observed
- Has received extensive restorative treatment before
- Low-protein, high-carbohydrate diet
- Poor oral hygiene habits, with little adult supervision
- Uses toothpaste containing fluoride
- Optimal water fluoridation levels
- No history of trauma

G. Extra-oral Exam
- No significant findings

H. Intra-oral Exam
Soft Tissues
- Plaque-induced gingivitis

Hard Tissues
- No significant findings

Occlusal Evaluation of Mixed Dentition
- Class 1 molars and canines

Other
- Generalized plaque accumulation
- Several teeth with extensive restorations
- Extensive caries present in the maxillary primary second molars, maxillary first permanent molars, and all mandibular molars

I. Diagnostic Tools
- Two bitewings; radiographic lesions could also be seen clinically (Figure 3.5.2a-b)
- Periapical radiograph of the lower right first permanent molar was not taken. The patient did not present signs nor symptoms to suspect the presence of periapical pathology

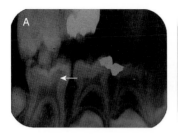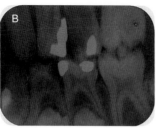

Figure. 3.5.2a–b. Pre-op bitewing radiographs. A. Pre-op right bitewing radiograph (arrow at deep lesion), B. Pre-op left bitewing radiograph

J. Differential Diagnosis

- Deep, carious lesion in the mandibular right first permanent molar with possible:
  - Reversible pulp inflammation
  - Irrreversible pulp inflammation
  - Partial pulp necrosis
  - Total pulp necrosis

K. Diagnosis and Problem List
Diagnosis

- Based on the history of pain, the clinical examination, and the radiographic findings, the most probable diagnosis is extensive carious lesion with reversible pulp inflammation

Problem List

- High caries risk due to several factors (cariogenic diet, poor oral hygiene with extensive plaque accumulation)
- Deep, untreated carious lesion (Figure 3.5.2a arrow)
- Poor compliance with dental appointments
- Early loss of maxillary right primary first molar: space maintenance
- Behavior management: Extremely apprehensive

L. Comprehensive Treatment Plan

- Urgent treatment of the carious lesion of the mandibular right first permanent molar
- Explanation to the mother of the importance of maintaining the first permanent molar for a proper occlusion
- Behavioral management considerations: Nitrous oxide analgesia
- Comprehensive treatment of other carious lesions
- Establishment of a caries prevention plan
- Follow-up care including:
  - Post-op and home care instructions
  - Appropriate prevention and recall plans

BACKGROUND INFORMATION 1
Partial Pulpotomy for Young Permanent Posterior Teeth

- A partial pulpotomy is indicated in a young permanent tooth for a small (<2 mm) carious exposure in which the pulpal bleeding can be controlled in one to two minutes. The tooth must be vital, with a diagnosis of normal pulp or reversible pulpitis. The procedure is usually reserved for teeth with little or no history of pain, absence of radiographic signs of pathology, percussion sensitivity, swelling, or mobility (American Academy of Pediatric Dentistry 2011–2012)

- The procedure involves the removal of pulp tissue beneath the exposure site judged to be inflamed (usually 1 to 3 mm) to reach healthy tissue below (see Case 2). Pulpal bleeding must be controlled quickly and the site should be covered with calcium hydroxide or mineral trioxide aggregate (MTA), followed by a restoration that seals the tooth from microleakage

- Before initiating treatment, it is critical to evaluate the degree of pulp inflammation in an attempt to distinguish between reversible and irreversible pulpitis. Vital pulp therapy in permanent teeth with history of pain has traditionally been considered contra-indicated. Although the correlation between clinical and histologic evaluation is poor, young permanent teeth are good candidates for this conservative treatment because of their rich blood supply that enhances the healing ability. Because the loss of the pulp in teeth with immature apices is so devastating, it seems advisable to attempt the partial pulpotomy procedure. If failure occurs, apexification can always be performed (Camp and Fuks 2006, Fuks and Heling. 2005)

- Any necessary consultations (orthodontic, endodontic, oral surgery, etc.)

M. Radiographic Follow-up

- Post-operative radiographs at nine months (Figure 3.5.3): A dentin bridge can be seen under the amputated pulp horn in the mandibular right permanent first molar (arrow). The two left mandibular primary molars were treated with

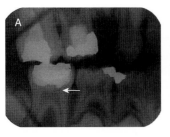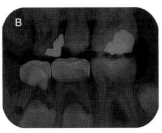

Figure 3.5.3a–b. Post-op bitewing radiographs. A. Post-op right bitewing radiograph (arrow at dentin bridge), B. Post-op left bitewing radiograph

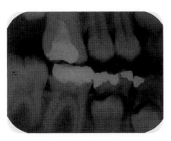

Figure 3.5.4. 3 years 10 months post-op right bitewing radiograph

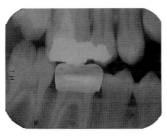

Figure 3.5.5. 4 years 9 months post-op right bitewing radiograph

formocresol pulpotomies followed by stainless steel crowns (SSC), and the maxillary left primary second molar was extracted
- Post-operative radiographs at 3 years, 10 months (Figure 3.5.4): The pulp appears within normal limits but there are signs of breakdown of the restoration on the mandibular right first permanent molar
- Post-operative radiograph at four years, nine months (Figure 3.5.5): The treated tooth has been restored with an SSC

N. Prognosis and Discussion
- Long-term studies have shown very high success rates of pulp capping and partial pulpotomy with respect to pulp survival. Radiographic evidence of hard tissue closure of the perforation can be seen three months after pulp capping in this case
- Mejare and Cvek (1993) reported a success rate of 91% (29/31) in cases with no clinical or radiographic signs of pathology after a follow-up of 24 to 140 months. The same study reported that four of six cases with temporary pain and radiographic signs of minor periapical involvement responded successfully. Another study (Mass and Zilberman 1993) also reported a success rate of 91% in 35 cases followed for 12 to 48 months
- Cvek and co-workers (1978, 1982) have reported 96% success with pulp capping and pulpotomy using Ca(OH)2 on traumatically exposed permanent pulps. The size of the exposure or time between injury and treatment was not critical as long as the superficially inflamed pulp tissue was removed before capping. These studies included both mature teeth and teeth with immature roots. Subsequent investigations have verified these findings.
- Histological examination of pulps from teeth successfully treated with partial pulpotomy and removed for restorative purposes showed no significant pathological changes. (Cvek et al. 1982)

O. Common Complications and Alternative Treatment Plans
- Unsuccessful partial pulpotomy in an immature permanent molar might result in pulp necrosis and eventually a periapical abscess. These cases must be followed by an apexification or apical barrier.

Self-study Questions

1. What are the indications for a partial pulpotomy in a young permanent tooth?
2. What are the contra-indications for a partial pulpotomy?
3. Why are young carious permanent molars good candidates for conservative treatments such as partial pulpotomy?
4. What are the complications of a partial pulpotomy failure in an immature permanent molar?
5. Why is bleeding control a diagnostic tool for the diagnosis of the pulp condition?

Answers are located at the end of the case.

Bibliography

American Academy of Pediatric Dentistry. 2011–2012. Guideline on pulp therapy for primary and young permanent teeth. *American Academy of Pediatric Dentistry Reference Manual*. pp. 212–19.

Camp J, Fuks AB. 2006. Pediatric endodontics: Endodontic treatment for the primary and young, permanent dentition. In: *Pathway of the Pulp*, 9th edition. Cohen S., Hargreaves KM (eds) Elsevier: St. Louis, pp. 822–882.

Cvek M. 1978. A clinical report on partial pulpotomy and capping with calcium hydroxide in permanent incisors with complicated crown fractures. *J Endod* 4:232–7.

Cvek M, Cleaton-Jones P, Austin J, Andreasen JO. 1982. Pulp reactions to exposure after experimental crown fractures or grinding in adult monkeys. *J Endod* 8:391–7.

Fuks AB, Heling I. 2005. Pulp therapy for the young permanent dentition. In: *Pediatric Dentistry, Infancy Through Adolescence*, 4th Edition. Pinkham JR, Casamassimo PS, McTigue DJ, Fields HW Jr., Nowak AJ (eds). Elsevier Saunders: St. Louis, pp. 577–92.

Mejare I, Cvek M. 1993. Partial pulpotomy in young permanent teeth with deep carious lesions. *Endod Dent Traumatol* 9:238–42.

Mass E, Zilberman U. 1993. Clinical and radiographic evaluation of partial pulpotomy in carious exposures of permanent molars. *Pediatr Dent* 15:257–9.

SELF-STUDY ANSWERS

1. A partial pulpotomy is indicated in a young permanent tooth for a small (<2 mm) carious exposure in which the pulpal bleeding must be controlled in one to two minutes. The tooth must be vital, with a diagnosis of normal pulp or reversible pulpitis

2. A partial pulpotomy is contra-indicated in a young permanent tooth with a large (>2 mm) carious exposure in which the pulpal bleeding cannot be controlled in one to two minutes (signs of an irreversible pulpitis)

3. Young permanent teeth are good candidates for this conservative treatment because of their rich blood supply that enhances the healing ability

4. Failure of a partial pulpotomy may result in pulp necrosis and/or a periapical abscess. Because the apex is not closed it is necessary to start an apexification procedure

5. Usually when bleeding does not stop after one to two minutes there is hyperemia or pulp inflammation, decreasing the prognosis of the partial pulpotomy.

Case 6

Pulpotomy With MTA in an Immature Permanent Molar

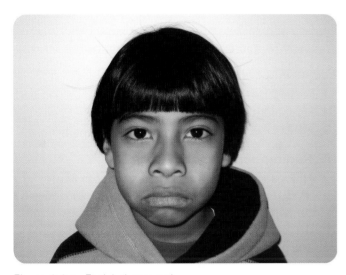

Figure 3.6.1. Facial photograph

A. Presenting patient
- 8-year-, 8-month-old male

B. Chief Complaint and History of Present Injury
- The patient was referred by a dentist for root canal treatment (RCT) of the mandibular right permanent first molar. At the initial appointment at his dentist, the tooth was asymptomatic but upon caries removal pulp exposure occurred. The dentist placed a Ca(OH)$_2$ paste over the exposure site with a temporary intermediate restorative material (IRM) filling and referred him to the endodontic clinic

C. Social History
- Youngest of five children
- Middle to high socio-economic class

D. Medical History
- G6PD deficiency, otherwise healthy
- No known drug or food allergies, no medications, vaccinations up to date

E. Medical Consult
- N/A

F. Dental History
- Has dental home
- Low-carbohydrate diet
- Good oral hygiene habits, brushes twice a day with adult supervision
- Uses toothpaste containing fluoride
- Optimal water fluoridation levels
- No history of trauma
- Cooperative

G. Extra-oral Exam
- No significant findings

H. Intra-oral Exam
Soft Tissues
- No significant findings

Hard Tissues
- No significant findings

Occlusal Evaluation of Mixed Dentition
- No significant findings

Other
- Slight accumulation of plaque
- Several teeth with restorations, including pulp therapy
- The mandibular right permanent first molar presented hypoplastic enamel areas and caries on the mesial surface. The tooth has physiologic mobility and shows no sensitivity to percussion, electric pulp test, and cold test

I. Diagnostic Tools
- Periapical radiograph (Figure 3.6.2.)
- Radiographic findings:
  - Radiopaque restoration in the mesial side of the tooth

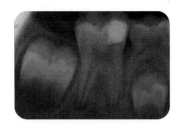

Figure 3.6.2. Pre-op mandibular right periapical radiograph

- Wide pulp chamber with prominent pulp horns
- Immature roots
- Round radiolucent area at the periapex surrounded by a radiopaque zone

J. Differential Diagnosis

- Pulp
  - Reversible pulpitis
  - Irreversible pulpitis
  - Complete or partial necrosis of the pulp
- Periapex
  - Normal: Dental sac
  - Chronic apical periodontitis

K. Diagnosis and Problem List

Diagnosis

- Based on the clinical examination and radiographic findings, the probable diagnosis is reversible pulpitis

Problem List

- The extent of the exposure is unknown
- Cold tests and electric pulp tests are unreliable in immature teeth
- It is difficult to differentiate between radiographic appearance of a dental sac and chronic apical periodontitis
- It is difficult to assess the extent of inflammation in the exposed pulp

L. Comprehensive Treatment Plan

- Treatment of mandibular right permanent first molar with mineral trioxide aggregate (MTA) pulpotomy
- Explanation to the parents about the importance of maintaining vitality of an immature permanent molar

Technique

- Local anesthesia and rubber dam
- Removal of temporary restoration and pulp capping material

- Removal of inflamed pulp tissue from the pulp chamber up to the level of the radicular pulp
- Irrigation with 2.5% sodium hypochlorite
- Hemostasis of the radicular pulp with a wet cotton pellet
- Coverage of the radicular pulp stump with MTA
- Temporary restoration with Coltosol and IRM

Other Treatment Options

- Two appointments: Place a wet cotton pellet over the MTA and on the second appointment verify the setting of the MTA and place a permanent restoration.
- One appointment: Place glass Ionomer liner over the MTA and do a permanent restoration

Follow-up Care

- Post-op instructions
- Permanent restoration
- Recall after 3, 6, and 12 months post-operatively

M. Radiographic Follow-up

- At subsequent follow-up visits the tooth is asymptomatic and the radiographic appearance of the periapices is similar to the contra-lateral tooth. The lack of response to vitality tests can be explained by the absence of coronal pulp tissue (Figures 3.6.3 to 3.6.6)

N. Prognosis and Discussion

- The goal of pulp treatment should be to maintain vitality and function at least until completion of full root development. Pulp tissue in teeth with deep caries is chronically inflamed but can still maintain its healing potential. Clinically, it is asymptomatic and thus diagnosed as reversible pulpitis. Vital pulp therapy should not be done in symptomatic teeth with sensitivity to percussion, swelling, or other obvious signs of pulpal necrosis
- The pulp may be exposed during caries removal and cavity preparation. Conservative treatment options include:
  - Direct pulp capping in mature and immature teeth
  - Partial pulpotomy in immature teeth if bleeding can be controlled
  - Cervical pulpotomy when bleeding can not be controlled at the entrance of the canal
- The radical options in immature teeth are apexification with Ca(OH)$_2$ or apical closure with MTA. In mature teeth, conventional RCT should be performed

BACKGROUND INFORMATION 1
Mineral Trioxide Aggregate

- Mineral trioxide aggregate (MTA) was first introduced for endodontic use in the early 1990s. This material was reported to be similar to Portland cement. It has a smaller mean particle size, contains fewer toxic heavy metals, has a longer working time, and appears to have undergone additional purification than regular Portland cement. It contains oxides, approximately 65% being CaO, which turns into $Ca(OH)_2$ when immersed in water (Tomson et al. 2007).

- The powder should be mixed with sterile water in 3:1 powder/liquid ratio. It is recommended that a moist cotton pellet may be temporarily placed in direct contact with the material and left until a follow-up appointment. Upon hydration, MTA forms a colloidal gel that solidifies to a hard structure in approximately three to four hours. Moisture from the surrounding tissues assists in the setting reaction.

- Hydrated MTA has an initial pH of 10.2, which rises to 12.5 three hours after mixing (Sarkar et al. 2005). MTA presented less microleakage than traditional materials in most of bacteria–based microleakage studies. Compared with $Ca(OH)_2$, MTA has demonstrated a greater ability to maintain the integrity of pulp tissue, producing a thicker dentinal bridge, less inflammation, less hyperemia, and less pulpal necrosis than $Ca(OH)_2$ (Roberts et al. 2007).

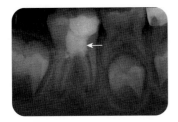

Figure 3.6.3. Immediate post-op periapical radiograph showing MTA in pulp chamber (arrow) and IRM restoration

O. Common Complications and Alternative Treatment Plans

- If the pulpotomy outcome is not favorable, the patient may present with pain and/or a periapical radiolucency, in which case an RCT should be done. Endodontic treatment is more complex in

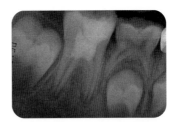

Figure 3.6.4. Three months post-op radiograph

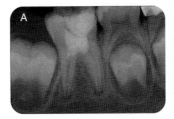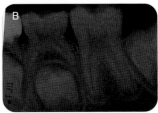

Figure 3.6.5a–b. Fifteen months post-op and contralateral radiographs

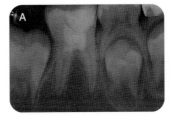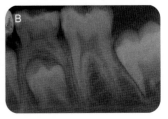

Figure 3.6.6a–b. Twenty-nine months post-op and contralateral radiographs

teeth with immature roots, and apexification or apical closure with MTA will have to be initiated. Apexification procedures with $Ca(OH)_2$ are long in duration and may result in a weaker root structure, because $Ca(OH)_2$ dressing frequently decreases the strength of the root (Andreasen, Munksgaard, and Bakland, 2006). Loss of vitality before root completion leaves thin dentin walls and a poor crown-root ratio

- Another complication from vital pulp therapy is accelerated dentin apposition with subsequent pulp canal obliteration (PCO). It is a well known complication in permanent teeth following direct trauma; clinically, it also may occur after pulpotomy. The treatment of permanent teeth with PCO is controversial. While some clinicians advocate RCT as soon as the process is detected, others favor a more conservative approach with intervention only in cases showing clear signs of pulp necrosis. Although the incidence of pulp necrosis in teeth displaying PCO seems to increase over time, prophylactic endodontic intervention on a routine basis does not seem justified (Kats-Sagi et al. 2004).

BACKGROUND INFORMATION 2
Pulpotomy

- The pulpotomy procedure involves removing part of the pulp tissue that is profusely bleeding or has degenerative changes, leaving intact the remaining vital tissue. The depth to which the tissue is removed is determined by clinical judgment. The pulp stump is then covered with a pulp capping agent, the aim of which is to promote reparative dentin formation at the amputation site. In multi-rooted teeth, the procedure is done by removing the pulp tissue to the orifices of the root canals (Camp and Fuks 2006).

- $Ca(OH)_2$ has been traditionally used for pulpotomies with relatively good results. When used over healthy pulp tissue, it stimulates dentin bridge formation. Due to its high alkalinity, $Ca(OH)_2$ causes superficial tissue necrosis and stimulation of tertiary dentin formation, together with an antibacterial effect (Witherspoon, Small, and Harris 2006).

- Recent studies have demonstrated that the dentin matrix is a reservoir of growth factors and other bio-active molecules that have been sequestered during dentinogenesis. These molecules may be released into the pulp tissue and contribute to dentin repair and regeneration. The beneficial effect of $Ca(OH)_2$ is probably due to its effect on releasing growth factors from the dentin matrix (Tomson et al. 2007). Another material with a similar mechanism of action is MTA (see Background Information 1).

Self-study Questions

1. *What are the possible treatment options for a pulpotomy on a young permanent molar using MTA?*

2. *What is the goal of vital pulp therapy?*

3. *What are the conservative treatment options when the pulp is exposed during caries removal or cavity preparation?*

4. *What are the advantages of MTA?*

5. *What is the treatment option if the pulpotomy fails in teeth with immature roots?*

Answers are located at the end of the case.

Bibliography

Andreasen JO, Munksgaard EC, Bakland LK. 2006. Comparison of fracture resistance in root canals of immature sheep teeth after filling with calcium hydroxide or MTA. *Dent Traumatol* 22:154–6.

Camp JH, Fuks AB. 2006. Pediatric endodontics: endodontic treatment for the primary and young permanent dentition. In: *Pathways of the Pulp*, 9th edition. Cohen S, Hargreaves KM (eds) Mosby: St. Louis.

Kats-Sagi H, Moskovitz M, Moshonov J, Holan G. 2004. Pulp canal obliteration in an unerupted permanent incisor following trauma to its primary predecessor: a case report. *Dent Traumatol* 20:181–3.

Roberts HW, Toth JM, Berzins DW, Charlton DG. 2007. Mineral trioxide aggregate material use in endodontic treatment: a review of the literature. *Dent Mater* 20:1–16.

Sarkar NK, Caicedo R, Ritwik P, Moiseyeva R, Kawashima I. 2005. Physicochemical basis of the biologic properties of mineral trioxide aggregate. *J Endodon* 31:97–100.

Tomson PL, Graver LM, Lumley PJ, Sloan AJ, Smith AJ, Cooper PR. 2007. Dissolution of bio-active dentine matrix components by mineral trioxide aggregate. *J Dent* 35:636–42.

Witherspoon DE, Small JC, Harris GZ. 2006. Mineral trioxide aggregate pulpotomies: a case series outcomes assessment. *JADA* 137:610–8.

SELF-STUDY ANSWERS

1. (a) Coverage of the radicular pulp stump with MTA, followed by a temporary restoration with Coltosol and IRM; (b) placement of a wet cotton pellet over the MTA and on the second appointment verification of the setting of the MTA and placement of a permanent restoration; (c) placement of glass ionomer liner over the MTA and permanent restoration of the tooth

2. The goal is to maintain pulp vitality and function, at least until completion of full root development.

3. (a) Direct pulp capping in mature and immature teeth; (b) partial pulpotomy in immature teeth if bleeding can be controlled; (c) cervical pulpotomy when bleeding can be controlled at the entrance of the canal

4. Its biocompatibility, strong seal when set, and indissolubility in fluids

5. Apexification or apical closure with MTA, followed by RCT

Case 7

Root End Closure—Apexification With Ca(OH)₂

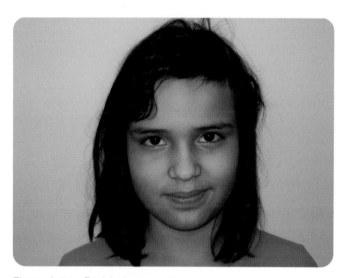

Figure 3.7.1. Facial photograph

A. Presenting Patient
- 10-year old female of Yemenite origin

B. Chief Complaint and History of Present Injury
- The patient was referred by her dentist for root canal treatment (RCT) of the maxillary left permanent central incisor which was laterally luxated nine months ago when she fell off her bike
- History of treatment: At the initial appointment in the dental office, the tooth did not respond to sensitivity tests and a radiolucent area was observed at the periapex. It was then diagnosed as having chronic apical periodontitis. A Calcium Hydroxide (Ca(OH)₂) dressing was placed in the canal and the access cavity was sealed with a temporary filling (intermediate restorative material; IRM)

C. Social History
- Third of five siblings
- Low to middle class family

D. Medical History
- Review of medical history revealed no significant findings, no known drug or food allergies, no medications, vaccinations up to date

E. Medical Consult
- N/A

F. Dental History
- Has a dental home
- Eats a regular balanced diet
- Good oral hygiene habits, brushes her teeth at least once a day, unsupervised
- Uses a fluoride-containing toothpaste
- Lives in an optimally fluoridated area
- Dental trauma nine months ago
- Cooperative

G. Extra-oral Exam
- No significant findings

H. Intra-oral Exam
Soft Tissues
- No significant findings

Hard Tissues
- No significant findings

Occlusal Evaluation of Mixed Dentition
- Class I molars, anterior crowding

Other
- Minimal plaque
- Caries-free
- First permanent molars with amalgam restorations

I. Diagnostic Tools
- A periapical radiograph of the maxillary left permanent central incisor (Figure 3.7.2) showed radiopaque material in the root canal, wide root canal with thin walls, immature tooth with wide open apex

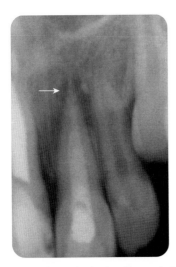

Figure 3.7.2. Diagnostic periapical radiograph (arrow at radiolucent area)

and a radiolucent area (Figure 3.7.2 arrow), and radiopaque material in the periapical area

- Clinical examination revealed temporary filling; 1-mm pocket; physiologic mobility; no sensitivity to percussion, electric pulp test (EPT), and cold test; slight tenderness on palpation; no sinus tract; no swelling

J. Differential Diagnosis

- N/A

K. Diagnosis and Problem List

Diagnosis

- Immature tooth with chronic periapical periodontitis and $Ca(OH)_2$ overfill

Problem List

- Remnants of $Ca(OH)_2$ beyond the apex may delay repair
- Difficult to establish correct working length in immature teeth
- Risky to file a tooth with thin root canal walls
- Cold test and EPT are unreliable in immature teeth
- Difficult to differentiate between the radiographic appearance of a dental sac and chronic apical periodontitis

L. Comprehensive Treatment Plan

- Explanation to the parents of the difficulties in treating an immature permanent tooth
- Apexification of the maxillary left permanent central incisor, followed by RCT and final restoration
- Follow-up care should include:
  - Immediate post-op and home care instructions after each appointment

FUNDAMENTAL POINT 1
Disinfection of the Root Canal

- An endodontic irrigant should ideally exhibit powerful antimicrobial activity, dissolve organic tissue remnants, flush out debris from instrumented root canals, provide lubrication, and be without cytotoxic effect on the periradicular tissues (Harrison 1984).
- Sodium hypochlorite solution is the most common irrigant due to its broad antimicrobial spectrum and unique capacity to dissolve necrotic tissue remnants (Hasselgren, Olsson, and Cvek 1988). It is used in concentrations ranging from 0.5% to 5.25% but it has a cytotoxic effect when injected into the periapical tissues (Tanomaru et al. 2002).
- Despite its usefulness for irrigation, chlorhexidine, in concentrations up to 2%, cannot be advocated as the main irrigant because it will not to dissolve necrotic tissue remnants (Naenni, Thoma, and Zehnder 2004). Chlorhexidine (2% concentration) causes less inflammatory response than 0.5% sodium hypochlorite (Tanomaru et al. 2002).
- $Ca(OH)_2$ is used as an intracanal medicament requiring a disinfection period of seven days. Combining it with other medicaments may enhance its efficacy in eliminating residual bacteria from the root canal system (Siqueira and Lopes 1999). Its high pH and low solubility keep the antimicrobial effect for a long period of time (Siqueira and Lopes 1999). It also assists in the debridement of the root canal, increasing the dissolution of necrotic tissue.

- Recall after one year, followed by yearly clinical and radiographic examination for five years

Dental Treatment

- First appointment
  - Local anesthesia, rubber dam, and removal of the IRM
  - Working length established using a radiograph and the paper point method. The new generation of paper points with markings is an effective mean for measurements
  - Copious irrigation with 0.5% chlorhexidine, followed by minimal mechanical instrumentation

of the root canal walls and additional irrigation with ultrasonic activation

- Because there was no apical stop, placement of a Ca(OH)$_2$ paste was done using a syringe with a small-gauge needle, followed by an IRM temporary filling
- Second appointment, two weeks later
  - Copious irrigation with 0.5% chlorhexidine
  - Root canal was packed with a thick paste of Ca(OH)$_2$ using endodontic pluggers. Verification of the density of the Ca(OH)$_2$ packing by a radiograph. Access cavity sealed with IRM
- Third appointment, three months later
  - No apical stop evident; therefore, repeat of the apexification procedure
- Fourth appointment, three months later
  - Presence of an apical barrier, so the root canal was dried and obturated with Gutta Percha and a sealer. Coronal access cavity double-sealed with Coltosol (Coltene Whaledent) and IRM. Patient referred back to pediatric dentist for the final restoration (Figures 3.7.3. and 3.7.4.)

M. Clinical and Radiographic Follow-up

- The tooth was asymptomatic and functional 12 months post-operatively (Figure 3.7.5.). The chronic periapical periodontitis healed

N. Prognosis and Discussion

- Apexification is a procedure that usually requires many appointments to change the Ca(OH)$_2$ dressing. Therefore, high compliance of the patient and parents is needed.
- Due to their thin dentinal walls, these teeth are prone to fracture; thus, a mouth guard is suggested to decrease the risk of injury in risky situations (sports, biking, etc). Nonetheless, the

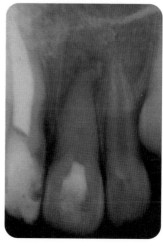

Figure 3.7.3. Radiograph showing apexification with Ca(OH)$_2$. Note the similar radiopacity of the canal and the dentin

---

BACKGROUND INFORMATION 1

Apexification

- The aim of apexification is to allow the formation of an apical barrier in immature teeth in which root growth and development cease due to pulp necrosis. Traditionally, apexification has been performed using Ca(OH)$_2$ dressing in a paste consistency. Its relatively good success rate has been attributed to its (a) high pH, (b) calcium ions, (c) hydroxyl ions, and (d) antibacterial effect (Fava and Saunders 1999).

- Ca(OH)$_2$ dressing should be placed in the first appointment and the second appointment should be scheduled two weeks to a month later. The aim of the second visit is to complete the debridement and remove the tissue remnants (Hasselgren, Olsson, and Cvek 1988). At this time, a thick paste of CA(OH)$_2$ is packed in the root canal using endodontic pluggers (Rafter 2005). At the next appointment, if the barrier is incomplete and the

patient feels the touch of a file, the apexification procedure is repeated until a complete barrier is formed. When an apical barrier is formed, a root canal filling is performed using either lateral condensation with Gutta Percha point or using the warm Gutta Percha technique (Rafter 2005).

- Apexification includes a coronal access that should be wide enough to include the pulp horns to prevent future contamination and discoloration. The preparation of the root canal is similar for both Ca(OH)$_2$ and MTA root end closure. The length of the root canal in immature teeth can be determined radiographically and by using the paper point method. The debridement of the root canal should be done with minimal instrumentation to prevent damage to the thin dentin walls. Irrigation with disinfecting solutions should be done carefully, avoiding pushing the solutions beyond the apex.

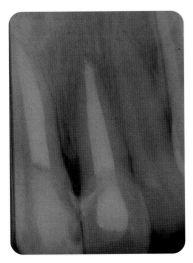

Figure 3.7.4. Radiograph showing obturation of the root canal

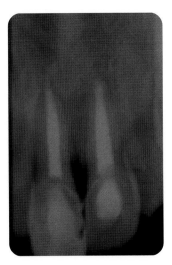

Figure 3.7.5. Twelve months post-op radiograph

caretakers and the patient should bear in mind that this tooth may be lost in the future.

O. Common Complications and Alternative Treatment Plans

Common Complications

- After apexification, the crown-root ratio is not favorable because the root is shorter than in a mature tooth; therefore, the prognosis of the tooth may be hampered. Post placement (if needed) is

difficult due to the width of the root canal and placement of a permanent crown should be delayed due to patient's continuous growth

Alternative Treatment Plans

- Another option is an apical closure with MTA, also called one-step apexification. Root canal filling can be carried out a few days later, after the MTA is set

BACKGROUND INFORMATION 2

Ca(OH)$_2$ in Apexification

- Chosak, Sela, and Cleaton-Jones (1997) demonstrated in an animal study that, after the initial filling with Ca(OH)$_2$, a repeated filling is not necessary for at least 6 months. It was assumed that the size of the blunderbuss apex before treatment influenced the type and time of closure (Yates 1988). Although repeated filling may not be necessary, one drawback of Ca(OH)$_2$ apexification is the frequency of cervical root fractures. Cvek (1992) reported that a significantly higher rate of root fractures was observed in immature than in mature teeth after a Ca(OH)$_2$ dressing and a root canal filling with Gutta Percha. The frequency of

fractures among immature teeth ranged from 77% in teeth with the least developed roots to 28% in teeth with the most developed roots.

- Recent studies have shown that long-term Ca(OH)$_2$ dressing, as required in apexification procedures, markedly decreases dentin fracture strength with time (Rosenberg, Murray, and Namerow 2007; Andreason, Munksgaard, and Bakland 2006). Thus, the use of Ca(OH)$_2$ in apexification should be re-evaluated. The prognosis may be further compromised by the placement of a temporary coronal seal (Tronstad et al. 2000).

Self-study Questions

1. *Is the stage of root development coherent with the child's age?*

2. *What special care should be taken in performing irrigation during root canal treatment of an immature tooth?*

3. *What are the suggested methods to determine working length in teeth with an open apex?*

4. *How can you verify that the Ca(OH)$_2$ paste filled the canal to its entire length?*

5. *What is the suggested technique for obturation in such case?*

Answers are located at the end of the case.

Bibliography

Andreasen JO, Munksgaard EC, Bakland LK. 2006. Comparison of fracture resistance in root canals of immature sheep teeth after filling with calcium hydroxide or MTA. *Dent Traumatol* 22:154–6.

Chosack A, Sela J, Cleaton-Jones P. 1997. A histological and quantitative histomorphometric study of apexification of nonvital permanent incisors of vervet monkeys after repeated root filling with a calcium hydroxide paste. *Endod Dent Traumatol* 13:211–7.

Cvek M. 1992. Prognosis of luxated non-vital maxillary incisors treated with calcium hydroxide and filled with gutta percha. A retrospective study. *Endod Dent Traumatol* 8:45–55.

Fava LR, Saunders WP. 1999. Calcium hydroxide pastes: classification and clinical indications. *Int Endod J* 32:257–82.

Harrison JW. 1984. Irrigation of the root canal system. *Dent Clin North Amer* 4:797–808.

Hasselgren G, Olsson B, Cvek M. 1988. Effects of calcium hydroxide and sodium hypochlorite on the dissolution of necrotic porcine muscle tissue. *J Endod* 14:125–7.

Naenni N, Thoma K, Zehnder M. 2004. Soft tissue dissolution capacity of currently used and potential endodontic irrigants. *J Endod* 30:785–7.

Rafter M. 2005. Apexification: a review. *Dent Traumatol* 21:1–8.

Rosenberg B, Murray PE, Namerow, K. 2007. The effect of calcium hydroxide root filling on dentin fracture strength. *Dent Traumatol* 23:26–9.

Siqueira JF Jr, Lopes HP. 1999. Mechanisms of antimicrobial activity of calcium hydroxide: a critical review. *Int Endod J* 32:361–9.

Tanomaru Filho M, Leonardo MR, Silva LAB, Anibal EF, Faccioli LH. 2002. Inflammatory response to different endodontic irrigating solutions. *Int Endod J* 35:735–9.

Tronstad L, Asbjørnsen K, Døving L, Pedersen I, Eriksen HM. 2000. Influence of coronal restorations on the periapical health of endodontically treated teeth. *Endod Dent Traumatol* 16:218–21.

Yates JA. 1988. Barrier formation time in non-vital teeth with open apices. *Int Endod J* 21:313–9.

SELF-STUDY ANSWERS

1. The central incisor erupts at 7 years of age and its root is completed three years later. Considering the fact that the trauma occurred nine months prior to the time she was referred to treatment (around age 9), the stage of root development is reasonable

2. Copious irrigation is performed carefully so as to not pass solutions beyond the apex and to avoid the risk of cytotoxic effect on periapical tissues

3. Using an apex locator in such cases is limited; hence, the paper point method confirmed by a radiograph is suggested

4. $Ca(OH)_2$ packing must be verified by a radiograph; all of the root canal should have the same opacity as the dentin

5. One way is to use the custom cone technique in which an "imprint" of the canal is taken using softened Gutta Percha. An alternative is to use warm vertical condensation; however, a complete apical barrier is necessary to avoid overfilling

Case 8

Root End Closure with MTA

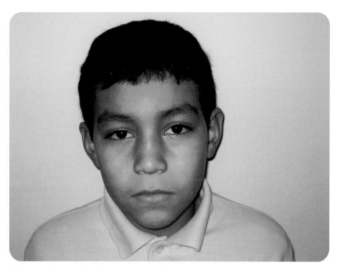

Figure 3.8.1. Facial photograph

A. Presenting Patient
- 9-year-old male

B. Chief Complaint and History of Present Injury
- The patient was referred by his dentist for root canal treatment (RCT) of the maxillary right permanent central incisor after a traumatic injury of unknown type to the anterior teeth at the age of 7
- History of treatment: At the emergency appointment, the patient presented with a large facial swelling diagnosed as an acute periradicular abscess originating from the maxillary right permanent central incisor. Upon accessing the root canal, there was pus drainage. The dentist placed a Ca(OH)$_2$ dressing in the canal, sealed it with a temporary filling (intermediate restorative material; IRM), and prescribed amoxicillin 250 mg/5 cc tid for one week

C. Social History
- Single child
- Middle-class family

D. Medical History
- No significant findings, no known drug or food allergies, no medications, vaccinations are up to date

E. Medical Consult
- N/A

F. Dental History
- Has a dental home
- Eats a regular balanced diet
- Fair oral hygiene habits, brushes his teeth twice a day unsupervised
- Uses a fluoride-containing toothpaste
- Lives in an optimally fluoridated area
- Dental trauma at age 7
- Cooperative

G. Extra-oral Exam
- No significant findings

H. Intra-oral Exam
Soft Tissues
- No significant findings

Hard Tissues
- No significant findings

Occlusal Evaluation of Mixed Dentition
- Class I permanent molars and primary canines, anterior crowding, overjet: 5 mm, overbite: 50%

Dental Exam
- Minimal plaque
- Caries free
- First permanent molars with amalgam restorations

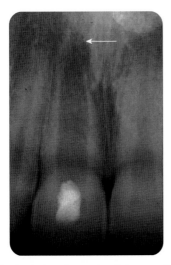

Figure 3.8.2. Periapical radiograph of the maxillary right permanent central incisor (arrow at radiolucent area)

BACKGROUND INFORMATION 1
Mineral Trioxide Aggregate
Mineral trioxide aggregate (MTA) is a powder that consists of hydrophilic particles which set in the presence of moisture; it reacts with tissue fluids to form a hard tissue apical barrier. MTA is the first restorative material that consistently allows over-growth of cementum and it may facilitate the regeneration of the periodontal ligament (Torabinejad et al. 1997, Schwartz et al. 1999). Obturation of the root canal can be done with a vertical condensation of warm Gutta Percha in the remainder of the canal.

I. Diagnostic Tools

- Periapical radiograph of the maxillary right permanent central incisor (Figure 3.8.2) showed temporary filling, wide root canal with thin walls, immature tooth with open apex, round radiolucent periapical area (Figure 3.8.2, arrow) surrounded by a radiopaque zone
- Clinical examination showed temporary filling; 2-mm pocket; physiologic mobility; no sensitivity to percussion, electrical pulp test (EPT), and cold test; slight tenderness on palpation; no sinus tract; no swelling

J. Differential Diagnosis

- Remnants of the dental sac
- Periapical true cyst
- Non-odontogenic lesion

K. Diagnosis and Problem List

Diagnosis

- Immature pulpless tooth with chronic apical periodontitis

Problem List

- Difficult to establish correct working length in immature teeth
- Risky to file a tooth with thin root canal walls
- Obturation of a tooth with wide open apex may result in overfilling
- Cold test and EPT are unreliable in immature teeth
- Difficult to differentiate between the radiographic appearance of a dental sac and chronic apical periodontitis

L. Comprehensive Treatment Plan

- Explain to the parents the difficulties in treating an immature permanent tooth
- Establish an apical barrier with mineral trioxide aggregate (MTA), followed by RCT and the final restoration
- Follow-up care should include:
  - Immediate post-op and home care instructions after each appointment
  - Recall after one year, followed by yearly clinical and radiographic examination for five years

Dental Treatment

- First appointment
  - Local anesthesia, rubber dam, and removal of the IRM temporary filling
  - Working length established using a radiograph in conjunction with the paper point method
  - Copious irrigation with 0.5% chlorhexidine, followed by minimal mechanical instrumentation of the root canal walls and additional irrigation with ultrasonic activation
  - Because there was no apical stop, a Ca(OH)$_2$ paste was placed using a syringe with a small-gauge needle, followed by an IRM temporary filling
- Second appointment, two weeks later
  - Copious irrigation with 0.5% chlorhexidine
  - Apical barrier created with MTA
  - Wet paper point and wet cotton pellet placed over the MTA plug followed by a temporary filling with IRM (Figure 3.8.3.)

- Third appointment, one week later
  - Setting of the MTA plug verified
  - Root canal space irrigated with 0.5% chlorhexidine and dried
  - Canal was obturated with warm injectable Gutta Percha (Figure 3.8.4.)
  - Coronal access double sealed with Coltosol and IRM
  - Patient referred back to dentist for final restoration

M. Clinical and Radiographic Follow-up

- The tooth is asymptomatic and functional 12 months post-operatively (Figure 3.8.5.). The size of the periapical radiolucency diminished; full healing is expected

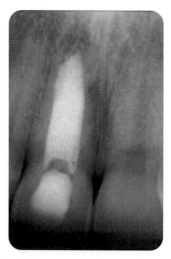

Figure 3.8.5. Twelve-month post-op radiograph

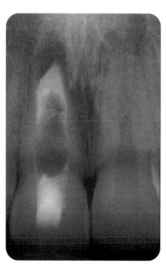

Figure 3.8.3. Radiograph showing closure of the apex with an MTA plug

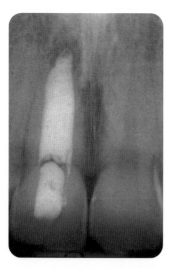

Figure 3.8.4. Radiograph showing obturation of the root canal

FUNDAMENTAL POINT 1
Ca(OH)$_2$ vs. MTA

- In comparison to Ca(OH)$_2$ apexification, apical closure with mineral trioxide aggregate (MTA) is more predictable along with reduction in treatment time, number of appointments, and radiographs. The tooth can be restored with minimal delay, preventing the risk of root fracture and re-infection. Use of MTA can also avoid the detrimental effects on the mechanical strength of dentin found with prolonged exposure to Ca(OH)$_2$.

N. Prognosis and Discussion

- Due to their thin dentinal walls, these teeth are prone to fracture. Therefore, a mouth guard is suggested to decrease the risk of injury in risky situations (sports, biking, etc.) Nonetheless, the caretakers and the patient should bear in mind that this tooth may be lost in the future.
- Traditional methods of restoration using metal posts and pins are often unsatisfactory. The post only retains the core and crown, but does not strengthen the tooth itself (Davy, Dilley, and Krejci 1981). Immature root filled teeth are often compromised by inappropriate post space preparation, coronal leakage, and secondary caries around prefabricated posts, or too large custom posts. It may be advantageous to use a light transmitting post and composite resin to internally strengthen the tooth (Sapir et al. 2004).

O. Common Complication and Alternative Treatment Plans

Common Complications

- After apexification, the immature root is short and the crown:root ratio is not favorable. Post placement (if needed) is difficult due to the size and irregular shape of the root canal, and placement of a permanent crown should be delayed due to the patient's continuous growth and maturing of the gingival tissues.

Alternative Treatment Plans

- Apexification with Ca(OH)$_2$
- Revascularization

Self-study Questions

1. **What are the main problems in endodontic treatment of immature teeth?**

2. **What are the problems in establishing working length in immature teeth?**

3. **What are the reasons for preferring a single-visit root closure with MTA rather than apexification with Ca(OH)$_2$?**

4. **How is the formation of an apical barrier verified in Ca(OH)$_2$ apexification?**

Answers are located at the end of the case.

Bibliography

Davy DT, Dilley GL, Krejci RF. 1981. Determination of stress patterns in root-filled teeth incorporating various dowel designs. *J Dent Res* 60:1301–10.

Sapir S, Mamber E, Slutzky-Goldberg I, Fuks AB. 2004. A novel multidisciplinary approach for the treatment of an intruded immature permanent incisor. *Pediatr Dent* 26:421–5.

Schwartz RS, Mauger M, Clement DJ, Walker WA 3rd. 1999. Mineral trioxide aggregate: a new material for endodontics. *JADA* 130:967–75.

Torabinejad M, Pitt Ford TR, McKendry DJ, et al. 1997. Histologic assessment of mineral trioxide aggregate as a root-end filling in monkeys. *J Endod* 23:225–8.

SELF-STUDY ANSWERS

1. Immature teeth have a wide open apex; therefore, it is impossible to seal the root canal without overfilling beyond the apex. Furthermore, after filling with $Ca(OH)_2$ these teeth are more prone to fracture

2. The exact position of the biologic apex in teeth with blunderbuss apex is not apparent. It is advisable to use a paper point to measure the exact length of the root canal. Bleeding at the end of the paper point or a wet paper point indicates overextension

3. (a) $Ca(OH)_2$ apexification is more time consuming than creating an apical barrier with MTA; (b) $Ca(OH)_2$ was shown to make these teeth more prone to fracture, whereas MTA strengthens the root; (c) it is assumed that MTA creates a better biologic seal; (d) root end closure with MTA is also more predictable

4. A Gutta Percha point is gently pushed toward the apex, until a barrier is felt. The patient should not feel anything. This should then be radiographically verified.

Case 9

Revascularization of Necrotic Immature Permanent Tooth With Apical Periodontitis

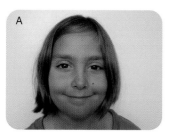 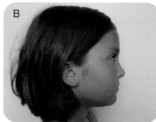

Figure 3.9.1a–b. Facial photographs

A. Presenting Patient
- 7-year-old Caucasian female
- New patient presenting as an emergency

B. Chief Complaint and History of Present Injury
- Her father stated that the patient "has had excruciating pain in the upper front tooth since yesterday"
- Trauma history: One month ago patient was playing with a ball, slipped, and fractured the maxillary left permanent central incisor. A few days later a composite coronal restoration was placed at a private dental clinic. The morning before this emergency visit, the patient complained of mild pain. She was then examined by an endodontist who recommended a follow-up. During the day and the following night the pain became unbearable, with some relief by nonsteroidal anti-inflammatory drugs

C. Social History
- Youngest of five children
- Low socio-economic class

D. Medical History
- No significant findings, no known food or drug allergies, no medications, vaccinations are up to date

E. Medical Consult
- N/A

F. Dental History
- Has a dental home
- Eats a balanced diet, not fond of sweets, loves salty snacks, and drinks mostly tap water
- Poor oral hygiene, brushes without supervision twice a day
- Uses toothpaste containing fluoride
- Water fluoridation level is 0.5 ppm

G. Extra-oral Exam
- Bilaterally enlarged submandibular lymph nodes
- Slightly incompetent lips

FUNDAMENTAL POINT 1
Obtaining a Trauma History
- Obtain information about the history and nature of the trauma (see Chapter 4)

Ask Questions Regarding:
- Any additional trauma to the teeth
- The nature of the present trauma:
  - Pain or tenderness to percussion
  - Tooth mobility
  - Bleeding from the gingival crevice or the surrounding tissues
  - Crown discoloration
  - Sensitivity to cold/hot stimulus
  - Information from previous dentists

H. Intra-oral Exam

Soft Tissues

- Generalized gingivitis

Hard Tissues

- Maxillary left permanent central incisor (Figure 3.9.2) showed composite restoration, mobility class II, very tender to touch and to very gentle tapping, tender to palpation, no crown discoloration, no response to electric pulp test (EPT) and cold test

Occlusal Evaluation of Mixed Dentition

- Class II molars, primary canines in crossbite, overjet: 4 mm, overbite: 4 mm

Other

- Extensive plaque accumulation
- Several primary and permanent teeth with extensive carious lesions

I. Diagnostic Tools

- Periapical radiograph of the maxillary left permanent central incisor (Figure 3.9.3) showed composite restoration, wide root canal with thin dentin walls, immature root with open apex, round radiolucent area around the apex

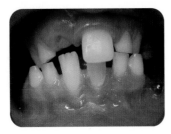

Figure 3.9.2. Pre-op intra-oral photo

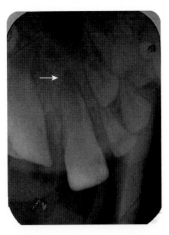

Figure 3.9.3. Pre-op periapical radiograph (arrow at radiolucent area)

J. Differential Diagnosis

- Acute periradicular periodontitis (pulp necrosis)
- Acute periradicular abscess (pulp necrosis)
- Normal dental sac

K. Diagnosis and Problem List

Diagnosis

- The pulp is necrotic. Because there is no clear evidence of periradicular radiolucency on the radiograph, the most probable diagnosis is acute periradicular periodontitis
- Carious lesions in the primary and permanent dentition

Problem List

- Difficult to establish correct working length in immature teeth
- Risky to file a tooth with thin root canal walls
- Obturation of a tooth with wide open apex may result in overfilling
- Cold test and EPT are unreliable in immature teeth
- Difficult to differentiate between the radiographic appearance of a dental sac and chronic apical periodontitis
- Possibility of root fracture (due to the thin dentin walls)
- Unfavorable crown-root ratio
- Untreated carious lesions in primary and permanent teeth
- Poor behavior

L. Comprehensive Treatment Plan

- Explanation to the parents of difficulties in treating an immature permanent tooth
- Behavioral management using nitrous oxide

FUNDAMENTAL POINT 2
Periradicular Pathology Definitions

- Acute periradicular (apical) periodontitis: Inflammation usually of the apical periodontium producing clinical symptoms including painful response to biting and percussion (American Association of Endodontists 2003)

- Acute periradicular (apical) abscess: An inflammatory reaction to pulpal infection and necrosis characterized by rapid onset, spontaneous pain, tenderness of the tooth to pressure, pus formation, and eventually swelling of associated tissues (American Association of Endodontists 2003)

BACKGROUND INFORMATION 1
Revascularization of Necrotic Immature Permanent Tooth*

Indications

- Permanent tooth
- Immature tooth (the wider the apical foramen the better the chance for revascularization)
- Necrotic pulp (chronic periradicular periodintitis or sinus tract may be present)
- No known allergy to any of the antibiotics used

Technique

- First step: Disinfect the root canals
  - Make a conservative access opening, followed by a length measurement (radiograph with an endodontic file or a Gutta Percha point). The file should be inserted 2 to 3mm short of the apical foramen to prevent damage to vital apical tissues (Figure 3.9.4.)
  - DO NOT instrument the root canal walls
  - Gently and carefully rinse the canal with 10ml of 5.25% NaOCl followed by 10ml of 2% chlorhexidine. The needle should be inserted 2 to 3mm short of the apical foramen
  - Dry the canal with sterile paper points
  - Introduce a Munce Canal Projector (CJM Engineering, Santa Barbara, CA) (three sizes available) through the access into the orifice of the canal (Reynolds, Johnson, and Cohenca 2009)
  - Build up the space between the projector and the access walls of the chamber using flowable composite; polymerize the material followed by removal of the Munce projector
  - Mix equal parts of ciprofloxacin, minocycline, and metronidazole with sterile saline
  - Insert the tri-antibiotic paste (3mix) into the canal using a sterile lentulo spiral in a slow-speed handpiece or a sterile syringe with a 20-gauge needle (2 to 3mm short of the apical foramen)
  - Clean the access cavity thoroughly of any residues from the 3mix (to the cementoenamel junction [CEJ] level) and seal the tooth temporarily with a sterile cotton pellet and a temporary sealing material
- Second step (four weeks later): Create a scaffold and seal the canal orifice
  - Ensure that the tooth is asymptomatic and without clinical signs of pathology (i.e., sinus tract)
  - Apply a rubber dam; remove the temporary restoration and cotton pellet
  - Rinse the 3mix out from the canal with 10ml of 5.25% NaOCl followed by 10ml of sterile saline
  - Dry the canal with sterile paper points
  - Insert a sterile endodontic hand file or an endodontic explorer past the canal terminus into the periapical tissues to induce bleeding to fill the canal spaces (irritate the tissue gently) (Figure 3.9.3a-b)
  - Stop the bleeding at a level of 2 to 3mm below the level of the CEJ with a moist cotton pellet (sterile saline); leave it for 15 minutes so that the blood will clot at that level
  - Place mineral trioxide aggregate (MTA) carefully over the blood clot, followed by a wet cotton pellet and a temporary sealing material
  - Take a radiograph to ensure correct placement of the MTA
- Third step (two weeks later): Seal the access cavity
  - Remove the temporary restoration and make sure the MTA is set
  - Place final coronal restoration with bonded composite resin
  - Reschedule the patient for follow-up appointments

*Banchs and Trope (2004)

- Emergency treatment of acute apical periodontitis, i.e., first step of revascularization
- Completion of the revascularization procedure and treatment of other teeth
- Follow up care includes:
- Oral hygiene instructions
- Caries prevention plan
- Orthodontic consultation
- Recalls at 3, 6 and 12 months after the revascularization, and once a year thereafter (Figures 3.9.5–7)

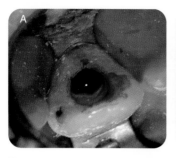
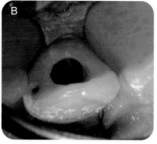

Figure 3.9.4a–b. A. Blood filling the root canal space, B. blood clot 2 to 3 mm below the cementoenamal junction

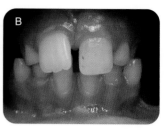
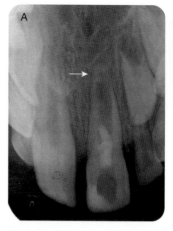

Figure 3.9.6a–b. A. Six-month post-op radiograph (arrow at closed apex), B. six-month post-op intra-oral photo

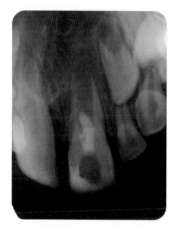

Figure 3.9.5. Three-month post-op radiograph

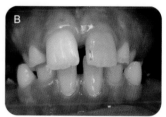
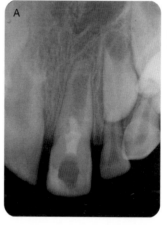

Figure 3.9.7a–b. A. 12-month post-op radiograph, B. 12-month post-op intra-oral photo

M. Clinical and Radiographic Follow-up

- At three-month follow-up the radiograph (Figure 3.9.5) shows a slight elongation of the root and the tooth has no clinical nor radiographic evidence of pathology. There is no sensitivity to cold test and EPT due to the presence of the composite and MTA. The temporary sealing material was replaced by a composite resin restoration
- At the six-month follow-up visit (Figure 3.9.6) there is continuous elongation of the root and thickening of the canal walls. The apex is closed (Figure 3.9.6, arrow) with a continuous periodontal ligament. The tooth has no clinical nor radiographic signs of pathology.
- At the one-year follow-up the tooth has no clinical nor radiographic signs of pathology (Figure 3.9.7)

N. Prognosis and Discussion

- Pulp necrosis following traumatic injuries is mainly related to the type and severity of the injury as well as to the stage of root development. Endodontic intervention is indicated when the pulp is necrotic or when there are clinical and radiographic signs of infection (Barnett 2002).

- The best treatment option for necrotic immature permanent teeth is regeneration of the pulp. The advantage of pulp revascularization is the possibility of further root development and strengthening of the dentin walls by deposition of hard tissue (Banchs and Trope 2004, Chueh and Huang 2006). Regeneration of pulp tissue in a necrotic infected tooth with apical periodontitis was thought to be impossible. However, recent research suggests that creating the unique circumstances that exist in revascularized avulsed cases allows regeneration of tissue to take place.
- The mixture of antibiotics used has been demonstrated to be effective in killing endodontic bacteria in the root canal and inside dentinal tubules *in vitro* and *in vivo* (Sato et al. 1996, Windley et al. 2005).

- More research is needed to improve this procedure and evaluate its efficacy and predictability

O. Common Complications and Alternative Treatment Plans

Complications

- Green-gray discoloration of the crown is sometimes evident after using 3 mix, which presents an esthetic problem
- Drug tolerance is a potential risk and, as a result, the disinfecting action will be impaired

- A systemic allergic reaction to the antibiotics can be life threatening

Alternative Treatment Plans

- When signs of pulp infection are persistent after the use of the 3 mix (i.e., sinus tract, continuous pain and sensitivity), Ca(OH)$_2$ can be used for apexification, or mineral trioxide aggregate (MTA) can be placed to create an apical barrier

Self-study Questions

1. **What are the indications for the revascularization procedure?**

2. **What should be used to disinfect the canal space in the revascularization procedure?**

3. **What are the advantages of using the revascularization procedure in necrotic immature permanent teeth?**

4. **When is endodontic intervention indicated after a traumatic injury?**

5. **What are possible complications of the revascularization procedure?**

Answers are located at the end of the case.

Bibliography

American Association of Endodontists. 2003. *An Annotated Glossary of Terms Used in Endodontics*, 7th edition. Chicago.

Banchs F, Trope M. 2004. Revascularization of immature permanent teeth with apical periodontitis: New treatment protocol? *J Endod* 30:196–200.

Barnett F. 2002. The role of endodontics in the treatment of luxated permanent teeth. *Dent Traumatol* 18:47–56.

Chueh LH, Huang GT. 2006. Immature teeth with periradicular periodontitis or abscess undergoing apexogenesis: A paradigm shift. *J Endod* 32:1205–13.

Reynolds K, Johnson J, Cohenca N. 2009. Pulp revascularization of necrotic bilateral bicuspids using a modified novel technique to eliminate potential coronal discolouration: a case report. *Int Endo J* 42:84–92.

Sato I, Ando-Kurihara N, Kota K, Iwaku M, Hoshino E. 1996. Sterilization of infected root-canal dentine by topical application of a mixture of ciprofloxacin, metronidazole and minocycline *in situ*. *Int Endod J* 29:118–24.

Windley W 3rd, Teixeira F, Levin L, Sigurdsson A, Trope M. 2005. Disinfection of immature teeth with a triple antibiotic paste. *J Endod* 31:439–43.

SELF-STUDY ANSWERS

1. Permanent, immature tooth (the wider the apical foramen the better the chance for revascularization), necrotic pulp (chronic periradicular periodontitis or sinus tract may be present), no known allergy to any of the antibiotics used

2. 5.25% NaOCl followed by 2% chlorhexidine followed by a mixture of antibiotics (ciprofloxacin, metronidazole, and minocycline) in the root canal for about four weeks

3. The advantages of pulp revascularization lie in the possibility of further root development and reinforcement of dentinal walls by deposition of hard tissue

4. When the pulp is necrotic or when there are clinical and radiographic signs of infection

5. Green-gray discoloration of the crown is sometimes evident after using 3 mix, which presents an esthetic problem. Drug tolerance is a potential risk and, as a result, the disinfecting action will be impaired. A systemic allergic reaction to the antibiotics can be life-threatening

4

Orofacial Trauma

Dennis J. McTigue and S. Thikkurissy

Clinical Cases in Pediatric Dentistry, First Edition. Edited by Amr M. Moursi.
© 2012 Blackwell Publishing Ltd. Published 2012 by Blackwell Publishing Ltd.

Case 1

Intrusion Injury to Primary Dentition

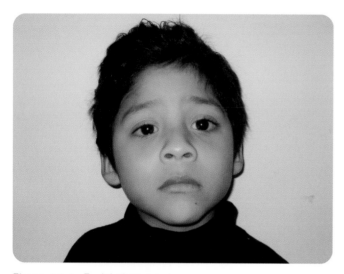

Figure 4.1.1. Facial photograph

A. Presenting Patient
- 2-year-, 7-month-old male
- New patient presenting as an emergency

B. Chief Complaint and History of Present Injury
- Mother stated, "My son was running and hit the stairs in our house"
- Child was running in home, fell and hit cement stairs three hours ago. Injury was witnessed by mother, who said that child "spit up food" after injury. No loss of consciousness
- Child was taken to local emergency room and cleared of any closed head trauma
- Child is in no distress

C. Social History
- Patient is only child
- Mother is the primary caregiver and stays at home
- Low socio-economic status

> **FUNDAMENTAL POINT 1**
> **Obtaining a Trauma History**
> - Confirm that tetanus immunizations are up to date. If last tetanus booster was five or more years prior and wound is contaminated with soil/debris, another tetanus toxoid booster is indicated (Broder et al. 2006, McTigue and Thikkurissy 2011)
> - Rule out closed head injury and refer for medical consult if patient is positive for any of the following (CDC 2007):
>   - Amnesia
>   - Nausea/vomiting
>   - Headache
>   - Lethargy/irritability/confusion
>   - Loss of consciousness
> - The preschool years represent a peak in incidence of dental trauma, with some reports citing incidence as high at 35% (Hargreaves et al. 1999)

D. Medical History
- History of recurrent otitis media infections per mother
- No known drug or food allergies, no medications, vaccinations are up to date

E. Medical Consult
- Completed at the emergency room

F. Dental History
- No dental home
- Fair oral hygiene; mother states she brushes his teeth every day
- Age-appropriate diet

- Uses toothpaste containing fluoride
- Optimally fluoridated water
- No history of trauma before today
- Child is acting age-appropriately, resisting being separated from mother

G. Extra-oral Exam

- Soft tissue injuries: Bruising noted on lip
- No other significant findings

H. Intra-oral Exam

Soft Tissues

- No significant findings

Hard Tissues

- No significant findings

Occlusal Evaluation of Primary Dentition

- Mesial step molar and class I canines

Other

- Minimal plaque accumulation noted
- Caries-free dentition
- Maxillary right primary lateral incisor: Slight mobility, brown discoloration noted middle third
- Maxillary right primary central incisor: Slight mobility
- Maxillary left primary central incisor: Intruded to gingival margin (Figure 4.1.2.)
- Maxillary left primary lateral incisor: Slight mobility, brown discoloration noted middle third

I. Diagnostic Tools

- Radiographs not possible due to very poor patient cooperation
- Vitality tests deferred

J. Diagnosis and Problem List

Diagnosis

- Maxillary right primary lateral incisor, right primary central incisor, and left primary lateral incisor: Subluxation
- Maxillary left primary central incisor: Intrusion

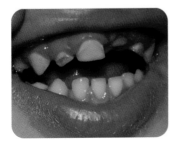

Figure 4.1.2. Intra-oral photo showing intrusion of maxillary left primary central incisor

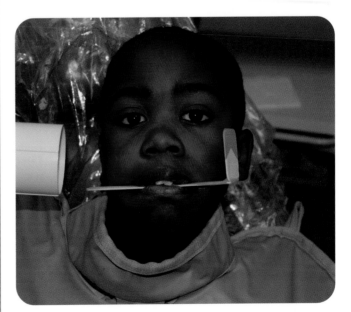

Figure 4.1.3. Example of technique for extra-oral lateral occlusal radiograph

Problem List
- No dental home
- Complete intrusion maxillary left primary central incisor

K. Treatment
- No treatment is indicated at this time (see Flowchart A at the end of this chapter)
- Advise parent of potential damage to permanent tooth bud, including potential hypocalcifications
- Discharge instructions
  - Avoid incising on injured segment until instructed otherwise
  - Watch for clinical signs such as presence of parulis or fistula
- Follow-up treatment
  - Patient was seen for follow-up at one and two months with minimal re-eruption noted
  - Four-month follow-up: Per mother, patient is asymptomatic; the maxillary left primary central incisor has fully re-erupted into position

L. Prognosis and Discussion
- The overall prognosis for this tooth is based on the observation that it did re-erupt. The four-month post-op radiograph demonstrated no periapical resorption or radiolucency. The full understanding of the impact of the trauma is limited to the two-dimensional radiograph, and the successful eruption of the permanent incisor is a benchmark for the overall success of treatment

M. Complications and Alternative Treatment Plan
- If the root tip had become exposed through gingival tissues, extraction would be indicated due to the poor healing prognosis
- If the tooth failed to re-erupt after six months of evaluation, an extraction would be the recommended course of treatment because any partial ankylotic changes could impede the path of eruption of the permanent incisor
- It is not unusual to have a concomitant root fracture on a primary incisor. If the coronal fractured segment poses any type of aspiration risk, then the recommendation is extraction of the coronal segment while leaving the apical segment alone

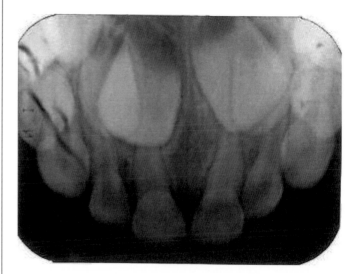

Figure 4.1.5. Radiograph showing no periapical resorption or radiolucency associated with the maxillary left primary central incisor

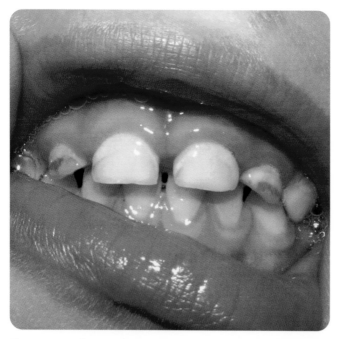

Figure 4.1.4. Intra-oral photo showing re-eruption of maxillary left primary central incisor

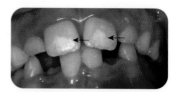

Figure 4.1.6. Example of hypoplastic defects (arrows) of the permanent successors following intrusion trauma to the primary incisors

FUNDAMENTAL POINT 3

Trauma Complications

- Trauma to primary teeth can lead to developmental or hypoplastic defects in permanent successors (Figure 4.1.6) (Sennhenn-Kirchner and Jacobs 2006)

- The majority of intruded primary incisors are displaced in a labial direction (Holan and Ram 1999)

- All teeth involved in injury must be re-assessed for potential pulpal injury, which may not surface immediately (Flores et al. 2007)

- The majority of intruded primary incisors (88% in some reports) will re-erupt within six months (Holan and Ram 1999)

- When there is no impingement on the permanent tooth bud, or the facial cortical plate has not been fractured, a wait-and-watch approach may be most prudent because most incisors will re-erupt within six months

Self-study Questions

1. *What are instances in which immediate extraction of intruded primary incisors would be indicated?*

2. *How long should one wait and watch intruded primary incisors to re-erupt?*

3. *If the intruded tooth is asymptomatic at one week post injury, is the pulp healthy?*

4. *If a root fracture was present in the apical one-third of the root, is it recommended to surgically extract the remaining root tip?*

Answers are located at the end of the case.

Bibliography

Broder K, Cortese M, et al. 2006. Preventing tetanus, diphtheria, and pertussis among adolescents: Use of tetanus toxoid, reduced diphtheria toxoid and acellular pertussis vaccines. Recommendations of the CDC Advisory Committee on Immunization practices. *MMWR.* Feb. 23, 2006, 55:1–43. www.cdc.gov/mmwr/preview/ mmwrhtml/rr55e223a1.htm and http://www.cdc.gov/ vaccines/vpd-vac/tetanus/default.htm.

Centers for Disease Control and Prevention (CDC). 2007. Heads Up. *Facts for Physicians about Mild Traumatic Brain Injury (MTBI).* http://www.cdc.gov/ncipc/tbi/Facts_for_ Physicians_booklet.pdf.

Flores MT et al. 2007. Guidelines for the management of traumatic dental injuries. III. Primary teeth. *Dent Traumatol* 23:196–202.

Garcia-López M, Martinez-Blanco M, Martinez-Mir I, Palop V. 2001. Amoxycillin-clavulanic acid-related tooth discoloration in children. *Pediatrics.* Sep;108(3):819.

Hargreaves JA, Cleaton-Jones PE, Roberts GJ, Williams S, Matejka JM. 1999. Trauma to primary teeth of South African pre-school children. *Endod Dent Traumatol* Apr;15(2):73–6.

Holan G, Ram D. 1999. Sequelae and prognosis of intruded primary incisors: a retrospective study. *Pediatr Dent* Jul-Aug;21(4):242–7.

McTigue D, Thikkurissy S. 2011. Trauma. In: *The Handbook of Pediatric Dentistry*, 4th Edition. Nowak AJ, Casamassimo PS (eds). American Academy of Pediatric Dentistry: Chicago. pp. 109–17.

Pugliesi DM, Cunha RF, Delberm AC, Sundefeld ML. 2004. Influence on the type of dental trauma on the pulp vitality and the time until treatment: a study in patients ages 0–3 years. *Dent Traumatol* Jun;20(3).139–42.

Sennhenn-Kirchner S, Jacobs HG. 2006. Traumatic injuries to the primary dentition and effects on permanent successors—a clinical follow-up study. *Dent Traumatol* Oct;22(5):237–41.

SELF-STUDY ANSWERS

1. If a radiograph, such as a lateral occlusal, indicates that the primary tooth is intimately associated with the permanent tooth bud, extraction may be indicated. Any potential aspiration risk to the child is also an indication for extraction. Extraction of the intruded incisor does not necessarily spare the successor from possible damage

2. While reports note that the majority of intruded primary incisors will re-erupt within six months, re-eruption should be assessed monthly and teeth should demonstrate significant re-eruption (although not necessarily complete) by two months. If there is no evidence of re-eruption, then a careful clinical and radiographic examination must be completed to re-assess treatment options such as extraction

3. No. In the instance of any traumatic injuries, the pulp may provide false-positive responses clinically for up to three weeks post injury. Sequelae such as replacement resorption may not be apparent until six weeks post injury.

4. If the remaining root tip is intimately related to the permanent tooth bud, then any treatment must be approached with the understanding that there is potential for damaging the permanent tooth as well

Case 2

Root Fracture in the Primary Dentition

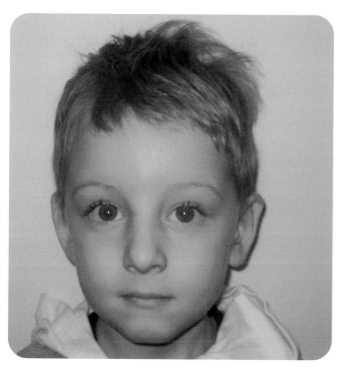

Figure 4.2.1. Facial photograph

A. Presenting Patient

- 4-year-, 6-month-old Caucasian male
- New patient presenting as an emergency

B. Chief Complaint and History of Present Injury

- Mom states, "My son knocked his teeth yesterday, and now they look brownish." The child was playing at the mall playground and fell. The injury was witnessed by the mother. There was no loss of consciousness and no complaint of pain

C. Social History

- Patient has no siblings
- Mother is the primary caregiver and stays at home
- Low socio-economic status

BACKGROUND INFORMATION 1
Trauma Prevention

- While many parents may believe that their children are taking preventive measures to avoid injury, such as bicycle helmets, the truth is that reports by children often reveal that when unsupervised, injury prevention measures are often not followed (Ehrlich et al. 2001)

- Studies have revealed that mouth guards are an effective primary protective measure at reducing the rate of dento-alveolar injuries, yet in some instances only 1% to 5% of children participating in sports actually wear mouth guards during practices (Spinas and Savasta 2007, Fakhruddin et al. 2007).

- Falls are typically the most common type of injury, and while the anecdotal belief is that increased supervision will prevent injuries, reports in the literature cite that only about 20% of parents believe increased supervision will prevent falls/injuries (Eberl et al. 2009)

- There is a reported peak in incidence of dental trauma during preschool years of as high as 35% (Hargreaves et al. 1999)

D. Medical History

- History of recurrent otitis media infections
- No known drug or food allergies, no medications, vaccinations are up to date

E. Medical Consult

- N/A

F. Dental History

- Child has seen dentist since 18 months of age

- Confirm that tetanus immunizations are up to date. If the last tetanus booster was five or more years prior and the wound is contaminated with soil/debris, another tetanus toxoid booster is indicated (Broder et al. 2006, McTigue and Thikkurissy 2011)

- Rule out closed head injury and refer for medical consult if the patient is positive for any of the following (CDC 2007):
  - Amnesia
  - Nausea/vomiting
  - Headache
  - Lethargy/irritability/confusion
  - Loss of consciousness

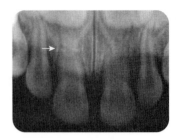

Figure 4.2.3. Radiograph showing root fractures of maxillary right (arrow) and left primary central incisors

- Take adequate radiographs to clearly image all involved teeth.

- Rule out other injuries, e.g., soft tissue lacerations, alveolar fractures, etc. (Flores et al. 2007)

- Vitality testing is of questionable value on primary teeth, and recognition of pulpal necrosis is typically based on clinical presentation (Pugliesi et al. 2004)

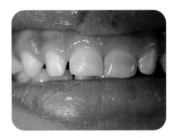

Figure 4.2.2. Intra-oral photo of maxillary right and left primary central incisors

- Fair oral hygiene with little adult supervision. Mild plaque accumulation on buccal surfaces of maxillary molars
- Diet is age appropriate
- Uses toothpaste containing fluoride twice daily
- Lives in optimally fluoridated area
- No history of trauma before today
- Child's behavior is age appropriate, and he is curious about dental instruments

G. Extra-Oral Exam
- Soft tissue injuries: mild contusions on upper lip

H. Intra-Oral Exam
Soft Tissues
- No significant findings

Hard Tissues
- Traumatized teeth: Maxillary right and left primary central incisors—class I mobility

Occlusal Evaluation of Primary Dentition
- No significant findings

Other
- Caries-free dentition

I. Diagnostic Tools
- Periapical radiograph shows root fracture in the middle third of the maxillary right and left primary central incisors
- Vitality tests deferred

J. Diagnosis and Problem List
Diagnosis
- Maxillary right and left primary lateral incisors: subluxation
- Maxillary right and left primary central incisors: middle root fractures

K. Treatment
- No treatment is indicated at this time (see Flowchart B at the end of this chapter)
- Discharge instructions: Avoid incising on injured segment until instructed otherwise. Watch for clinical signs such as presence of parulis or fistula

- Follow-up treatment: Follow up within four weeks to reassess healing and potential need for future treatments.

L. Prognosis and Discussion

- Root fractures located on the apical third present a good prognosis. Teeth with root fractures in the middle segment should be observed closely as in the case presented. The more coronal the fracture is, the worse the prognosis. Cases in which there is significant mobility of the coronal segment and/or mobility of the coronal segment result in poor outcomes

M. Complications and Alternative Treatment Plan

- If the fracture had been located in the coronal third, the recommendation would be to remove the coronal segment because the prognosis is poor. There is some controversy as to whether apical segments need to be removed. Direct visualization of the apical segment would facilitate extraction, while poor or no visualization could result in damage to permanent tooth bud

---

BACKGROUND INFORMATION 2
Dental Root Fractures

- Root fractures traditionally heal by one of four means:
  1. Calcified tissue (bony healing)
  2. Interposition of connective tissue
  3. Interposition of bone and connective tissue
  4. Interposition of granulation tissue
- The most common forms of root fracture healing are calcified tissue and interposition of connective tissue (Cvek et al. 1995)
- Splinting primary teeth should be attempted only after careful risk:benefit analysis, including:
  1. Patient cooperation
  2. Ability to provide adequate isolation if a resin splint is used
  3. Parental compliance with needed follow-up care
- While some studies have shown success with primary tooth splinting, medico-legal considerations must be discussed with caregivers

---

FUNDAMENTAL POINT 3
Complications of Dental Trauma

- Tooth discoloration is a common post-traumatic complication
- Dark gray discoloration of primary incisors soon after injury may fade and does NOT warrant immediate treatment
- Discoloration noted soon after injury is not representative of definitive pulpal diagnosis (Holan 2004)
- Tooth discoloration that first appears well after the trauma may be indicative of changes in pulp vitality and potential necrosis (Soxman et al. 1984)
- All teeth involved in injury must be re-assessed for potential pulpal injury (Flores et al. 2007)

Self-study Questions

1. **What are the situations in which extraction of tooth and/or segments is warranted?**
2. **Would management differ if discoloration had occurred 26 months after injury?**

3. **When is splinting of primary teeth indicated?**

Answers are located at the end of the case.

Bibliography

Broder K, Cortese M, et al. 2006. Preventing tetanus, diphtheria, and pertussis among adolescents: Use of tetanus toxoid, reduced diphtheria toxoid and acellular pertussis vaccines. Recommendations of the CDC Advisory Committee on Immunization practices. *MMWR.* Feb. 23, 2006, 55:1–43. www.cdc.gov/mmwr/preview/mmwrhtml/rr55e223a1.htm and http://www.cdc.gov/vaccines/vpd-vac/tetanus/default.htm.

Centers for Disease Control and Prevention (CDC). 2007. *Heads Up. Facts for Physicians about Mild Traumatic Brain Injury* (MTBI). http://www.cdc.gov/ncipc/tbi/Facts_for_Physicians_booklet.pdf.

Cvek M, Andreasen JO, Borum MK. 1995. Healing of 208 intra-alveolar root fractures in patients aged 7–17 years. *J Endod* Jul;21(7):391–3.

Eberl R, Schalamon J, Singer G, Ainoedhofer H, Petnehazy T, Hoellwarth ME. 2009. Analysis of 347 kindergarten-related injuries. *Eur J Pediatr* 168:163–6.

Ehrlich PF, Longhi J, Vaughan R, Rockwell S. 2001. Correlation between parental perception and actual childhood patterns of bicycle helmet use and riding practices: implications for designing injury prevention strategies. *J Pediatr Surg* May;36(5):763–6.

Fakhruddin KS, Lawrence HP, Kenny DJ, Locker D. 2007. Use of mouthguards among 12- to 14-year-old Ontario schoolchildren. *J Can Dent Assoc* Jul-Aug;73(6):505.

Flores MT, et al. 2007. Guidelines for the management of traumatic dental injuries. III. Primary Teeth. *Dent Traumatol* 23:196–202.

Hargreaves JA, Cleaton-Jones PE, Roberts GJ, Williams S, Matejka JM. 1999. Trauma to primary teeth of South African pre-school children. *Endod Dent Traumatol* Apr;15(2):73–6.

Holan G. 2004. Development of clinical and radiographic signs associated with dark discolored primary incisors following traumatic injuries: a prospective controlled study. *Dent Traumatol* Oct;20(5):276–87.

McTigue D, Thikkurissy S. 2011. Trauma. In: *The Handbook of Pediatric Dentistry*, 4th Edition. Nowak AJ, Casamassimo PS (eds) American Academy of Pediatric Dentistry: Chicago. pp. 109–17.

Pugliesi DM, Cunha RF, Delberm AC, Sundefeld ML. 2004. Influence on the type of dental trauma on the pulp vitality and the time until treatment: a study in patients ages 0–3 years. *Dent Traumatol* Jun;20(3).139–142.

Soxman JA, Nazif MM, Bouquot J. 1984. Pulpal pathology in relation to discoloration of primary anterior teeth. *ASDC J Dent Child* Jul–Aug;51(4):282–4.

Spinas E, Savasta A. 2007. Prevention of traumatic dental lesions: cognitive research on the role of mouthguards during sport activities in paediatric age. *Eur J Paediatr Dent* Dec;8(4):193–8.

SELF-STUDY ANSWERS

1. As the fracture is placed more coronally, the prognosis worsens for the tooth. Furthermore, the aspiration risk must be assessed. Parents should be made aware of the possibility for the need to remove the coronal and/or entire segment at a later date if no treatment is immediately rendered

2. Per the 2007 International Association of Dental Traumatology (IADT) guidelines (http://www.iadt-dentaltrauma.org), transient discoloration immediately following injury is not uncommon. This discoloration is most often reddish or grayish. Discoloration that occurs well after the traumatic injury may be indicative of pulpal necrosis and result in inflammatory resorption despite the patient remaining asymptomatic

3. Splinting primary teeth should be attempted only after careful risk:benefit analysis, including patient cooperation and behavior, ability for adequate isolation if a resin splint is used, and parental compliance and understanding of the need for follow-up care. While some studies have demonstrated success with splinting primary teeth, full medico-legal considerations need to be discussed with parents/caregivers

Case 3

Complicated Crown Fracture, Permanent Tooth

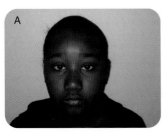
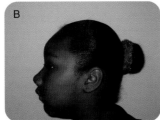

Figure 4.3.1a–b. Facial photographs

A. Presenting Patient

- 8-year-, 7-month-old African-American female
- New patient presenting as an emergency

B. Chief Complaint and History of Present Injury

- Mother reports, "My daughter fell off her bicycle and broke her tooth."
- Child fell while riding her bike at her grandmother's house about three and a half hours ago. The grandmother had no transportation so the patient waited until her mother returned home from work to come to the clinic. The accident was witnessed by her 12-year-old cousin. There was no loss of consciousness.

C. Social History

- Patient is in third grade
- Lives at grandmother's house with mother, one younger sibling, and two cousins
- Mother works two jobs and provides for all in household; the grandmother is the primary care provider
- Low socio-economic status

D. Medical History

- No significant findings, no known food or drug allergies, no medications, vaccinations are up to date

FUNDAMENTAL POINT 1
History for Trauma

- Rule out closed head injury and refer for medical consult if patient is positive for any of the following (CDC 2007):
  - Amnesia
  - Nausea/vomiting
  - Headache
  - Lethargy/irritability/confusion
  - Loss of consciousness
- Ask patient and parent if they know where the broken tooth fragment is. Rule out aspiration or impaction of the fragment in soft tissue wounds of the lips or tongue
- Confirm that tetanus immunizations are up to date if there are soft tissue injuries contaminated with soil (Broder et al. 2006)

E. Medical Consult

- N/A

F. Dental History

- No dental home
- Mother reports infrequent dental exams through local school program
- Diet high in refined carbohydrates
- Poor oral hygiene
- Child reports brushing with fluoridated toothpaste once per day
- Community water is optimally fluoridated
- No previous history of dental trauma

G. Extra-oral Exam

- No significant findings

H. Intra-oral Exam

Soft Tissues

- No significant findings

Hard Tissues

- No obvious carious lesions
- Traumatized tooth: Maxillary right permanent central incisor—complicated fracture (pulp exposure), class II mobility (Figure 4.3.2)

Occlusal Evaluation of Mixed Dentition

- No significant findings

Other

- Poor oral hygiene with extensive plaque accumulation

I. Diagnostic Tools

- Periapical radiograph demonstrates immature apices of maxillary incisors (Figure 4.3.3)
- Percussion tests
  - Maxillary permanent lateral incisors: Negative
  - Maxillary permanent central incisors: +2
- Vitality tests: Deferred

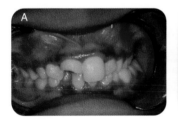 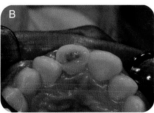

Figure 4.3.2a–b. Intraoral photos showing maxillary right permanent central incisor—complicated fracture (pulp exposure)

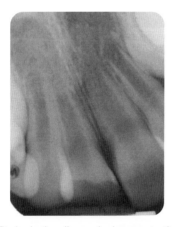

Figure 4.3.3. Periapical radiograph demonstrating immature apices of maxillary incisors

J. Diagnosis and Problem List

Diagnosis

- Maxillary right permanent central incisor: Complicated crown fracture with subluxation

---

FUNDAMENTAL POINT 2
Examination for Crown Fracture Injuries

- Take adequate radiographs that clearly show all involved teeth, including periapices
- Note apical development because it impacts treatment selected (see Flowchart C at end of this chapter) and prognosis. Pulp survival is more likely in luxated teeth with immature apices. Pulp canal obliteration is the most common sequela to luxation injuries to immature permanent teeth
- Rule out other injuries, e.g., root fractures, alveolar fractures
- Vitality tests frequently yield false-negative results for up to three months following an injury

(Flores et al. 2007)

BACKGROUND INFORMATION 1
Treatment for Crown Fractures

- Optimal care indicates treatment as soon as possible after the injury. Patient behavior, lack of availability of facilities and materials, or management of more serious injuries may delay treatment. Successful outcomes have been reported when treatment of complicated crown fractures is delayed up to several days, so the clinician may elect to defer treatment until the following morning, if necessary, to assure optimal treatment
- The treatment objective is to complete a debridement of inflamed or infected pulp tissue while maintaining healthy pulp tissue. This is particularly important in immature teeth in order for complete root maturation (apexogenesis) to occur

(Cvek 1978, Flores et al. 2007)

K. Comprehensive Treatment

- See Flowchart C at the end of the this chapter
- Maxillary right permanent incisor: Partial pulpotomy (Cvek technique, see Fundamental Point 3)
  - Isolate tooth with rubber dam
  - Gently remove 1.5 to 2 mm of pulp tissue with sterile bur and copious irrigation with water (Figure 4.3.4)
  - Use wet cotton pellet to control hemorrhage.
  - Cover pulp with calcium hydroxide, followed by glass ionomer
  - Assure an excellent seal with composite resin provisional restoration (Figure 4.3.5). Final restoration may be completed at same appointment if it can be done atraumatically. However, final restoration should be deferred if tooth is mobile
  - Suture gingival lacerations (if indicated). Prescribe over-the-counter acetaminophen or ibuprofen for pain, as needed

Discharge Instructions

- Avoid incising on injured tooth until tenderness resolves
- Instruct parents to watch for clinical signs including tooth discoloration and presence of parulis or fistula
- Instruct child to report increased pain or mobility

Follow-up Treatment

- Two-week post-op visit
  - Clinical exam: Assess vitality with cold and electric pulp tests; assess color, mobility, and pain to percussion

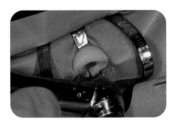

Figure 4.3.4. Partial pulpotomy technique

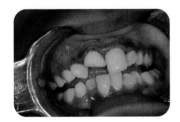

Figure 4.3.5. Composite resin provisional restoration

- Complete final restoration of tooth if not done at first appointment
- Six-week post-op visit
  - Clinical exam: Repeat assessment above
  - Radiographic exam: Assess for signs of pulp necrosis, periapical radiolucency, or inflammatory resorption, and for continuing root development
- Repeat same post-op assessments at six months and one year.

L. Prognosis and Discussion

- Prognosis depends on maintaining vitality of the pulp in the maxillary right permanent central incisor. The goal is to achieve full root maturation by removing inflamed pulp tissue while retaining healthy pulp in the root canal and crown. While a direct pulp cap may be simpler and quicker to perform than a partial pulpotomy, the consequences of failure (pulp necrosis) are dire in a tooth with an immature apex. Lacking a vital pulp makes the chances of the tooth achieving complete root maturation markedly decreased. A false-negative response to vitality tests is possible for up to three months. Continuing root development in immature teeth is a sign of a positive treatment outcome (Flores et al. 2007)

M. Common Complications and Alternative Treatment Plans

- An excellent seal is required to prevent bacterial contamination of the pulp tissue by saliva. Fracture lines extending subgingivally and lack of tissue fluid control can complicate placement of a secure, sealed restoration. Pulp necrosis will inevitably

---

FUNDAMENTAL POINT 3
Partial Pulpotomy

- Only a superficial layer of inflamed pulp tissue is removed, leaving healthy pulp tissue in the coronal chamber and root canal space
- Copious irrigation and a sharp, sterile bur are used to minimize injury to the remaining pulp
- The access preparation is deep enough (1.5 to 2 mm) to contain the wound dressing (CaOH or mineral trioxide aggregate [MTA]) and glass ionomer seal

(Cvek 1978, Flores et al. 2007)

occur if the restoration is not completely sealed. Close follow-up is critical because inflammatory resorption can rapidly destroy the thin root if the pulp becomes necrotic

- In cases of an immature permanent incisor with a necrotic pulp, a partial pulpotomy is not indicated because it is a vital technique. In immature teeth, revascularization can be attempted by first disinfecting the root canal space with antibiotic paste and then stimulating bleeding to form a scaffold for the ingrowth of healthy connective tissue. If successful, this technique enables the root to mature physiologically (apexogenesis). Another option is to induce apexification, which is the placement of a mechanical barrier at the root apex against which root canal filling materials are placed. The use of mineral trioxide aggregate (MTA) enables the clinician to perform this apexification procedure in one step

Self-study Questions

1. **How quickly must a partial pulpotomy be performed to assure optimal healing?**
2. **What complications compromise the success of a partial pulpotomy?**
3. **Can a tooth treated by a partial pulpotomy be completely restored immediately?**
4. **What are the options for treatment of an immature permanent incisor with a totally necrotic pulp?**

Answers are located at the end of the case.

Bibliography

Broder K, Cortese M, et al. 2006. Preventing tetanus, diphtheria, and pertussis among adolescents: Use of tetanus toxoid, reduced diphtheria toxoid and acellular pertussis vaccines. Recommendations of the CDC Advisory Committee on Immunization practices. *MMWR.* Feb. 23, 2006, 55:1–43. www.cdc.gov/mmwr/preview/ mmwrhtml/rr55e223a1.htm and http://www.cdc.gov/ vaccines/vpd-vac/tetanus/default.htm

Centers for Disease Control and Prevention (CDC). 2007. Heads Up. *Facts for Physicians about Mild Traumatic Brain Injury* (MTBI). http://www.cdc.gov/ncipc/tbi/Facts_for_ Physicians_booklet.pdf

Cvek M. 1978. A clinical report on partial pulpotomy and capping with calcium hydroxide in permanent incisors with complicated crown fractures. *J. Endo* 4:232–7.

Flores MT, et al. 2007. Guidelines for the management of traumatic dental injuries. I. Fractures and luxations of permanent teeth. *Dent Traumatol* 23:66–71.

SELF-STUDY ANSWERS

1. Optimal healing occurs if the partial pulpotomy is performed soon after the injury. However, positive outcomes have been reported when this treatment was delayed days to weeks after the injury. Best practice is to complete the procedure as soon as adequate assistance and facilities are available. This may mean deferring treatment until the following day

2. To succeed, a partial pulpotomy must be performed as aseptically as possible. Primary causes of failure include inadequate isolation and lack of an absolute seal by the temporary restoration

3. It may be possible to complete the final restoration on a tooth treated with a partial pulpotomy; however, since luxation injuries frequently accompany such severe crown fractures, deferring the final restoration until the periodontal ligament (PDL) has healed is recommended

4. A partial pulpotomy is a vital technique and is not indicated when the pulp is totally necrotic. In immature teeth, revascularization can be attempted by first disinfecting the root canal space with antibiotic paste and then stimulating bleeding to form a scaffold for the ingrowth of healthy connective tissue. If successful, this technique enables the root to mature physiologically (apexogenesis). Another option is to induce apexification, which is the placement of a mechanical barrier at the root apex against which root canal filling materials are placed. The use of mineral trioxide aggregate (MTA) enables the clinician to perform this apexification procedure in one step.

Case 4

Dentoalveolar Luxation Injury to Permanent Dentition

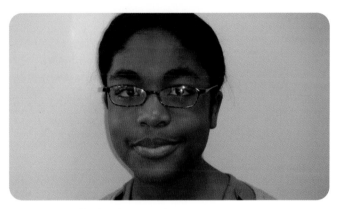

Figure 4.4.1. Facial photograph

A. Presenting Patient

- 13-year-, 6-month-old African-American female
- New patient presenting as an emergency

B. Chief Complaint and History of Present Injury

- Mom states, "My daughter's tooth was knocked crooked"
- Child was playing soccer, tripped, and fell on another child 45 minutes ago. Injury was witnessed by friends. No loss of consciousness or vomiting was noted
- Patient is in mild discomfort

C. Social History

- Mother is the primary caregiver and works full-time
- Middle class family
- Patient has a 7-year-old sister
- Patient plays basketball and soccer

D. Medical History

- No significant findings, no known food or drug allergy, no medications, vaccinations are up to date

E. Medical Consult

- N/A

F. Dental History

- Has dental home, sees dentist every six months
- Fair oral hygiene, unsupervised according to mother
- Age-appropriate diet
- Uses toothpaste containing fluoride
- Optimally fluoridated water
- No history of trauma before today
- Patient is cooperative and acting age-appropriate

G. Extra-oral Exam

- Soft tissue: Swollen upper lip
- Lip incompetence

H. Intra-oral Exam

Soft Tissues

- Gingival and upper labial mucosa abrasions

Hard Tissues

- Alveolar fracture of the segment containing the maxillary left permanent central and lateral incisors (Figure 4.4.2) Maxillary right permanent lateral and central incisors: Mobility class I
- Maxillary left permanent central incisor: Palatal displacement of approximately 6 mm
- Maxillary left permanent lateral incisor: Palatal displacement of approximately 4 mm

Occlusal Evaluation of Permanent Dentition

- Class II molar and class II canine relationships bilaterally, moderate maxillary crowding

Other

- Minor plaque accumulation on mandibular incisors
- Caries-free dentition

FUNDAMENTAL POINT 1
History for Trauma

- Confirm that tetanus immunizations are up to date. If last tetanus booster was five or more years prior and wound is contaminated with soil/debris, another tetanus toxoid booster is indicated (Broder et al. 2006, McTigue and Thikkurissy 2011)
- Rule out closed head injury and refer for medical consult if the patient is positive for any of the following (CDC 2007):
  - Amnesia or loss of consciousness
  - Nausea/vomiting
  - Headache
  - Lethargy/irritability/confusion
- Studies have noted that an overjet greater than 3 mm and/or Angle Class II malocclusion are significant risk factors for dental trauma. Increased overjet and class II malocclusion are often associated with lip incompetence, another significant risk factor for dental trauma. About 30% of dental trauma is caused by sports injuries (Cornwell 2005)
- According to the American Dental Association, the ideal recommendations for a mouth guard include:
  - Be properly fitted to the wearer's mouth and accurately adapted to his or her oral structures
  - Be made of resilient material and cover all remaining teeth on one arch, customarily the maxillary
  - Stay in place comfortably and securely
  - Be physiologically compatible with the wearer
  - Be relatively easy to clean
  - Have high-impact energy absorption and reduce transmitted forces upon impact
- Studies support the reduction of sports-based oral injuries with the use of a custom mouth guard (Labella et al. 2002)

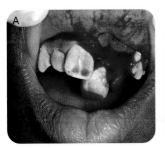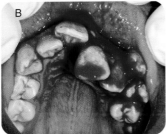

Figure 4.4.2a–b. Intra-oral photos showing soft tissue and dental trauma

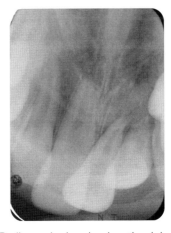

Figure 4.4.3. Radiograph showing luxation injury

I. Diagnostic Tools

- Periapical radiograph demonstrates displacement of the maxillary left permanent central and lateral incisors with apparent complete apical development
- Vitality tests deferred

J. Diagnosis and Problem List

Diagnosis

- Maxillary right permanent lateral and central incisors: Subluxation
- Maxillary left permanent central and lateral incisors: Lateral luxation with associated alveolar fracture. Due to extent of the luxation and the stage of apical development, there is a high likelihood that both teeth will become necrotic. Alveolar segments need to be re-approximated as closely as possible to facilitate healing

Problem List

- Displaced maxillary permanent central incisors
- Alveolar fracture
- Soft tissue laceration

FUNDAMENTAL POINT 2
Examination for Dental Trauma

- Take adequate radiographs to clearly image all involved teeth

- Note apical development because it impacts the treatment selected and prognosis

- Rule out other injuries, e.g., root fractures, alveolar fractures

- Vitality tests are not indicated on day of injury and even up to three weeks post-trauma because they provide unreliable information (Flores et al. 2007)

- Trauma often occurs to multiple teeth; therefore, the entire dentition must be assessed for potential injury (Wright et al. 2007)

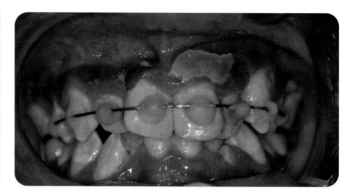

Figure 4.4.4. Intra-oral photo showing splint

K. Treatment

- See Flowchart D at the end of this chapter
- Maxillary left permanent central and lateral incisors: Reposition corresponding alveolar segment and verify positioning radiographically. Suture gingival lacerations as indicated
- Stabilize with splint fixation for four weeks. The splint should be passive and allow physiologic movement; materials such as fishing line (40 lb test) or a light stainless steel orthodontic wire (0.16 to 0.18)

Discharge Instructions

- Prescribe over-the-counter pain medications
- Avoid incising on injured segment until instructed otherwise
- Watch for clinical signs, including tooth discoloration, presence of parulis or fistula
- Patient to report if splint becomes dislodged

Follow-up Treatment

- Two-week post-op evaluation
  - Maxillary right permanent lateral and central incisors: Normal response to cold, responsive to electric pulp test (EPT)
  - Maxillary left permanent central and lateral incisors: Non-responsive to cold, non-responsive to EPT.

FUNDAMENTAL POINT 3
Alveolar Fracture

- Once reduced, the fractured alveolar segments should be stabilized with splinting such as 40 pound test fishing line or a light stainless steel orthodontic wire to allow for optimal physiologic healing

- An occlusal change due to misalignment of fractured segment is often noted (Flores et al. 2007)

- Periodontal evaluation of teeth in injured alveolar segment should be performed once osseous healing has stabilized, usually six to eight weeks after the injury (Andreasen 1993)

- All teeth involved in injury must be re-assessed for potential pulpal injury, which may not surface immediately (Flores et al. 2007)

- Treatment
  - Removal of pulp tissue of the maxillary left permanent central and lateral incisors and placement of Ca(OH)$_2$ as an interim medicament (see Flowchart D at the end of this chapter)

L. Prognosis and Complications

- Initial prognosis depends heavily upon when the pulp tissue is removed. The likelihood of inflammatory resorption increases when no treatment is provided within two weeks of the injury
- After severe trauma in which the root surface is damaged, the direct contact between osteoclasts and mineralized dentin/cementum may lead to replacement resorption, also known as ankylosis

M. Complications and Alternative Treatment Plan

- If the alveolar segment cannot be immediately reduced, controlled pressure may be applied in an occlusal or coronal direction to facilitate repositioning. If still unsuccessful, an open reduction approach may be required, involving laying a flap for direct visualization (see Fundamental Point 3)

- If excessive bleeding prevents successful application of a splint, alternatives such as suture splints may need to be considered
- In teeth with immature apices, pulp therapy may be deferred, because these teeth present with a greater ability to revascularize

Self-study Questions

1. **Why was the pulp removed at the two-week follow-up?**
2. **Can the patient's malocclusion (class II) be considered a risk factor for this type of injury?**
3. **What information does a negative response to cold thermal testing the day of injury indicate?**

4. **At what point should periodontal probing of traumatized teeth in a displaced alveolar segment take place?**

Answers are located at the end of the case.

Bibliography

Andreasen FM, Steinhardt U, Bille M, Munksgaard EC. 1993. Bonding of enamel-dentin crown fragments after crown fracture. An experimental study using bonding agents. *Endod Dent Traumatol* Jun;9(3):111–4.

Broder K, Cortese M, et al. 2006. Preventing tetanus, diphtheria, and pertussis among adolescents: Use of tetanus toxoid, reduced diphtheria toxoid and acellular pertussis vaccines. Recommendations of the CDC Advisory Committee on Immunization practices. *MMWR*. Feb. 23, 2006, 55:1–43. www.cdc.gov/mmwr/preview/mmwrhtml/rr55e223a1.htm and http://www.cdc.gov/vaccines/vpd-vac/tetanus/default.htm.

Centers for Disease Control and Prevention (CDC). 2007. Heads Up. *Facts for Physicians about Mild Traumatic Brain Injury* (MTBI). http://www.cdc.gov/ncipc/tbi/Facts_for_Physicians_booklet.pdf.

Cornwell H. 2005. Dental trauma due to sport in the pediatric patient. *J Calif Dent Assoc* Jun;33(6):457–61.

Flores MT, et al. 2007. Guidelines for the management of traumatic dental injuries. I. Fractures and luxations of permanent teeth. *Dent Traumatol* 23:66–71.

Labella CR, Smith BW, Sigurdsson A. 2002. Effect of mouthguards on dental injuries and concussions in college basketball. *Med Sci Sports Exerc* Jan;34(1):41–4.

McTigue D, Thikkurissy S, 2011. Trauma. In: *The Handbook of Pediatric Dentistry*, 4th Edition. Nowak AJ, Casamassimo PS (eds). American Academy of Pediatric Dentistry: Chicago. pp. 109–17.

Wright G, Bell A, McGlashan G, Vincent C, Welbury RR. 2007. Dentoalveolar trauma in Glasgow: an audit of mechanism and injury. *Dent Traumatol* Aug;23(4):226–31.

SELF-STUDY ANSWERS

1. The first signs of pulpal necrosis typically present at two weeks in a tooth with a closed apex and a significant alveolar fracture, making the chances for natural revascularization very low. If pulp removal is delayed, it could precipitate inflammatory resorption, which reduces the overall prognosis of the tooth

2. Yes. Studies have noted that an overjet of more than 3 mm and/or class II malocclusion is a significant risk factor for dental trauma. Increased overjet and class II malocclusion are often associated with lip incompetence, another significant risk factor for dental trauma

3. None. Pulp vitality tests are often foregone on the day of the trauma, and up to three weeks afterwards because results are often false and unreliable

4. Traumatized teeth located within a displaced alveolar segment should not be periodontally probed until osseous healing has occurred, which may take six to eight weeks

Case 5

Permanent Tooth Root Fracture and Extrusive Luxation

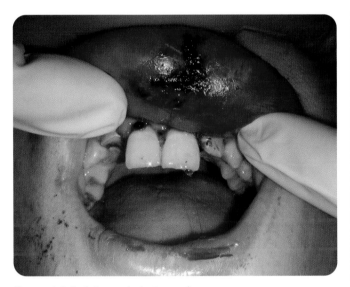

Figure 4.5.1. Intra-oral photograph

A. Presenting Patient

- 14-year-, 1-month-old Caucasian male
- Presenting as an emergency

B. Chief Complaint and History of Present Injury

- Mother reports, "My son fell off a skateboard last night"
- The patient fell yesterday while skateboarding in small town approximately 75 miles from the office. He was examined in the emergency department (ED) of the local hospital, where a laceration on his upper lip was sutured. There were no witnesses but the patient reported no loss of consciousness

C. Social History

- Patient is in 9th grade. He is an only child who lives at home with both parents
- Middle class family

FUNDAMENTAL POINT 1
Dental History

- Confirm that tetanus immunizations are up to date. If last tetanus booster was five or more years prior and wound is contaminated with soil/debris, another tetanus toxoid booster is indicated (Broder et al. 2006, McTigue and Thikkurissy 2011)
- Rule out closed head injury and refer for medical consult if the patient is positive for any of the following (CDC 2007):
  - Amnesia
  - Nausea/vomiting
  - Headache
  - Lethargy/irritability/confusion
  - Loss of consciousness

D. Medical History

- ADHD, otherwise non-significant
- Medications: Adderall 15 mg PO QID, but patient is not compliant
- No drug or food allergies, vaccinations are up to date, last tetanus booster was 18 months ago

E. Medical Consult

- Completed in the ED last night

F. Dental History

- Has dental home
- Fair oral hygiene. Brushes twice daily, unsupervised
- Diet is high in carbohydrates and sweetened soft drinks
- History of approximately one new occlusal surface carious lesion/year; has multiple white spot lesions on smooth surfaces of teeth

- Uses toothpaste containing fluoride
- Lives in an area with optimally fluoridated water
- No previous history of dental trauma
- Personable and cooperative for treatment

G. Extra-oral Exam

- Soft tissues: 2.5-cm laceration on upper lip sutured in ED last night; swollen lip

H. Intra-oral Exam

Soft Tissues

- 5-mm vertical laceration on interdental papilla between the maxillary permanent central incisors

Hard Tissues and Dental Exam (Figure 4.5.1)

- No bone fractures
- Conservative composite occlusal restorations on first molars, sealants on second molars. Multiple white spot lesions on smooth surfaces
- Maxillary right permanent lateral incisor: Complicated fracture with pulp exposed, mobility class I
- Maxillary right permanent central incisor: Possible root fracture, coronal fragment extruded 2 mm, mobility class III
- Maxillary left permanent central incisor: Extruded 3 mm, mobility class III
- Maxillary left permanent lateral incisor: Uncomplicated crown fracture, enamel and dentin, mobility class I

Occlusal Evaluation of Permanent Dentition

- Class I molar and class I canines; 4mm overjet, 50% overbite

Other

- Moderate generalized plaque accumulation

I. Diagnostic Tools

- Maxillary anterior periapical radiograph revealed:
  - Mature root formation of anterior teeth with closed apices

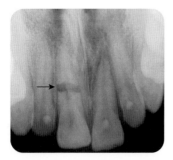

Figure 4.5.2. Radiograph of maxillary right permanent central incisor root fracture (arrow at fracture)

- Complicated fracture with pulp exposure on the maxillary right permanent lateral incisor
- Middle third root fracture of the maxillary right permanent central incisor (Figure 4.5.2., arrow)
- Extruded maxillary left permanent central incisor
- Uncomplicated crown fracture on the maxillary left permanent lateral incisor
- Percussion test:
  - Maxillary right permanent canine: Negative
  - Maxillary right permanent lateral incisor: Positive
  - Maxillary right and left permanent central incisors: Deferred
  - Maxillary left permanent lateral incisor: Positive
  - Maxillary left permanent canine: Negative
- Vitality test
  - Deferred

J. Diagnosis and Problem List

Diagnosis

- Dental and soft tissue trauma

Problem List

- Maxillary right permanent lateral incisor: Complicated crown fracture with subluxation
- Maxillary right permanent central incisor: Middle third root fracture
- Maxillary left permanent central incisor: Extruded. Neurovascular pulp tissue likely severed at apex and pulpectomy is indicated to prevent inflammatory resorption
- Maxillary left permanent lateral incisor: Uncomplicated fracture of enamel and dentin

K. Treatment

- Maxillary right permanent lateral incisor: See Chapter 4, Case 3 for clinical management
- Maxillary right permanent central incisor: See Flowchart B at the end of this chapter. Reposition the tooth fragments with digital pressure. Apply flexible splint using 50 lb. monofilament fishing line or light orthodontic wire for four weeks. Verify tooth position radiographically
- Maxillary left permanent central incisor: See Flowchart D at the end of this chapter. Reposition the extruded tooth with finger pressure. Apply flexible splint using 50 lb. monofilament fishing line or light orthodontic wire for two weeks. The periodontal ligament (PDL) re-attachment process is not complete at that time so normal mobility may not yet be reached. Evidence indicates that

FUNDAMENTAL POINT 2

Root Fractures

- Multiple radiographic projections and angulations improve diagnostic accuracy. Occlusal and 90° horizontal views are recommended

- Luxated teeth and coronal fragments should be repositioned as soon as possible (Flores et al. 2007-l)

- Types of root fracture healing include:

  - Healing with hard tissue: Fragments in close contact with fracture line barely visible

  - Interposition of hard and soft tissue between fragments: Fragments surrounded by periodontal ligament (PDL) are separated by an ingrowth of bone

  - Interposition of soft tissue only: Fragments are close but separated by PDL space

- The prognosis for root fracture healing is good, 60% to 78%. The prognosis is better for mid and apical third fractures than for fractures in the coronal third

- Factors favoring healing include:

  - Immature root development

  - Limited displacement of the coronal fragment: 1mm or less

  - Repositioning to optimal position, i.e., close approximation of fragments

  - Flexible splinting: Significantly better healing rates occur when light splints are applied with minimal manipulation of the fragments

- Middle and apical third root fractures are splinted for four weeks

- Longer splint time recommended for root fractures in the cervical third, up to four months

- Systemic antibiotics do not appear to promote healing and their use is questionable

Andreasen et al. 2004a,b, Cvek et al. 2001, Andreasen et al. 1999

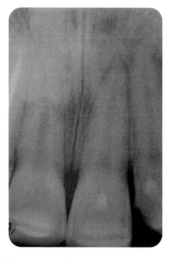

Figure 4.5.3. Follow-up radiograph

healing is improved under these conditions and the patient is instructed to avoid biting on the injured teeth until normal mobility has returned. Using composite resin to attach the splint to the teeth allows the clinician to release some teeth while keeping others splinted

- Maxillary left permanent lateral incisor: Tooth should be monitored clinically and radiographically for pulp vitality and pulpectomy performed if it becomes non-vital

- Suture gingival lacerations (if indicated). Prescribe over-the-counter acetaminophen or ibuprofen for pain as needed

Discharge Instructions

- Chlorhexidine mouth rinse for two weeks

- Soft diet and avoid incising on injured tooth until tenderness resolves

- Maintain good oral hygiene by gentle toothbrushing after meals

Follow-up Treatment

- Maxillary right permanent central incisor: Remove splint after four weeks. Monitor pulpal and periodontal healing clinically and radiographically for at least one year. Root canal therapy up to the level of the fracture line is indicated if pulpal necrosis develops

- Maxillary left permanent central incisor: Remove this tooth from the splint after two weeks. Complete pulpectomy at that time. Fill canal with calcium hydroxide $(CaOH)_2$ for two to four weeks and then obturate with Gutta Percha if no evidence of root resorption

L. Prognosis and Discussion

- Maxillary right permanent central incisor: The prognosis for healing in this root-fractured tooth is favorable. The fracture occurred in the middle third and excellent repositioning was achieved. Though treatment was delayed almost 24 hours, evidence indicates that positive healing outcomes are still probable. The tooth should be carefully monitored and endodontics initiated only if pulp necrosis is evident. If pulp necrosis occurs, it is almost always in the coronal fragment. Treatment is to complete root canal therapy on the coronal fragment only

- Maxillary left permanent central incisor: The prognosis for survival of this tooth is good, provided the pulp is removed within two weeks. The neurovascular pulpal tissue is surely severed at the apex when a tooth is extruded. Immature teeth with open apices have the potential to revascularize, so monitoring them for several weeks is appropriate prior to beginning root canal treatment. On the other hand, mature teeth with closed apices are very unlikely to revascularize and their pulps should be extirpated within three weeks to prevent inflammatory resorption

Self-study Questions

1. **Can one wait and watch an extruded permanent incisor until signs of pulpal necrosis are observed?**

2. **How is pulpal necrosis managed in a root-fractured tooth?**

3. **What are important principles regarding splinting root-fractured teeth?**

4. **Will extruded teeth have normal mobility when the splint is removed?**

5. **What clinical and radiographic signs indicate successful healing of root-fractured teeth?**

Answers are located at the end of the case.

Bibliography

Andreasen J, et al. 2004a. Healing of 40 intra-alveolar root fractures. 1. Effect of pre-injury and injury factors such as sex, age, stage of root development, fracture type, location of fracture and severity of dislocation. *Dent Traumatol* 20:192–202.

Andreasen J, et al. 2004b. Healing of 40 intra-alveolar root fractures. 2. Effect of treatment factors such as treatment delay, repositioning, splinting type and period and antibiotics. *Dent Traumatol* 20:2–3–211.

Andreasen JO, Andreasen FM, Bakland LK, Flores MT. 1999. *Traumatic dental injuries—a manual.* Munksgaard: Copenhagen, pp. 26–7.

Broder K, Cortese M, et al. 2006. Preventing tetanus, diphtheria, and pertussis among adolescents: Use of tetanus toxoid, reduced diphtheria toxoid and acellular pertussis vaccines. Recommendations of the CDC Advisory Committee on Immunization practices. *MMWR.* Feb. 23, 2006, 55:1–43. www.cdc.gov/mmwr/preview/mmwrhtml/rr55e223a1.htm and http://www.cdc.gov/vaccines/vpd-vac/tetanus/default.htm

Centers for Disease Control and Prevention (CDC). 2007. Heads Up. *Facts for Physicians about Mild Traumatic Brain Injury (MTBI).* http://www.cdc.gov/ncipc/tbi/Facts_for_Physicians_booklet.pdf

Cvek M, Andreasen JO, Borum MK. 2001. Healing of 208 intra-alveolar root fracture in patients aged 7–17 years. *Dental Traumatol* 17:52–62.

Flores MT, et al. 2007. Guidelines for the management of traumatic dental injuries. I. Fractures and luxations of permanent teeth. *Dent Traumatol* 23:66–71.

McTigue D, Thikkurissy S, 2011. Trauma. In: *The Handbook of Pediatric Dentistry*, 4th Edition. Nowak AJ, Casamassimo PS (eds). American Academy of Pediatric Dentistry: Chicago. pp. 109–17.

SELF-STUDY ANSWERS

1. The neurovascular pulpal tissue is surely severed at the apex when a tooth is extruded. Immature teeth with open apices have the potential to revascularize, so monitoring them for several weeks is appropriate prior to beginning root canal treatment. On the other hand, mature teeth with closed apices are very unlikely to revascularize and their pulps should be extirpated within three weeks to prevent inflammatory resorption

2. The pulps of approximately three-quarters of root-fractured teeth survive, but when they fail, it is almost always in the coronal fragment. Treatment is to complete root canal therapy on the coronal fragment only

3. Recent evidence indicates that flexible splints applied for shorter periods of time than previously thought favor healing. Four weeks is recommended for fractures in the middle and apical thirds. Two to three months of splinting time is indicated for fractures in the coronal third

4. Extruded teeth are splinted for two weeks. The PDL re-attachment process is not complete at that time, so normal mobility may not yet be reached. Evidence indicates that healing is improved under these conditions and the patient is instructed to avoid biting on the injured teeth until normal mobility has returned

5. Root-fractured teeth may heal with a hard tissue union, with interposition of connective tissues or with interposition of bone and connective tissues. Radiographic signs of success indicate presence of lamina dura and no signs of bone or root resorption

Case 6

Permanent Incisor Intrusion

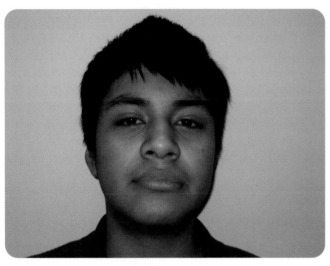

Figure 4.6.1. Facial photograph

A. Presenting Patient

- 12-year-, 7-month-old male
- New patient presenting for an emergency

B. Chief Complaint and History of Present Injury

- Foster dad reports, "He fell while running and pushed his tooth up"
- Patient fell while playing dodge-ball at home approximately 45 minutes ago. Foster dad brought him immediately to the hospital dental clinic. There was no loss of consciousness but patient could not remember anything about the injury, which was witnessed by two friends. He said his head hurt and that he felt sick to his stomach. The dentist sent him to the emergency department (ED) immediately to be examined for closed head injury. He returned to the dental clinic 90 minutes later

C. Social History

- Patient is in seventh grade, age appropriate
- Child is currently in foster care due to abuse at home
- Upper-middle class family

D. Medical History

- No significant findings, no known drug or food allergies, no medications, vaccinations are up to date

E. Medical Consult

- Completed in the ED

F. Dental History

- Child is patient of a local dentist who was not available to provide care
- Has received limited orthodontic treatment; has retention wire on lingual surfaces of maxillary incisors
- Foster father reports that patient eats "everything put in front of him." He particularly likes chips, soda, and fried foods
- Oral hygiene is good; patient is unsupervised
- Uses fluoridated toothpaste
- Lives in an optimally fluoridated community and rarely drinks bottled water
- No history of previous dental injury

G. Extra-oral Exam

- No significant findings

H. Intra-oral Exam

Soft Tissues

- Attached gingiva lacerated adjacent to intruded maxillary right permanent central incisor

Hard Tissues

- No bone fractures

- Rule out closed head injury and refer for medical consult if the patient is positive for any of the following (CDC 2007):
  - Amnesia
  - Nausea/vomiting
  - Headache
  - Lethargy/irritability/confusion
  - Loss of consciousness
- Confirm that tetanus immunizations are up to date. If last tetanus booster was five or more years prior and wound is contaminated with soil/debris, another tetanus toxoid booster is indicated (Broder et al. 2006, McTigue and Thikkurissy 2011)
- Secure informed consent for treatment from a person authorized by the court to make decisions about children in foster care. That may not be the foster parent, so the agency should be contacted to verify consent procedures. Specific rules vary among states.

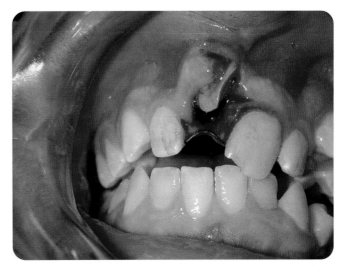

Figure 4.6.2. Intra-oral photo showing soft tissue and dental trauma

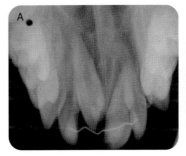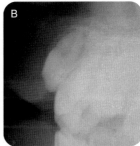

Figure 4.6.3a–b. Radiographs showing dental trauma

Occlusal Evaluation of Permanent Dentition
- Class I canines, class I molars; 4 mm overjet, 20% overbite

Other
- Moderate plaque
- Dentition is caries-free

Dental Exam Findings
- Maxillary right permanent lateral incisor: Class I mobility
- Maxillary right permanent central incisor: Intruded approximately 10 mm, no mobility, uncomplicated mesioincisal crown fracture (enamel and dentin)
- Maxillary left permanent central incisor: Class I mobility, uncomplicated mesioincisal crown fracture (enamel and dentin)

I. Diagnostic Tools
- Intra-oral periapical radiographs of maxillary anterior area:
  - Demonstrate mature root formation of anterior teeth and closed apices

- The maxillary right permanent central incisor is intruded approximately 10 mm and labially luxated with concomitant fracture of alveolar plate
- The periodontal ligament (PDL) space is obliterated on the occlusal radiographic image (Figure 4.6.3)
- Panoramic radiograph
  - Normal development
  - No fractures or displacements of skeletal tissues
- Percussion tests
  - Maxillary right permanent lateral incisor: Positive
  - Maxillary right permanent central incisor: Negative, high metallic sound
  - Maxillary left permanent central incisor: Positive
  - Maxillary left permanent lateral incisor: Negative
- Vitality tests
  - Deferred because results are not reliable at the time of injury

FUNDAMENTAL POINT 2
Complications with Intrusion Injuries

- False-negative response to vitality tests possible for up to three months

- Intruded teeth yield a high-pitched, metallic sound upon percussion and demonstrate loss of periodontal ligament (PDL) space, radiographically (Flores 2007)

- Healing complications (pulp necrosis, root resorption, and marginal bone loss) occur more frequently in teeth with completed root development than in immature teeth

- Associated crown fractures with exposed dentin increase the risk for pulp necrosis in intruded teeth (Andreasen, et al. 2006)

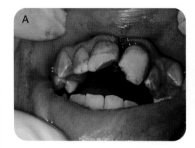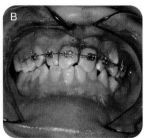

Figure 4.6.4a–b. Intra-oral photos showing repositioning of intrusion and splint

FUNDAMENTAL POINT 3
Intrusion Injuries

- Teeth intruded 6mm or less can be repositioned with light orthodontic forces. This may improve the chance of optimal healing

- Immature teeth with open apices and intruded 6mm or less can be allowed to reposition spontaneously. Rapidly reposition orthodontically if no movement is noted within three weeks

- Systemic antibiotic administration does not improve healing in intrusion injuries.

Andreasen, et al. 2006, Flores, et al. 2007

J. Diagnosis and Problem List
Diagnosis

- Maxillary right permanent central incisor: Intrusion/ lateral luxation and uncomplicated mesioincisal crown fracture. Intruded permanent teeth are at high risk for pulp necrosis, marginal bone loss, and inflammatory and replacement root resorption, particularly when intruded greater than 7mm.

- Maxillary left permanent central incisor: Uncomplicated mesioincisal crown fracture

K. Treatment

- See Flowchart A at the end of this chapter

- Maxillary right permanent central incisor: Surgically reposition as soon as possible and splint with 40lb. monofilament fishing line or light orthodontic wire for three to four weeks

- Maxillary left permanent central incisor: Apply glass ionomer or composite resin temporary restoration on fracture to cover exposed dentin (Figure 4.6.4.)

Discharge Instructions

- Prescribe over-the-counter acetaminophen or ibuprofen for pain as needed

- Chlorhexidine mouth rinse for two weeks

- Soft diet and avoid incising on injured tooth until tenderness resolves

- Maintain good oral hygiene by gentle toothbrushing after meals

Follow-up Treatment

- Maxillary right permanent central incisor: Complete pulpectomy within three weeks of injury. Fill canal

with Ca(OH)$_2$ for two to four weeks. Because this tooth is likely to ankylose and undergo replacement resorption, do not place Gutta Percha unless healing is indicated by presence of lamina dura and no signs of resorption. Remove splint after four weeks and complete final composite restoration

- Maxillary left permanent central incisor: Complete final composite restoration after splint is removed

L. Prognosis and Discussion

- Maxillary right permanent central incisor: The short-term prognosis for this tooth is favorable because the tooth was repositioned quickly and the pulp was extirpated before it could become necrotic and initiate inflammatory resorption. The root is also mature, having achieved complete root length and substantial root wall thickening. The long-term prognosis for tooth retention is guarded due to the severity of the intrusion injury which surely caused severe damage to the periodontal ligament. This tooth is at great risk for ankylosis and replacement resorption, which would become clinically and radiographically apparent within two to three months. Clinical signs included loss of physiologic mobility, high-pitched, metallic sound on percussion, and relative infraocclusion as the child's maxilla grows. Radiographic signs include loss of PDL space and bony infringement

- Maxillary left permanent central incisor: The long-term prognosis appears good because the tooth did not appear to be luxated but it should be closely monitored clinically and radiographically for up to two years.

M. Complications and Alternative Treatment Plans

- The most damaging complication would be ankylosis and replacement resorption of the

intruded right central incisor. Because the patient is only 12 years old, significant future maxillary growth is anticipated. This tooth will then begin to infraocclude, causing periodontal defects and an esthetic dilemma. Extracting the tooth at this age would result in substantial loss of alveolar bone support in that area, necessitating bone grafting prior to implant placement or restoration with a fixed prosthesis. A better alternative would be to surgically remove the crown below the level of the alveolar bone (decoronation) to maintain alveolar bone height and breadth in advance of the final restoration after maxillary growth is completed

Self-study Questions

1. **What are the most common complications of an intrusion injury?**
2. **How do I assess the neurologic status of an injured patient?**
3. **How does the management of an intruded immature (open apex) permanent tooth differ from that of a mature tooth?**
4. **In children in the early stages of the mixed dentition, it is sometimes hard to know if an**

incisor was intruded or if it had just not erupted completely. What clinical tests improve the diagnosis of an intrusion injury?
5. **What clinical and radiographic signs indicate successful treatment of intrusion injuries?**

Answers are located at the end of the case.

Bibliography

Andreasen, et al. 2006. Traumatic intrusion of permanent teeth. Part 2. A clinical study of the effect of preinjury and injury factors, such as sex, age, stage of root development, tooth location, and extent of injury including number of intruded teeth on 140 intruded permanent teeth. *Dent Traumatol* 22:90–8.

Broder K, Cortese M, et al. 2006. Preventing tetanus, diphtheria, and pertussis among adolescents: Use of tetanus toxoid, reduced diphtheria toxoid and acellular pertussis vaccines. Recommendations of the CDC Advisory Committee on Immunization practices. *MMWR.* Feb. 23, 2006, 55:1–43. www.cdc.gov/mmwr/preview/

mmwrhtml/rr55e223a1.htm and http://www.cdc.gov/vaccines/vpd-vac/tetanus/default.htm.

Centers for Disease Control and Prevention (CDC). 2007. Heads Up. *Facts for Physicians about Mild Traumatic Brain Injury (MTBI).* http://www.cdc.gov/ncipc/tbi/Facts_for_Physicians_booklet.pdf

Flores MT, et al. 2007. Guidelines for the management of traumatic dental injuries. I. Fractures and luxations of permanent teeth. *Dent Traumatol* 23:66–71.

McTigue D, Thikkurissy S. 2011. Trauma. In: *The Handbook of Pediatric Dentistry*, 4th Edition. Nowak AJ, Casamassimo PS (eds). American Academy of Pediatric Dentistry: Chicago pp. 109–17.

SELF-STUDY ANSWERS

1. Intrusions are serious injuries with a relatively poor prognosis because of the crushing of the PDL fibers, pulp tissue, and supporting bone. Ankylosis with resulting replacement root resorption is common, as is pulp necrosis and inflammatory root resorption

2. Serious closed head injury may accompany significant dental injuries in children. Symptoms of concussion included confusion, disorientation, memory loss, headache, nausea, and emotional liability. Medical consultation to rule out serious head injury is indicated immediately if the child is positive for these findings

3. Recent evidence indicates that immature teeth may reposition themselves spontaneously so they can be monitored for several weeks. If no movement occurs, repositioning with orthodontic forces should be initiated. Some clinicians recommend mildly luxating the tooth prior to applying the orthodontic force

4. Intruded teeth are displaced forcefully into the alveolar bone and will be completely immobile. A percussion test will yield a high-pitched hollow or metallic sound. The PDL space will not be visible on radiographic exam

5. The tooth is in normal position and responds normally to mobility and percussion tests. Radiographically, no replacement or inflammatory root resorption is occurring and intact lamina dura is evidenced around the root

Case 7

Permanent Tooth Avulsion

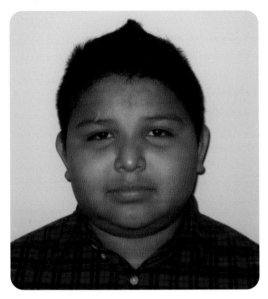

Figure 4.7.1. Facial photograph

A. Presenting Patient
- 11-year-, 5-month-old Hispanic male
- Presenting as an emergency

B. Chief Complaint and History of Present Injury
- Father reports, "My son took an elbow playing basketball and knocked out a tooth"
- Injury occurred at school approximately 60 minutes ago and was witnessed by coach and teammates. There was no loss of consciousness nor other injuries. The maxillary right permanent central incisor fell on the basketball court floor. The tooth was placed first in a cup with the patient's saliva and was transferred to a carton of milk within 10 minutes. The coach called the father at work, who then transported the patient to his dentist's office. Bleeding from the socket and lips was easily controlled with gauze pressure

C. Social History
- Patient is in sixth grade, age appropriate
- Lives at home with parents and younger sister
- Middle class family

D. Medical History
- Review of medical history reveals no significant findings, no known drug or food allergies, no medications, vaccinations are up to date

E. Medical Consult
- N/A

F. Dental History
- Routine recall exams every six months since age 4 in the same dental office
- Good oral hygiene and dietary habits
- Uses toothpaste containing fluoride
- Optimal water fluoridation
- No history of trauma before today

G. Extra-oral Exam
- No facial asymmetry
- No bony fractures
- Upper and lower lip lacerations and contusions
- Normal mandibular range of motion, intact temporomandibular joint (TMJ)
- Competent lips

H. Intra-oral Exam
Soft Tissues
- No significant findings

Hard Tissues
- Caries-free dentition
- Traumatized teeth (Figure 4.7.2)
  - Maxillary right permanent central incisor: Avulsed, mesioangular fracture of enamel and dentin

FUNDAMENTAL POINT 1

Reimplantaion and History of Dental Avulsion

- Immediate replantation is the best treatment for an avulsed tooth
  - The person answering the phone at the doctor's office should advise responsible person with the injured child to replant the tooth immediately
- Management of avulsed permanent teeth at injury site
  - Hold tooth by the crown, rinse gently with water, do not scrub root surface
  - Immediately replant tooth at site of injury, if possible. After replantation, bite on gauze or a clean towel to avoid tooth aspiration. If replantation is not possible, place tooth in Hank's Balanced Salt Solution, cold milk, saline, or saliva—in that order of preference—to maximize vitality of the root surface cells (Flores, et al. 2007)
- When patient with avulsed tooth arrives, ask parents:

1. How did the accident occur? Rule out closed head injury and refer for medical consult if the patient is positive for any of the following (CDC 2007):
   - Amnesia
   - Nausea/vomiting
   - Headache
   - Lethargy/irritability/confusion
   - Loss of consciousness
2. Where did the accident occur? Confirm that tetanus immunizations are up to date. If last tetanus booster was five or more years prior and wound is contaminated with soil/debris, another tetanus toxoid booster is indicated (Broder et al. 2006, McTigue and Thikkurissy 2011)
3. When did the accident occur?
   - Extra-oral dry time determines prognosis of replanted tooth
   - Dry time greater than 60 minutes leads to ankylosis and replacement resorption

BACKGROUND INFORMATION 1

Management of Avulsion Injuries

Transport Media for Avulsed Teeth

- Hank's Balanced Salt Solution (HBSS) is the most favorable storage medium but is rarely available
- Cold milk is the best option after HBSS. Tooth should be placed in a small cup of milk and then the cup placed in a bowl of ice
- Saline solution or saliva are the next options if cold milk is not immediately available
- Water is hypotonic and will quickly kill periodontal ligament cells

Flores, et al. 2007

Systemic Antibiotics

- Doxycycline (a semi-synthetic tetracycline) is the first choice due to potential anti-resorptive properties. It is contraindicated in children under

the age of 8 due to potential tooth discoloration. If the child is 8 years old and weights more than 45 kg, oral doxycycline (100 mg q 12 h first day, then 50 mg q 12 h days 2 to 10)

- In children 8 years old and younger, penicillinVK (20 to 50 mg/kg/d in four divided doses for seven days)

Teeth With Extra-oral Dry Time Greater Than 60 Minutes

- Poor prognosis for survival with ankylosis and replacement resorption is the expected outcome
- Soaking the tooth in fluoride for 20 minutes may delay but not prevent replacement resorption
- Decoronation of the tooth to preserve the alveolar bone is recommended if teeth become ankylosed and infrapositioned greater than 1 mm.

Cohenca A., et al. 2007

- Maxillary left permanent central incisor: Mesioangular fracture of enamel and dentin

Occlusal Evaluation of Early Permanent Dentition

- Canines and molars in class II, lower anterior crowding; overjet: 3 mm, overbite: 95%

I. Diagnostic Tools

- Radiograph deferred until tooth replanted to minimize extra-oral time
- Percussion tests
  - Maxillary right permanent lateral incisor: Negative
  - Maxillary right permanent central incisor: – +1
  - Maxillary left permanent lateral incisor: Negative
- Vitality tests
  - Deferred

J. Diagnosis and Problem List

Diagnosis

- Maxillary right permanent central incisor:—Avulsion and mesioangular fracture of enamel and dentin
- Maxillary left permanent central incisor: Subluxation and mesioangular fracture of enamel and dentin
- Lip lacerations
- Malocclusion

K. Comprehensive Treatment

- See Flowchart E at the end of this case
- Maxillary right permanent central incisor: Examine socket for alveolar fracture and reposition with end of mirror, if needed. Rinse root carefully with saline and replant with digital pressure (Figure 4.7.3.)
- Apply flexible splint, including some adjacent teeth, using 50 lb. monofilament fishing line or light, passive orthodontic wire for 10 to 14 days, using light or self-cured composite (Figure 4.7.4.).
- Verify tooth position radiographically
- Suture gingival/lip lacerations (if indicated)

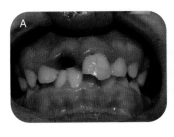 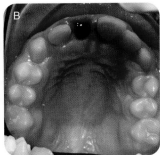

Figure 4.7.2a–b. Intra-oral photos showing avulsion and dental fracture

- Prescribe over-the-counter acetaminophen or ibuprofen for pain as needed
- Prescribe systemic antibiotics
  - If 8 years of age or older and 45 kg or more: Oral doxycycline (100 mg q 12 h first day then 50 mg q 12h days 2 through 10)
  - If under 8 years of age: Oral PenVK (20 to 50 mg/kg/d in four divided doses) for seven days

Discharge Instructions

- Chlorhexidine mouth rinse twice daily for two weeks
- Soft diet until splint is removed
- Maintain good oral hygiene
- Return to clinic within seven to 10 days of replantation for follow-up
- Perform pulpectomy if avulsed tooth has a closed apex: Fill canal with Ca(OH)$_2$ for two to four weeks, then obturate with Gutta Percha
- Close monitoring is indicated in first year

Follow-up Treatment

- Clinical exam in post-op months one, three, six, and 12
- Radiographic exam in six to eight weeks to rule out root resorption. Repeated at six and 12 months
- Restoration of involved teeth with composite
- Orthodontic consult
- Endodontic consult
- Continue dental recalls every six months

L. Prognosis and Discussion

- Maxillary right permanent central incisor (avulsed): Prognosis for long-term tooth survival depends on maintaining vitality of periodontal ligament (PDL) fibers on the root. Goal is to preserve PDL vitality by minimizing extra-oral time and storing tooth in physiologic media until replantation
- Maxillary left permanent central incisor (subluxated): Tooth should be monitored clinically and radiographically for pulp vitality and pulpectomy performed if it becomes non-vital

M. Common Complications and Alternative Treatment Plans

- Ankylosis with replacement root resorption is the most common complication in avulsed teeth. Signs include loss of mobility, high percussion tone, and radiographic disappearance of lamina dura and PDL space. Decoronation of the tooth to preserve alveolar bone is recommended if teeth become infrapositioned greater than 1 mm (Cohenca, et al. 2007)

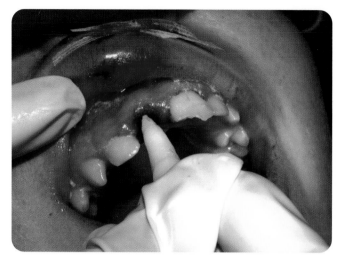

Figure 4.7.3. Intra-oral photos showing replantation of avulsed tooth

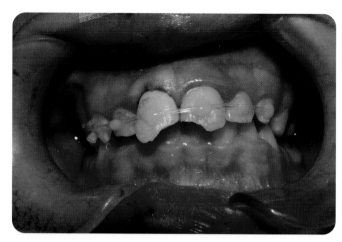

Figure 4.7.4. Intra-oral photo showing flexible splint

- Inflammatory root resorption can occur if the pulp is not extirpated from mature avulsed teeth within three weeks. Toxic byproducts of necrosis provoke an inflammatory reaction at the PDL that can destroy the root within weeks. Radiographic evidence of inflammatory resorption includes typically ragged resorption of lateral root surface

and possibly the apical area. The pulp canal should be thoroughly cleansed and disinfected. A calcium hydroxide dressing is then placed as an intracanal medicament for two months. Obturation of the canal with Gutta Percha is completed when radiographs confirm that the resorption is stopped

---

FUNDAMENTAL POINT 2

Possible Outcomes following avulsion

- Immature teeth with open apices may revascularize, so pulp extirpation should be deferred until clinical and radiographic signs of pulp necrosis are apparent (Flores, et al. 2007)

- Decoronation of the tooth to preserve alveolar bone is recommended if teeth become ankylosed and infrapositioned greater than 1 mm (Cohenca, et al. 2007)

- Revascularization of immature teeth is most likely to occur if replantation occurs within 15 minutes. Covering the root with topical minocycline hydrochloride microspheres (Arestin™) or soaking in a 1% doxycyline solution prior to replantation disinfects the apical tissues and enhances revascularization; however, the extra-oral period should not be extended if these are not immediately available (Flores, et al. 2007)

Self-study Questions

1. *When is tetanus prophylaxis indicated following a tooth avulsion/replantation?*

2. *What are the most important principles in the initial management of an avulsed permanent tooth?*

3. *How does the management of an avulsed immature (open apex) permanent tooth differ from that of a mature tooth?*

4. *How can the prognosis for revascularization of an avulsed immature incisor be improved?*

5. *What are important principles in the management of an ankylosed permanent tooth?*

Answers are located at the end of the case

Bibliography

Broder K, Cortese M, et al. 2006 Preventing tetanus, diphtheria, and pertussis among adolescents: Use of tetanus toxoid, reduced diphtheria toxoid and acellular pertussis vaccines. Recommendations of the CDC Advisory Committee on Immunization practices. *MMWR.* Feb. 23, 2006, 55:1–43. www.cdc.gov/mmwr/preview/mmwrhtml/rr55e223a1.htm and http://www.cdc.gov/vaccines/vpd-vac/tetanus/default.htm.

Centers for Disease Control and Prevention (CDC). 2007. Heads Up. *Facts for Physicians about Mild Traumatic Brain Injury (MTBI).* http://www.cdc.gov/ncipc/tbi/Facts_for_Physicians_booklet.pdf.

Cohenca A, Cohenca N, Stabholz A. 2007. Decoronation—a conservative method to treat ankylosed teeth for preservation of alveolar ridge prior to permanent prosthetic reconstruction: literature review and case presentation. *Dent Traumatol* 23:87–94.

Flores MT, et al. 2007. Guidelines for the management of traumatic dental injuries. II. Avulsion of permanent teeth. *Dent Traumatol* 23:130–6.

SELF-STUDY ANSWERS

1. If the patient has not had a tetanus toxin booster within five years

2. Maintaining the vitality of the periodontal ligament by minimizing the extra-oral period and providing immediate replantation if possible (preferred). If that is not possible, transporting the tooth to the dentist in physiologic media such as Hank's Balanced Salt Solution or cold milk with replantation as soon as possible

3. Besides maintaining the vitality of PDL fibers, an additional goal in managing avulsed immature incisors is to promote revascularization of the pulp canal with vital tissue to achieve complete root maturation (apexogenesis). Therefore, pulp extirpation should be deferred until clinical and radiographic signs of pulp necrosis are apparent

4. By minimizing the extra-oral period to less than 15 minutes and by soaking the tooth in a 1% Doxycycline solution for five minutes before replantation. This disinfects the apical tissues and significantly enhances the likelihood of revascularization

5. An ankylosed tooth in a growing child will become infrapositioned ("submerged") as the child grows. Decoronation should be considered in these cases to prevent a periodontal defect (including adjacent teeth) and to preserve alveolar bone

Case 8

Soft Tissue Injury Management

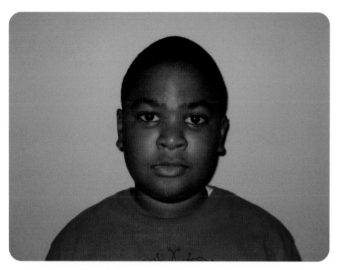

Figure 4.8.1. Facial photograph

A. Presenting Patient

- 7-year, 9-month-old African-American male
- Presenting as an emergency

B. Chief Complaint and History of Present Injury

- Father states, "My son fell at school and scraped his mouth"
- Child was running in halls at school and fell one hour ago. Injury was witnessed by classmates and teacher. There was no loss of consciousness

C. Social History

- Patient has two siblings, ages 12 and 16
- Mother is the primary caregiver and stays at home
- Middle class family

D. Medical History

- History of mild seasonal-induced asthma for which he takes a bronchodilator (β_2 agonist) as needed
- Allergic to penicillin
- No known food allergies, no current medications, vaccinations are up to date

E. Medical Consult

- N/A

F. Dental History

- Child has seen dentist every six months since age 2
- Good oral hygiene habits, with some adult supervision
- Normal diet
- Uses fluoridated toothpaste twice daily
- Lives in optimally fluoridated area
- No history of trauma before today
- Very cooperative for oral examination

G. Extra-oral Exam

- No significant findings
- Soft tissue injuries should only be addressed once any hard tissue (bony, dental) injuries have been ruled out (Armstrong 2000)

H. Intra-oral Exam

Soft Tissues

- Gingival degloving noted around the maxillary permanent central incisors (Figure 4.8.2.)

Hard Tissues

- No significant findings

Occlusal Evaluation of Mixed Dentition

- Class II molar

Other

- Caries-free dentition
- Maxillary right permanent central incisor was unerupted according to father
- Current pain rating per child 6/10 but he is playful and interactive

I. Diagnostic Tools

- Maxillary occlusal and periapical radiographs of maxillary permanent central incisors show no significant findings
- Vitality tests
  - Deferred
- Take adequate radiographs to clearly show all involved teeth
- Rule out other injuries, e.g., root fractures, alveolar fractures (Flores et al. 2007)

J. Diagnosis and Problem List

Diagnosis

- Avulsion of gingival tissue

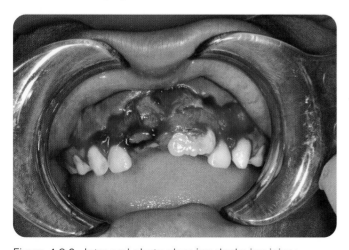

Figure 4.8.2. Intra-oral photo showing degloving injury

K. Treatment

- Mechanical cleansing of wound with sterile water

Discharge Instructions

- Avoid manipulation of injured segment until instructed otherwise. Watch for clinical signs such as presence of parulis or fistula
- Take over-the-counter analgesics as required
- Non-alcoholic chlorhexidine mouth rinse prescribed to keep tissues clean
- Child may continue to brush teeth as usual

Follow-up Treatment

- One-week post injury: All teeth test normally (Figure 4.8.3.)
- Five months post injury: All teeth test normally (Figure 4.8.4.)

L. Prognosis and Discussion

- Prognosis for uneventful and normal healing depends on adherence to basic soft tissue surgical principles, such as decontamination of area through irrigation, and good wound edge management. In this case, due to the avulsion of soft tissue, this wound was allowed to heal by secondary intention, which is the migration of granulation tissue to direct healing. Careful mechanical irrigation/debridement are of consequence in tissue healing. All teeth involved in injury must be re-assessed for potential pulpal injury, which may not surface immediately

M. Complications and Alternative Treatment Plan

- If this child had lost consciousness at school, medical clearance would be warranted prior to proceeding with treatment of dental injuries

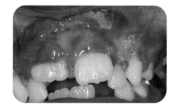

Figure 4.8.3. One-week follow-up intra-oral photo

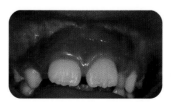

Figure 4.8.4. Five-month follow-up intra-oral photo

- If this child returned with a soft tissue infection, clinical signs observed could include purulent exudate from site of injury, localized tissue necrosis, and fever. Management would involve careful debridement of the local area and empirical use of antibiotics and analgesics for pain

---

BACKGROUND INFORMATION 1
Management of Oral Soft Tissue Trauma

- Parents and patients must be made aware that there is potential for localized tissue color change and contour change due to damage to melanocytes, as well as compromise of muscle attachments in deeper lesions (Essen et al. 2004)

- Adequate debridement of tissues and allowance for abscess drainage in conjunction with appropriate empirical antibiotic therapy are all basic principles of soft tissue infection management. Factors such as low oxygen tension can directly influence tissue healing (Fung et al. 2003)

- Soft tissue suturing prepares the wound for healing and promotes healing by primary intention (Peterson et al. 1993)

- Resorbable sutures, such as polygycolic gut or vicryl, are often used. Resorbable sutures may cause localized inflammatory reactions which can delay healing, and thus are not used or recommended on the skin (Peterson et al. 1993)

- There is no evidence indicating that the routine suturing of minor tongue lacerations has any positive effect on healing. Uncontrollable hemorrhage and potential for airway compromise are the only immediate reasons for suturing a tongue laceration (Ud-din and Gull 2007)

Self-study Questions

1. *In this case, is gingival repigmentation a clinical measure of successful treatment?*

2. *If the gingival tissue had merely been lacerated and an associated tooth luxation noted, which injury should be treated first?*

3. *What are some local factors that may influence soft tissue healing?*

Answers are located at the end of the case.

Bibliography

Armstrong BD. 2000. Lacerations of the mouth. *Emerg Med Clin North Am* 18:471–80.

Broder K, Cortese M, et al. 2006. Preventing tetanus, diphtheria, and pertussis among adolescents: Use of tetanus toxoid, reduced diphtheria toxoid and acellular pertussis vaccines. Recommendations of the CDC Advisory Committee on Immunization practices. *MMWR.* Feb. 23, 2006, 55:1–43. www.cdc.gov/mmwr/preview/ mmwrhtml/rr55e223a1.htm and http://www.cdc.gov/ vaccines/vpd-vac/tetanus/default.htm.

Centers for Disease Control and Prevention (CDC). 2007. Heads Up. *Facts for Physicians about Mild Traumatic Brain Injury (MTBI).* http://www.cdc.gov/ncipc/tbi/Facts_for_ Physicians_booklet.pdf.

Esen E, Haytac MC, Oz IA, Erdogan O, Karsli ED. 2004. Gingival melanin pigmentation and its treatment with the CO2 laser. *Oral Surg Oral Med Oral Pathol Oral Radiol Endod* Nov;98(5):522–7.

Flores MT, et al. 2007. Guidelines for the management of traumatic dental injuries. I. Fractures and luxations of permanent teeth. *Dent Traumatol* 23:66–71.

Fung HB, Chang JY, Kuczynski S. 2003. A practical guide to the treatment of complicated skin and soft tissue infections. *Drugs* 63(14):1459–80.

McTigue D, Thikkurissy S. 2011. Trauma. In: *The Handbook of Pediatric Dentistry*, 4th Edition. Nowak AJ, Casamassimo PS (eds). American Academy of Pediatric Dentistry: Chicago pp. 109–17.

Peterson L, Ellis E, Hupp J, Tucker M. 1993. *Contemporary Oral and Maxillofacial Surgery*, 2nd edition. Mosby: St. Louis.

Ud-din Z, Gull S. 2007. Should minor mucosal tongue lacerations be sutured in children? *Emerg Med* 24:123–4.

SELF-STUDY ANSWERS

1. No. Studies (Esen et al. 2004) have demonstrated that ablation of gingival melanocytes may result in loss of pigmentation. Melanocyte repopulation of traumatized tissues are thought to originate in the free gingivae. In this case, the avulsion of the marginal and free gingivae eliminate the potential source for melanocytes

2. All hard bony injuries should be treated first to give the practitioner a good perspective on the true extent of the soft tissue injury. Treating the soft tissue injury first also leads to the potential of tissue re-injury during treatment of tooth displacements

3. Local factors that may influence soft tissue healing include low oxygen tension to the region and corresponding ischemia, infection, and localized edema

Flowchart A: Intrusion Injuries

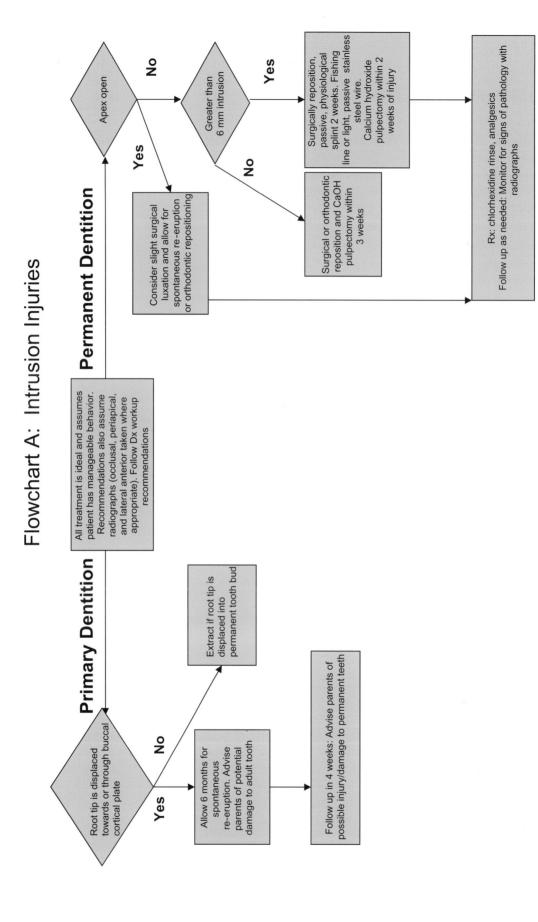

Flowchart A: Intrusion injuries. Reprinted with permission from McTigue D, Thikkurissy S. 2011. Trauma. In: *The Handbook of Pediatric Dentistry*, 4th Edition. Nowak AJ, Casamassimo PS (eds). American Academy of Pediatric Dentistry: Chicago. pp. 109–17.

Flowchart B: Root Fractures

Primary Dentition

Fracture located in coronal 1/3 of root or segment is aspiration risk (mobility III+)

- **Yes** → Extract coronal segment. Leave apical segment if not visible/easily removed
- **No** → Clinical and radiographic follow up in 4 weeks: Advise parents of possible injury/damage to permanent teeth NO SPLINT IS INDICATED

Permanent Dentition

All treatment is ideal and assumes patient has manageable behavior. Recommendations also assume appropriate pre-operative radiographic survey has been accomplished. Follow DX workup recommendations

Coronal segment is mobile

- **No** → No treatment required
- **Yes** → Re-approximate segments. If fracture is located in coronal 1/3 of root, splint for 2-3 months or consider decoronation and root submersion. Otherwise passive, physiologic splint (e.g. 40 - 50 pound test fishing line or light stainless steel) wire for 4 weeks

→ Rx: chlorhexidine rinse, analgesics Clinical and radiographic follow up: 4 weeks to monitor for signs of pathology

Flowchart B: Root fractures. Reprinted with permission from McTigue D, Thikkurissy S. 2011. Trauma. In: *The Handbook of Pediatric Dentistry*, 4th Edition. Nowak AJ, Casamassimo PS (eds). American Academy of Pediatric Dentistry: Chicago. pp. 109–17.

Flowchart C: Crown Fracture Injuries

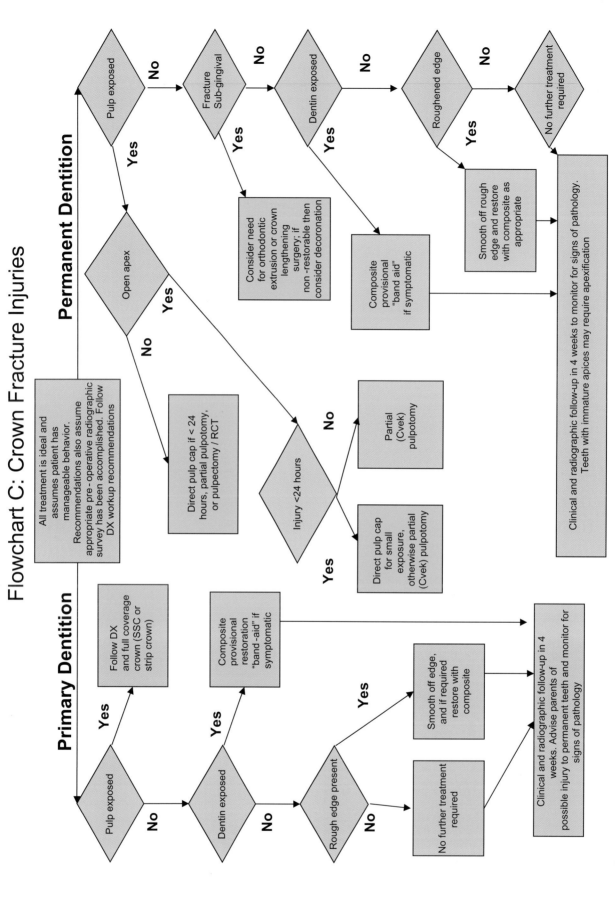

All treatment is ideal and assumes patient has manageable behavior. Recommendations also assume appropriate pre-operative radiographic survey has been accomplished. Follow DX workup recommendations

Permanent Dentition

Pulp exposed — No → Fracture Sub-gingival — No → Dentin exposed — No → Roughened edge — No → No further treatment required

Pulp exposed — Yes → Open apex
- Open apex — Yes → Direct pulp cap if < 24 hours, partial pulpotomy, or pulpectomy / RCT
- Open apex — No → Injury <24 hours
  - Injury <24 hours — No → Partial (Cvek) pulpotomy
  - Injury <24 hours — Yes → Direct pulp cap for small exposure, otherwise partial (Cvek) pulpotomy

Fracture Sub-gingival — Yes → Consider need for orthodontic extrusion or crown lengthening surgery; if non-restorable then consider decoronation

Dentin exposed — Yes → Composite provisional "band aid" if symptomatic

Roughened edge — Yes → Smooth off rough edge and restore with composite as appropriate

Clinical and radiographic follow-up in 4 weeks to monitor for signs of pathology. Teeth with immature apices may require apexification

Primary Dentition

Pulp exposed — Yes → Follow DX and full coverage crown (SSC or strip crown)

Pulp exposed — No → Dentin exposed

Dentin exposed — Yes → Composite provisional restoration "band-aid" if symptomatic

Dentin exposed — No → Rough edge present

Rough edge present — Yes → Smooth off edge, and if required restore with composite

Rough edge present — No → No further treatment required

Clinical and radiographic follow-up in 4 weeks. Advise parents of possible injury to permanent teeth and monitor for signs of pathology

Flowchart C: Crown fracture injuries. Reprinted with permission from McTigue D, Thikkurissy S. 2011. Trauma. In: *The Handbook of Pediatric Dentistry*, 4th Edition. Nowak AJ, Casamassimo PS (eds). American Academy of Pediatric Dentistry: Chicago. pp. 109–17.

Flowchart D: Lateral Luxation/Extrusion Injuries

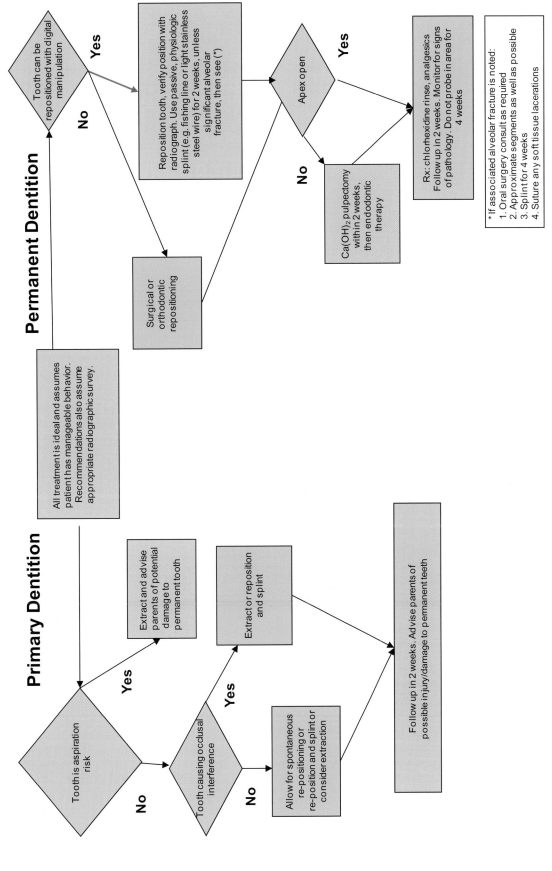

Flowchart D: Lateral luxation/extrusion injuries. Reprinted with permission from McTigue D, Thikkurissy S, 2011. Trauma. In: *The Handbook of Pediatric Dentistry*, 4th Edition. Nowak AJ, Casamassimo PS (eds). American Academy of Pediatric Dentistry: Chicago. pp. 109–17.

Flowchart E: Tooth Avulsion*[1]

[1] Source:Lee J. et al. 2001. Management of avulsed permanent incisors: a decision analysis based on changing concepts. Pediatr Dent 23:357–360

Apex Status

Open Apex

Closed Apex

Replant <15min or 15 min - 6 hrs EO time in HBSS or cold milk

No

Yes

15 min - 2 hrs in water/ saliva OR dry storage <60 min?

No

Yes

Dry storage >60 min?

Yes

Change transport media to HBSS if available

Soak in NaOCl or citric acid for 3 min and rinse; or debride and remove PDL gently with scaler

Place in NaF for 20 min

1. Replant
2. Obtain PA radiograph to verify proper position
3. Place flexible splint
4. Rx antibiotics
   - Chlorhexidine rinse for 10d
   - If >8 y/o and <45kg: doxycycline (4 mg/kg/day divided q 12 h first day, then 2 mg/kg/day divided q 12 h days 2 through 10)
   - If >8 y/o and >45 kg: doxycycline (100 mg q 12h first day, then 50 mg q 12 h days 2 through 10)
   - If <8 y/o: pen FLOWCHART V (2050mg/kg/d in four divided doses) for 7 days
5. Tetanus booster req'd if >5 years since booster
6. Post-op Instructions
   - Rx chlorhexidine, Rx antibiotic
   - soft food while splint on
   - OHI
   - avoid contact sports
   - if splint loose, contact dentist immediately
7. F/U 7-10 days
8. Monitor for apexification/RCT

(*) **Do not reimplant primary teeth.** Confirm complete avulsion with radiographic survey and assess area for alveolar fracture

Replanted <15 min EO time?

No

Yes

15 min-6 hrs EO time in HBSS or milk?

No

Yes

Soak in 1%Doxycycl. Solution for 5 min (50 mg Doxycycl. Capsule in 5 ml saline)

15min-2hrs in water or saliva?

No

Yes

Change transport media to HBSS if available

Dry storage <60 min?

No

Yes

Dry storage >60 min?

Yes

Re-implantation usually not indicated

Flowchart E: Tooth avulsion. Reprinted with permission from McTigue D, Thikkurissy S. 2011. Trauma. In: *The Handbook of Pediatric Dentistry*, 4th Edition. Nowak AJ, Casamassimo PS (eds). American Academy of Pediatric Dentistry: Chicago. pp. 109–17.

5

Infant Oral Health

Paul Casamassimo and Homa Amini

Clinical Cases in Pediatric Dentistry, First Edition. Edited by Amr M. Moursi.
© 2012 Blackwell Publishing Ltd. Pubished 2012 by Blackwell Publishing Ltd.

Case 1

Perinatal Oral Pathology

FUNDAMENTAL POINT 1

Obtaining a History

- Obtain a thorough history of the pregnancy and birth
- Obtain a thorough understanding of the child's natal teeth, including when first observed, associated complications with ventilator tubing, or infections

Cunha et al. (2001), Amini and Casamassimo (2010)

A. Presenting Patient

- 7-day-old male
- Consultative visit requested by neonatologist

B. Chief Complaint

- Neonatologist requests "evaluation of what appear to be teeth erupting on bottom jaw"

C. Social History

- First child
- 21-year-old single, immigrant mother
- Qualified for public assistance

D. Medical History

- Born two weeks prematurely
- On ventilator for two days
- Currently in pediatric intensive care unit (PICU)

E. Medical Consult

- N/A

F. Dental History

- Teeth present at birth

G. Extra-oral Exam

- Head misshapen
- Sparse hair

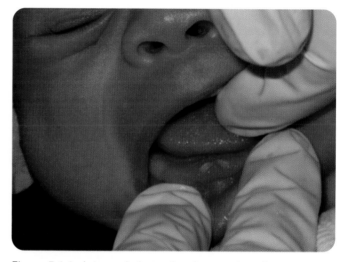

Figure 5.1.1. Intra-oral photo showing natal teeth

FUNDAMENTAL POINT 2

Clinical Exam: Significance of Findings

- Determine if the teeth present a problem for nursing due to irritation of child or mother. Also determine the potential risk of aspiration if teeth are mobile
- If removal is contemplated, use radiographic examination to determine whether teeth are supernumerary or prematurely erupting normal teeth

H. Intra-oral Exam

- Edentulous maxillary arch
- High maxillary frenum
- Palate intact
- Mandibular arch with teeth in O and P positions, partially erupted, brownish in color, rotated and firm to manipulation

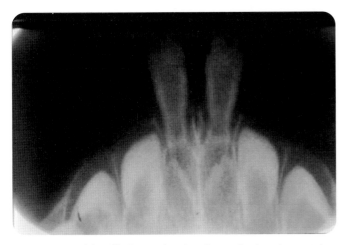

Figure 5.1.2. Mandibular occlusal radiograph showing natal teeth

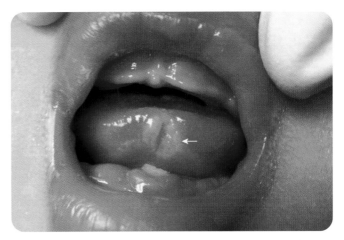

Figure 5.1.3. Traumatic ulcer (arrow) on the ventral surface of the tongue

BACKGROUND INFORMATION 1
Natal and Neonatal Teeth

- Teeth can be present at birth (natal teeth) or erupt shortly after birth (neonatal teeth)
- Most natal teeth are members of the normal complement of primary teeth
- Most natal teeth appear in the mandibular anterior region
- Natal teeth may be associated with other disorders, usually those involving the skin, bones, or ectoderm, such as chondroectodermal dysplasia. Therefore, careful systemic evaluation of children with natal teeth is necessary

I. Diagnostic Tools

- Occlusal radiograph of mandibular anterior region

J. Differential Diagnosis

- Other congenital neonatal pathology including Bohn's nodules, Epstein's pearls, and other retention phenomena

K. Diagnosis and Problem List

Diagnosis

- Natal teeth

Problem List

- Potential for nursing difficulty
- Potential for aspiration
- Potential for traumatic ulcer of the ventral surface of the tongue (Riga-Fede). See Figure 5.1.3 for an example of Riga-Fede
- Potential for trauma to the mucosa of the opposing arch

L. Treatment Plan

- Observe for mobility, ulcerations, nursing difficulty
- Extraction as indicated

M. Prognosis and Discussion

- No literature describes the risk of aspiration of natal teeth, so removal should be based primarily on the appearance, firmness, and likelihood of function of the tooth
- In the event the tooth is a member of the normal complement of primary teeth, parents should be made aware that the loss might result in alteration of spacing and alignment of the remaining primary teeth

N. Complications and Alternative Treatment Plan

- How would the treatment plan change if breastfeeding were negatively affected?
- How would the treatment plan change if the infant developed a ventral tongue surface ulcer?

Self-study Questions

1. What is the probability that natal teeth are members of the normal complement of primary teeth?

2. Where do natal teeth most often occur in the mouth?

3. What are reasons for removal of a natal tooth?

4. What is the difference between a natal and neonatal tooth?

5. What are characteristics of other neonatal oral lesions that would help differentiate a natal tooth?

Answers are located at the end of the case.

Bibliography

Amini H, Casamassimo PS. 2010. Prenatal dental care: a review. *General Dentistry* 58(3):176–80.

Cunha RF, Boe FAC, Torriani DD, Frossard WTG. 2001. Natal and neonatal teeth: review of the literature. *Pediatric Dentistry* 23:158–62.

Oral health care during pregnancy and early childhood. Practice guidelines. http://www.health.state.ny.us/publications/0824.pdf.

SELF-STUDY ANSWERS

1. The overwhelming probability is that a natal or neonatal tooth is a member of the 10 primary teeth in the arch, with fewer than 10% in most surveys being supernumeraries.

2. Most natal teeth occur in the mandibular arch in the incisor region, and more than half the time they occur in pairs.

3. Natal or neonatal teeth are removed if they present a risk of aspiration, are determined not to have functional integrity, if they present problems for the child in nursing, or if they are supernumerary teeth.

4. For definitional purposes, a natal tooth is one present at birth and a neonatal tooth is one that erupts after birth within the first 30 days of life.

5. The other congenital oral abnormalities, which might be mistaken for a natal tooth, include a keratin-filled body such as a Bohn's nodule or a mucous retention cyst. These are softer in consistency.

Case 2

First Dental Visit, Acquired Pathology

A. Presenting Patient
- 16-month-old Caucasian female

B. Chief Complaint
- Mom states, "My pediatrician said I should take my baby to a dentist to look at her teeth."

C. Social History
- First child
- Stay-at-home mother
- Medicaid coverage for medical and dental care

D. Medical History
- Allergies to nuts
- Gastroesophageal reflux (GERD)
- Medications: Pepcid AC

E. Medical Consult
- Contact allergist or primary care medical provider

F. Dental History
- Child has never been to a dentist
- Mother receives regular dental care
- Unfluoridated water system (private well)
- Oral hygiene is not performed
- Child is still on the bottle
- Child sucks thumb or pacifier when desired

G. Extra-oral Exam
- Normal weight and height for age
- Head and neck exam within normal limits

H. Intra-oral Exam
- Intra-oral soft tissues normal, with minor gingivitis
- Fourteen teeth present and within normal range for age
- Plaque on teeth with areas of cervical decalcification (Figure 5.2.2.)
- Incisal edges rounded and worn but not carious

FUNDAMENTAL POINT 1
Medical and Dental Histories

- Contact physician about nature of allergy: When it was first observed, intensity, therapy, how well controlled it is
- Note possible cross reactivity of various substances in patients with nut allergy, including some kinds of fluoride varnish
- Be aware of heightened risk of allergic responses to other materials used in dentistry, such as latex
- Determine the cause and extent of Gastroesophageal reflux (GERD) and efficacy of Pepcid therapy

---

I. Diagnostic Tools
- Caries Risk Assessment Tool
- Fluoride assessment of drinking water

J. Differential Diagnosis
- N/A

K. Diagnosis and Problem List
Diagnosis
- Normally developing child, with age appropriate oral development
- GERD
- High risk for dental caries

Problem List
- Still feeding from bottle, including at bedtime
- Indeterminate fluoride status
- No oral hygiene being practiced
- Dental erosion from GERD

BACKGROUND INFORMATION 1

Food Allergies and Gastroesophageal Reflux (GERD)

Food Allergies

- Food allergies occur in the first two years of life and are IgE-mediated
- Cow's milk, hen's eggs, soy, peanuts, tree nuts, wheat, fish, and shellfish account for 90% of food allergies
- Management is based on identification of the antigen and then avoidance of the food
- Children often outgrow milk, soy, egg, and wheat allergies, but have lifelong problems with nuts and shellfish

Allen, Hill, and Heine (2006)

Gastroesophageal Reflux (GERD)

- Gastroesophageal reflux disease (GERD) causes dental erosion in most afflicted dental patients to some degree
- Drug treatments include acid-neutralizers (milk of magnesia), histamine-2 blockers (ranitidine/Zantac), prokinetic agents (cisapride/Propulsid), and proton pump inhibitors (omeprazole/Prilosec)
- Surgical treatment may involve fundoplication (Nissan procedure)
- Soft tissue involvement can include chronic laryngitis, laryngeal ulcers, chronic sore throat

Barron, et al. (2003)

FUNDAMENTAL POINT 2

Dental History in Infant Oral Health

- In the dental history assessment, cover the six major areas of anticipatory guidance: stage of development, oral hygiene, fluorides, diet, habits, and injury prevention

AAPD (2011–12), Nowak and Casamassimo (1995)

L. Comprehensive Treatment Plan

- Provide parents with alternatives to bottle use and ways to eliminate sleeping with the bottle at night
- Perform an assessment of the fluoride content of the family's main source of drinking water and prescribe supplementation as needed

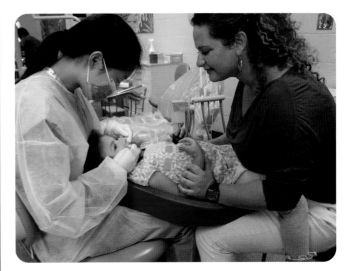

Figure 5.2.1. Knee-to-knee exam position

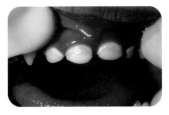

Figure 5.2.2. Intra-oral photo showing cervical decalcification

FUNDAMENTAL POINT 3

Intra-oral Exam in Infant Oral Health

- Plaque on teeth at this age and the surrogate measure of gingivitis are strong predictors of future dental caries (Alaluusua and Malmivirta 1994)
- Loss of anatomical definition is one indicator of dental erosion and at this age should be a warning sign (Barron et al. 2003)
- Oral erythema and gingivitis also may accompany GERD (Barron et al. 2003)

- Instruct parent on methods of oral hygiene with attention to frequency and use of a "smear" of fluoridated dentifrice since this child is at increased caries risk as well as the susceptibility of acid-exposed enamel to wear
- Include recommendation for next health supervision visit to determine compliance and

outcomes of preventive anticipatory guidance and progress of erosion

- Apply office-based fluoride
- Consider recommending a product containing amorphous calcium phosphate (ACP) to aid in remineralizing the teeth

M. Prognosis and Discussion

- Cessation of bottle feeding will hinge on providing the family with workable alternatives and strategies that fit into their lifestyle. Culture, family dietary habits, and stresses of daily life all need to be considered in recommendations because these are often listed as reasons why parents keep children on the bottle
- Fluoride assessment can be done through use of kits or by involving the local health department if it provides that service. The measure obtained must be from the main source of drinking water, but the clinician must also assess dietary habits and lifestyle issues, such as daycare, that may affect supplementation level. For example, a low-caries-risk child with other daily sources of optimally fluoridated water may not need supplementation

- Oral hygiene instruction requires consideration of location, timing, parents' manual skills, use of dentifrice, devices, and positioning. Each of these affect success and outcomes
- The decalcification and erosive effects on teeth must be monitored closely and treated with full-coverage restoration if they progress to cavitation
- Establish a more frequent recall schedule for the next health supervision visit to assess success and provide the next phase of anticipatory guidance

N. Common Complications and Alternative Treatment Plans

- Allergy to nuts may also include reaction to some fluoride varnish formulations. Care should be taken to check with manufactuers before applied in the office
- Should a fluoride supplement be prescribed, proper dosing and storage should be covered to prevent overuse or poisoning
- A careful distinction should be made between erosion and cavitation from caries. These two separate entities are sometimes confused, especially on posterior teeth
- One school of thought would be to immediately crown the affected teeth, but if erosion of enamel or cavitation occurs on other teeth, this would require a second procedure

Self-study Questions

1. **What are historical risk factors believed to be indicative of an elevated susceptibility to dental caries?**
2. **What are clinical risk factors believed to be indicative of an elevated susceptibility to dental caries?**
3. **What are some alternatives to a night-time bottle that can be offered to parents trying to break their child of a bedtime habit?**

4. **What may be factors that affect the amount of fluoride a very young child receives through dietary sources?**
5. **What are elements of a systematic approach to GERD in a child this age?**

Answers are located at the end of the case.

Bibliography

Alaluusua S, Malmivirta R. 1994. Early plaque accumulation: a sign for caries risk in young children. *Community Dentistry and Oral Epidemiology* 22:273–6.

Allen KJ, Hill DJ, Heine RG. 2006. Food allergy in childhood. *MJA* 185:394–400.

American Academy of Pediatric Dentistry. 2011–12. Guideline on Infant Oral Health. Reference Manual. *Pediatr Dent* 33(6):124–8.

Barron R, Carmichael R, Marcon M, Sandor G. 2003. Dental erosion in gastroesophageal reflux disease. *Journal of the Canadian Dental Association* 69(2):84–9.

Nowak A, Casamassimo P. 1995. Using anticipatory guidance to provide early dental intervention. *Journal of the American Dental Association* 126(8):1156–63.

SELF-STUDY ANSWERS

1. Many historical risk factors have been identified including low socio-economic status, low fluoride exposure, lack of oral hygiene, high frequency and amount of sugar exposure, medical problems or disabilities, and previous dental caries experience

2. The clinical risk factors which can be assessed on examination are poorly formed teeth or teeth with deep pits and fissures, existing dental caries including white spot lesions or decalcification, and plaque on teeth

3. To eliminate a bottle habit, parents can substitute water or gradually dilute the contents of the bottle over several nights with water. They can clean the teeth well and take the bottle away when the child falls asleep. A pacifier or other object can be substituted for the bottle. The parent can read or rock the child to sleep

4. A child living in a fluoridated community may still not receive adequate fluoride. The child may be breastfed, given bottled water without fluoride, given premixed formula or formula made with non-fluoridated water, the home may have a reverse osmosis water filteration system, or the child may spend most of the time outside the home in a non-fluoridated environment.

5. The immediate and long-term treatment plans hinge on successful medical management of GERD. Close interaction with the child's physician is necessary. A comprehensive assessment should be followed with medication or surgery as indicated. Depending on the stage of deterioration of the dentition, local non-invasive measures should be considered first, followed by definitive restorative care if needed. Fluorides figure prominently in this intervention to remineralize enamel.

Case 3

Early Childhood Caries Managed with Interim Therapeutic Restorations

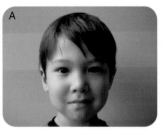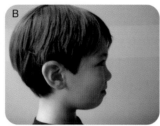

Figure 5.3.1a–b. Facial photographs

A. Presenting Patient
- 34-month-old Asian male

B. Chief Complaint
- Parents noticed "brown spots" on front teeth

C. Social History
- Second child
- Mother is primary caregiver
- Parents are married
- Both parents are employed and obtain regular dental care
- They have dental insurance

D. Medical History
- All systems normal
- No allergies
- Child has previously taken amoxicillin for otitis media

E. Medical Consult
- N/A

F. Dental History
- Child has not seen a dentist yet for a routine visit
- Parents brush patient's teeth once a day with a non-fluoridated dentifrice
- Family lives in a fluoridated community
- Child has ad lib access to sippy cup but does not use bottle

G. Extra-oral Exam
- Head and neck examination within normal limits
- Height and weight within normal limits for age

H. Intra-oral Exam
- Soft tissue within normal limits except for a few areas of gingival inflammation

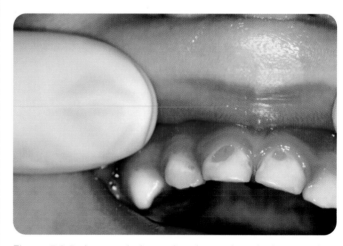

Figure 5.3.2. Intra-oral photo showing carious lesions on the facial surfaces of the anterior teeth

---

FUNDAMENTAL POINT 1
Treatment Planning for Interim Therapeutic Restorations (ITR)

- Carious lesions suited for ITR should be confined to dentin with sound enamel margins and no pulpal involvement
- A radiograph is useful in conforming the extent of caries, but may not be possible in the very young child

AAPD (2011–12a,b)

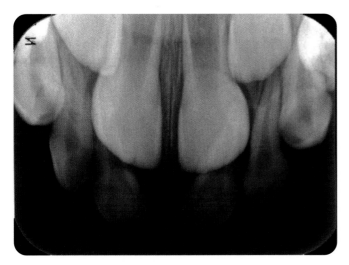

Figure 5.3.3. Maxillary periapical radiograph

- Eruption and occlusion of dentition within normal range for age with 16 teeth present
- Carious lesions noted on the facial surfaces of teeth D, E, and F (maxillary right lateral, right central, and left central)

I. Diagnostic Tools

- Radiographs: Maxillary periapical or occlusal
- Caries Risk Assessment Tool

J. Differential Diagnosis

- N/A

K. Diagnosis and Problem List

Diagnosis

- Dental caries involving dentin on teeth D, E, F

Problem List

- Infrequent oral hygiene
- Ad lib access to sippy cup containing juice
- Inability to cooperate for outpatient definitive dental restorations

L. Comprehensive Treatment Plan

- Oral hygiene instruction using brushing with smear of fluoridated dentifrice
- Dietary analysis and counseling with attention to sugar and frequency control
- Caries removal and restoration using interim therapeutic restoration (ITR) and glass ionomer cement
- Recall interval of three months to assess outcomes and reinforce caries protective factors
- Behavior management using parent-assisted immobilization
- Application of fluoride varnish to teeth

BACKGROUND INFORMATION 1
Interim Therapeutic Restorations

- Interim therapeutic restoration (ITR) is the proper term to describe treatment, in which follow-up and continued care are planned. Atraumatic or alternative restorative technique (ART) are terms to be reserved for situations in which this treatment may be the final therapy for the particular tooth
- ITR uses hand instruments to remove gross decay without local anesthetic. The cavity is restored with a glass ionomer cement (GIC)
- ITR is employed when conventional restoration and behavior management are not possible
- ITR can be followed by conventional restoration later
- GIC is the material of choice because of its ease of use, compatibility with slight moisture, fluoride release, and chemical adhesion to tooth structure

AAPD (2011–12a,b)

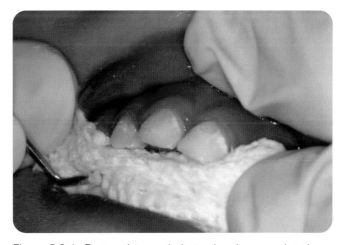

Figure 5.3.4. Post-op intra-oral photo showing completed treatment

M. Post-operative Intra-oral Photographs

- Note tooth-colored interim therapeutic restorations in Figure 5.3.4.

N. Prognosis and Discussion

- Oral hygiene should occur twice daily, once in the morning after breakfast and once before bed. The procedure should be done at a time and in a place that fits comfortably into this family's lifestyle. Because of the high caries risk, a small amount of fluoride dentifrice should be used when brushing for topical effect. No rinsing should follow brushing to allow retention of fluoride in the oral cavity.

- Juice should be eliminated from the child's diet along with other sources of sugar. Children at this age should have only a few ounces of juice per day, preferably at meal times.

- It is unlikely that this child would cooperate for traditional dental care in an outpatient setting. Therefore, the behavioral plan must include management of movement, so treatment can be completed. The child's age and weight make pharmacologic management through conscious sedation or general anesthesia risky and expensive. Fortunately, the nature of the treatment planned is such that it can be achieved with protective stabilization, preferably using the parent in the knee-to-knee position, in one visit.

- ITR is the treatment of choice for several reasons, including behavior. The minimal extent of caries and the well-defined lesions lend themselves to this technique. Glass ionomer cement has a fluoride-releasing property and can be of preventive, as well as restorative, benefit in this case.

O. Common Complications and Alternative Treatment Plans

- ITR-type restorations may be lost and require reapplication. This can be due to the incomplete removal of decay and the often poor isolation and excessive movement. Parents should be advised that this is usually not a definitive treatment and will require close follow-up and possible re-treatment

- An alternative treatment plan might be to use sedation or general anesthesia. Because of the child's age, these are both risky procedures, but are sometimes used. The minimal amount of treatment needed supports using ITR and protective stabilization.

- Teeth can also be definitively treated. If the child's movement is minimal, a local anesthetic can be used followed by rotary instruments to completely remove decay. If salivary contamination can be avoided the teeth can be restored with a composite or other definitive restorative material

Self-study Questions

1. *What are current recommendations for inclusion of fluoride dentifrice in toothbrushing for children under 3 years of age?*

2. *What are properties of glass ionomer cements that make them ideal for interim therapeutic restoration?*

3. *What are some characteristics of fluoride varnish that make it superior to traditional gels and foams for use in a child this age?*

4. *What recordkeeping entries are recommended when using protective stabilization for a child for dental treatment?*

5. *What characteristics of sugar in the diet that can contribute to caries should be discussed with parents when making recommendations for its reduction?*

Answers are located at the end of the case

Bibliography

American Academy of Pediatric Dentistry. 2011–12a. Guideline on pediatric restorative dentistry. Reference Manual. *Pediatr Dent* 33(6):205–11.

American Academy of Pediatric Dentistry. 2011–12b. Policy on interim therapeutic restorations (ITR). Reference Manual. *Pediatr Dent* 33(6):45–6.

ANSWERS

1. Recently, the recommendations for use of fluoride dentifrice have changed so that children at risk for caries should receive a small amount of fluoride dentifrice when their teeth are brushed. This is a smear at ages 1 to 2 years and a pea-sized amount at age 2 to 3 years

2. Glass ionomers have several properties that make them ideal for this procedure. They are less sensitive to moisture in the cavity, release fluoride, and are adherent to dentin, and some formulations can be light-cured. They are also tooth colored and can provide esthetic restorations

3. Current fluoride varnish formulations taste good, are tooth colored, have a high concentration of fluoride, stay on the teeth longer, and do not require a prolonged period of time without drinking as do other formulations

4. When protective stabilization is used, the operator should record the reason for its use, the additional consent provided by parents, the type of stabilization, how long it was used and any side effects, and its efficacy

5. Sugar intake counseling should examine the types (sucrose or other sugars), amounts (quantified in number of exposures), consistency (liquid or solid), frequency, patterns (meals or snacks), accompanying foods (milk and cookies), and attempts at clearance or removal (brushing or rinsing).

Case 4

First Dental Visit, Healthy Child

A. Presenting Patient
- 12-month-old African-American female

B. Chief Complaint
- Mom reports, "My pediatrician said I needed to bring her in for her first dental check-up"

C. Social History
- Lives with parents and two older siblings
- Mother is primary caregiver

D. Medical History
- Review of systems: Normal
- History of well-child visits and immunizations up to date in medical home

E. Medical Consult
- N/A

F. Dental History
- Never had a dental visit
- No toothbrushing performed at this time
- Fluoridated water supply is main source of drinking water
- Uses pacifier intermittently
- Still on the bottle for meals and snacks, but not ad lib

G. Extra-oral Exam
- Head, neck, and facial features normal
- Height and weight at 60% percentile
- Child marginally cooperative for knee-to-knee examination

H. Intra-oral Exam
- Soft tissues healthy
- Eight teeth present, developmentally within normal range for age but with crowding
- Plaque on teeth

FUNDAMENTAL POINT 1
Dental History in Infant Oral Health

- This child is on time for her first dental visit, which should occur by her first birthday (AAPD 2011–12a)
- Brushing should be occurring since she is dentate, with just a smear of fluoridated dentifrice (Nowak and Casamassimo 1995)
- Consider other forms of preventive therapy such as improving the oral hygiene of the mother and advising her to chew xylitol gum (Isokangas et al. 2000)
- The habits do not pose a problem at this age (See Chapter 6, Case 4 for more on oral habits)
- The mother should be weaning her at this time and transitioning her to a sippy cup or regular cup (Dietz and Stern 1999)
- The age 1 visit is an excellent opportunity to evaluate the risk of other non-carious conditions such as altered eruption, trauma, occlusion, nutrition and obesity, soft and hard tissue pathology, and child abuse (Casamassimo and Nowak 2009)

I. Diagnostic Tools
- Caries Risk Assessment Tool

J. Differential Diagnosis
- N/A

K. Diagnosis and Problem List
Diagnosis
- Well child, at moderate risk for dental caries

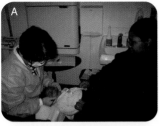
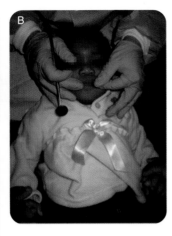
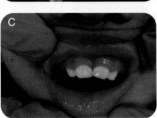

Figure 5.4.1a–c. A. Knee-to-knee exam, B. extra-oral exam, C. intra-oral exam

BACKGROUND INFORMATION 1
Caries Risk Assessment

- This child presents a few caries risk factors, according to the Caries Risk Assessment Tool of American Academy of Pediatric Dentistry, including lack of oral hygiene resulting in plaque accumulation and use of the bottle between meals

- She would be considered a moderate-to-high caries risk and preventive efforts in anticipatory guidance would be directed at beginning twice-daily oral hygiene with a smear of fluoride dentifrice and transitioning off the bottle

- Parental education should include an assessment of parental oral health. The association between maternal oral health and infant oral health should be discussed. The parent should also be advised of transmissibility of cariogenic bacteria and methods to reduce it. Avoiding the sharing of eating utensils is one way of reducing transmissibility

AAPD (2011–12b), Berkowitz (2003)

Problem List
- Lack of oral hygiene
- Still using bottle

L. Comprehensive Treatment Plan

- Prophylaxis and application of topical fluoride in varnish form because of the child's age and inability to manage trays and foams
- Use knee-to-knee positioning due to inability to cooperate
- Preventive anticipatory guidance on oral hygiene and weaning
- See child again in six months to assess compliance and effectiveness of home care

M. Prognosis and Discussion

- Oral hygiene success will depend upon the parents' ability to provide twice daily brushing for this child. With so few teeth, this should not be a major issue. Her age suggests that positioning will be important for oral hygiene delivery
- Bottle weaning takes some planning and effort. In this child's favor is the fact that she is not using the bottle at night and that her pediatrician will likely support this transition
- Pediatrician and parents should be complimented for establishing a dental home at the appropriate age. This should allow for prevention of caries and other disorders through anticipatory guidance and early intervention.

N. Common Complications and Alternative Treatment Plans

- N/A

Self-study Questions

1. **What areas should be covered in anticipatory guidance related to oral hygiene?**
2. **What is the dietary pattern that is considered normal for a child from six months to 12 months?**
3. **When do habits become a concern in the pre-school child?**
4. **What factors are considered when determining the recall interval in infant oral health?**
5. **What characteristics of fluoride varnish make it the preferred method of administration for this child?**

Answers are located at the end of the case.

Bibliography

American Academy of Pediatric Dentistry. 2011–2012a. Infant Oral Health Care, Reference Manual. *Pediatr Dent* 33(6):124–8.

American Academy of Pediatric Dentistry. 2011–12b. Guideline on Perinatal Oral Health Care, Reference Manual. *Pediatr Dent* 33(6):118–23.

Berkowitz RJ. 2003. Acquisition and transmission of Mutans streptococci. *J Calif Dent Assoc* 31(2):135–8.

Casamassimo PS, Nowak, AJ. 2009. Anticipatory guidance. In: *Early Childhood Oral Health*. Berg JH, Slayton, RL (eds). Wiley-Blackwell: Ames, IA.

Dietz WH, Stern L (eds). 1999. *American Academy of Pediatrics Guide to Your Child's Nutrition*. Villard Books: New York.

Isokangas P, Söderling E, Pienihäkkinen K, Alanen P. 2000. Occurrence of dental decay in children after maternal consumption of xylitol chewing gum: A follow-up from 0 to 5 years of age. *J Dent Res* 79(11):1885–9.

Nowak A, Casamassimo P. 1995. Using anticipatory guidance to provide early dental intervention. *Journal of the American Dental Association* 126(8):1156–63.

SELF-STUDY ANSWERS

1. A thorough coverage of oral hygiene includes frequency and duration, a technique demonstration with the child, review of devices, dentifrice use, location at home, positioning ideas, and problem solving such as how to fit oral hygiene into the family pattern

2. A child may be breast or bottle fed into six months of age. In the next six months, breastfeeding may be stopped or continued, depending on the needs and wishes of the mother and child. Some solid food is introduced in this period as well and bottle feeding ends with a transition to a cup at meal times. At 12 months, the child should be feeding himself and drinking from a cup on a trial basis since the process is initially messy

3. Habits are emotionally satisfying in the first few years of life and become detrimental when they cause dental changes, which can occur at any time. Allowing a habit to continue is a balance between its benefit to the child and any effect it may have on oral health. Most habits are lost by the third year of life. However, parents should be counseled on the potential effects of habits and be encouraged to wean the child from pacifiers or fingers as soon as is feasible

4. Caries risk factors not only determine anticipatory guidance information to be provided parents, but also how frequently a child is seen again. The reliance of a child on parental care makes it important to assess outcomes in areas such as oral hygiene and diet as well as anticipated parental compliance. No fixed interval is right for every child and the dentist should determine what is a reasonable amount of time to give parents to effect improvement

5. Fluoride varnish is ideal for the preschool child because it can be put on easily and requires minimal compliance. Today's formulations taste good, can be placed on semi-wet teeth, and are tooth colored. The effectiveness of fluoride varnish is well established, while the use of foams or gels in brush-on regimens enjoys little scientific support

Case 5

General Anesthesia, Restorative Case, Disability

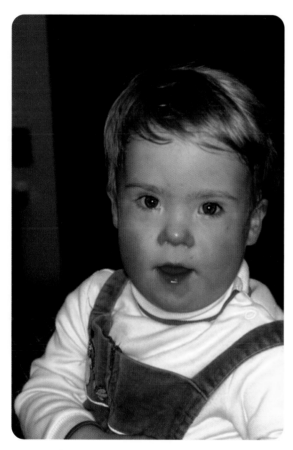

Figure 5.5.1. Facial photograph

A. Presenting Patient
- 28-month-old Caucasian male
- New patient visit

B. Chief Complaint
- Mom states, "My son has some bad teeth and his lip swelled up"

C. Social History
- Patient is in special preschool
- Parents are in their 40s, both employed

- No siblings
- Family lives in rural area
- Mother is the primary caregiver and works part-time
- Socio-economic status is mid-level

D. Medical History
- Down syndrome
- Tetralogy of Fallot
- Medications: Digitalis
- Tentative and resistive behavior for all health care given

E. Medical Consult
- Cardiologist and primary care physician regarding treatment. Discuss indication and contraindications for treatment under conscious sedation or general anesthesia, medication alteration, and any concerns about antibiotic coverage for infective endocarditis

F. Dental History
- No history of previous visit
- Optimal water fluoridation levels

BACKGROUND INFORMATION 1
Down Syndrome and Tetralogy of Fallot
Down Syndrome

- Down syndrome is a genetic disorder caused by Down syndrome trisomy 21.
- Down syndrome is associated with below average intellectual functioning, short stature, tendency toward obesity, immune dysfunction, low-set ears, and cardiac defects
- Oral findings in Down syndrome include open mouth, protruding tongue, hypoplastic maxilla, missing and conical teeth, and precocious periodontal disease
- Behavior management in the dental setting due to intellectual deficits may be a problem

Weddell et al. (2004)

Tetralogy of Fallot

- The four characteristics of Tetralogy are overriding aorta, ventriculoseptal defect, pulmonary stenosis, and right ventricular hypertrophy
- Tetralogy is considered a complex cardiac condition and requires antibiotic coverage for dental treatment
- Tet spells are transient and often unpredictable episodes of respiratory difficulty that can be life threatening

Wilson et al. (2007), (Bernstein 2007)

- Highly cariogenic diet
- Brushing by parents once per day

G. Extra-oral Exam
- Open mouth posture
- No other significant findings

H. Intra-oral Exam
- Soft tissue with moderate gingivitis (Figure 5.5.2.)
- Moderate plaque accumulation
- Oral hygiene is poor
- Primary dentition
- Dental caries in anterior and posterior teeth
- Occlusion: Class III primary molars, no crowding, class III canines

FUNDAMENTAL POINT 2
History and Exam in Down Syndrome Patients

- Behavior management alternatives must addressed. Strategies may be complicated by possible hearing problems that are often associated with Down syndrome
- Congenital heart conditions require antibiotic coverage
- Down Syndrome patients tend to be mouth breathers. This can lead to:
  - Reduction in salivary flow
  - Increased caries risk
  - Increased risk for gingivitis

Weddell et al. (2004)

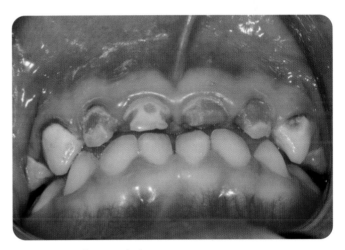

Figure 5.5.2. Intra-oral photo

I. Diagnostic Tools
- Radiographic survey
- Maxillary and mandibular occlusal radiographs
- Four periapical radiographs of posterior quadrants

J. Differential Diagnosis
- N/A

K. Diagnosis and Problem List
Diagnosis
- Down syndrome
- Tetralogy of Fallot
- Dental caries

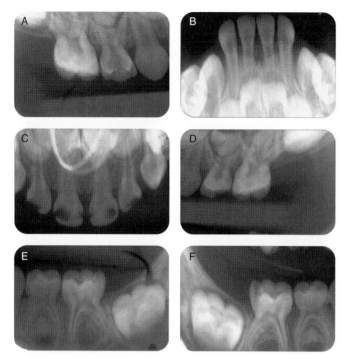

Figure 5.5.3a–f. Radiographs showing carious lesions

Problem List

- High caries risk due to existing caries and special needs
- Requires antibiotic coverage for any dental surgery
- Potentially uncooperative behavior
- Existing dental caries

L. Comprehensive Treatment Plan

- Establish a dental home
- Dental prophylaxis
- Fluoride treatment with fluoride varnish
- Review of oral hygiene (with parent and child)

- Restoration of all carious lesions under general anesthesia due to extent of decay and inability to cooperate for outpatient treatment
- Three-month recall
  - Re-evaluate caries risk
  - Re-evaluate oral hygiene status

M. Prognosis and Discussion

- The prognosis for caries is guarded due to poor oral hygiene and child's special needs. Prognosis could be improved with better oral hygiene and more frequent recall visits for preventive therapy
- The prognosis for improved behavior is also guarded due to the nature of the syndrome, with its lifelong limited intellectual functioning
- Dental treatment will continue to require antibiotic coverage due to the nature of the cardiac defect and its high risk for infective endocarditis

N. Complications and Alternative Treatment Plans

- How would the behavior management differ if the patient were cooperative for dental care, but with same disease levels?
- Would antibiotic coverage be required for preventive care?

Self-study Questions

1. *What are some important questions that need to be asked when taking a medical history with a patient who has severe cardiac disease?*
2. *What are some other cardiac conditions requiring infective endocarditis (IE) prophylaxis?*
3. *List five oral manifestations found in patients with Down syndrome.*

4. *What are considerations for radiographic examination in this patient?*
5. *What are the three categories of information used to make a caries risk assessment as defined by the American Academy of Pediatric Dentistry?*

Answers are located at the end of the case.

Bibliography

American Academy of Pediatric Dentistry. 2011–2012a. Guideline on Prescribing Dental Radiographs. Reference Manual. *Pediatric Dentistry* 33(6), pg. 289–91. www.aapd.org/media/Policies_Guidelines/E_Radiographs.pdf

American Academy of Pediatric Dentistry. 2011–2012b. Guideline on Caries-Risk Assessment. Reference Manual. *Pediatric Dentistry* 33(6) pp 110–17. www.aapd.org/media/Policies_Guidelines/P_CariesRiskAssess.pdf

American Academy of Pediatric Dentistry. 2011–2012c. Guideline on Management of Dental Patients with Special Health Care Needs. Reference Manual. *Pediatric Dentistry* 33(6), pp 142–6. www.aapd.org/media/Policies_Guidelines/G_SHCN.pdf

American Academy of Pediatric Dentistry. 2011–2012d. Guideline on Behavior Guidance for the Pediatric Dental Patient. Reference Manual. *Pediatric Dentistry* 33(6) pp. 142–6. www.aapd.org/media/Policies_Guidelines/G_BehavGuide.pdf

American Dental Association Council on Scientific Affairs. 2006. The use of dental radiographs: Update and Recommendations. *JADA* 137:1304–12. www.ada.org/prof/resources/topics/topics_radiography_examinations.pdf

Bay CA, Steele MW, Davis HW. 2007. Chapter 1: Genetic disorders and dysmorphic conditions. In: *Atlas of Pediatric Physical Diagnosis*, 5th edition. Zitelli BJ, Davis HW (eds). Elsevier: Philadelphia pp. 9–10.

Bernstein D. 2007. Congenital heart disease. In: *Nelson's Textbook of Pediatrics*, 18th edition. Kliegman RM, Behrman RE, Jenson HB, Stanton BF (eds) Elsevier: Philadelphia. pp. 1906–12.

Weddell JA, Sanders BJ, Jones JE. 2004. Dental problems of children with disabilities. In: *Dentistry for the Child and Adolescent*, 8th edition. McDonald RE, Avery DR, Dean JA (eds) Mosby: Philadelphia. pp. 524–56.

Wilson W, Taubert KA, Gevitz M, et al. 2007. Prevention of infective endocarditis: Guidelines from the American Heart Association. http://circ.ahajournals.org/cgi/reprint/CIRCULATIONAHA.106.183095.

SELF-STUDY ANSWERS

1. Description and name of the condition, previous treatment, cardiologist contact, limitations and other morbidity, medication(s) the patient takes and the frequency

2. The American Heart Association considers prosthetic valves, previous infective endocarditis, complex cyanotic heart disease, and surgically constructed shunts and conduits as high risk; acquired valvular dysfunction, hypertrophic cardiomyopathy, and mitral valve prolapse with regurgitation are considered moderate risk

3. Down syndrome patients tend to be mouth breathers, have a relative mandibular prognathism, small and conical teeth, retained primary teeth, large and protruding tongues, small maxilla, and precocious periodontal disease

4. Some of the factors considered in choosing a radiographic survey include cooperation, number and placement of teeth present, contacts between teeth, and existing disease

5. History, clinical evaluation, and supplemental professional assessment

6

Growth and Development

Jeffrey A. Dean

Clinical Cases in Pediatric Dentistry, First Edition. Edited by Amr M. Moursi.
© 2012 Blackwell Publishing Ltd. Pubished 2012 by Blackwell Publishing Ltd.

Case 1

Orthodontic Documentation, Evaluation, and Assessment

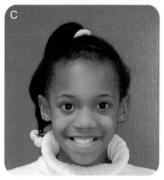

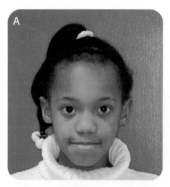

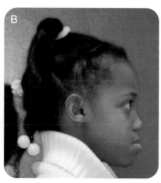

Figure 6.1.1a–c. Frontal, lateral, and frontal smiling extra-oral photos

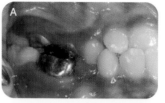

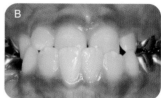

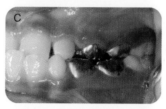

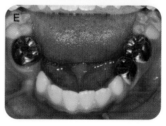

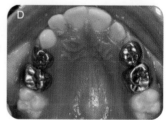

Figure 6.1.2a–e. Intra-oral photos showing all views

A. Presenting Patient

- 8-year-, 5-month-old African-American female

B. Chief Complaint

- Mom's complaint is that her daughter's "lower jaw is too far forward"

C. Social History

- Patient is an active middle school student
- Both parents are teachers in local middle school

D. Medical History

- Non-contributory

E. Medical Consult

- Not necessary at this time

F. Dental History

- Seen for routine dental maintenance visits by her pediatric dentist after having comprehensive restorative care as a preschooler
- Optimal water fluoridation levels (city water)
- Dietary assessment is satisfactory
- Supervised brushing

G. Extra-oral Exam

- Concave and forward sloping, facial profile secondary to apparent mandibular prognathia
- Otherwise, fairly symmetrical facial features

H. Intra-oral Exam

- Transitional dentition
- Overbite: 2 mm, with -3 mm overjet and anterior crossbite

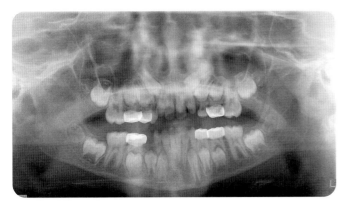

Figure 6.1.3. Panoramic radiograph

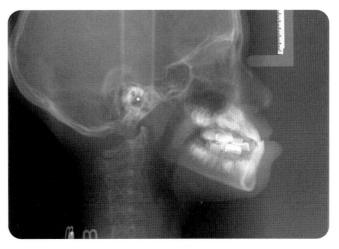

Figure 6.1.4. Cephalometric radiograph

- Soft tissue within normal limits
- Mild plaque accumulation
- Caries free, but multiple restorations

I. Diagnostic Tools
- Full mouth radiographs and panoramic view
- Lateral cephalometric radiograph
- Well trimmed orthodontic study models

J. Differential Diagnosis
- Maxillary deficiency or mandibular prognathia

K. Diagnosis and/or Problem List
Diagnosis
- Class III mixed dentition malocclusion

Problem List
- Class III skeletal and dental classification
- Anterior crossbite with significant negative overjet

FUNDAMENTAL POINT 1
Orthodontic Records

- Comprehensive orthodontic treatment requires a proper assessment to be done prior to initiation of care, including a questionnaire of the patient (medical/dental history, chief complaint, etc.), examination (oral health, function, and facial proportions) and diagnostic records

- Comprehensive diagnostic records include dental study models, an 8 series photographic collage, complete intra-oral radiographs, a cephalometric radiograph including tracing, and an anterior-posterior radiograph when indicated (for example, when there is a possible facial or occlusal asymmetry). Some adjustment in this standard will more than likely be forthcoming, with the use of cone beam computed tomography (CBCT) becoming more commonplace.

- Although it is generally understood that comprehensive orthodontic treatment requires this complete record documentation, questions often arise as to how many diagnostic records are needed for minor or interceptive treatment. While this can vary from case to case, the main concept is to ensure a full and complete diagnosis of the problem being evaluated so that the treatment addresses this problem and does not overlook confounding conditions. Dental versus skeletal crossbite correction is a good example. In the case of a simple, one-tooth anterior crossbite caused by dental tipping, dental study models or a photographic collage may be enough for documentation. However, if the patient appears to have an anterior crossbite because of a skeletal alignment problem, comprehensive diagnostic records are essential. When in doubt, a more thorough evaluation may be the most prudent approach

- See the American Academy of Pediatric Dentistry (AAPD) Guidelines on Management of the Developing Dentition and the American Board of Orthodontics Case Report Preparation

AAPD (2011–12a), Proffit et al. (2007)

BACKGROUND INFORMATION 1
Orthodontic Informed Consent

- Informed consent is basically a discussion and documentation of the treatment to be rendered, as well as the risks, benefits and alternatives to this treatment

- Common orthodontic treatment risks to be covered during consent include caries, root resorption, periodontal disease, necrotic pulp, discomfort, trauma, temporomandibular joint disorder (TMD) considerations, impacted teeth, length of treatment, prognosis, and relapse

- Many examples of orthodontic informed consent forms are readily available and should be used by practitioners prior to treatment. Inherent in the concept of *informed* consent, however, is that these forms must be reviewed with the patient by the practitioner to ensure an understanding by the patient and parent

- See The Orthodontic CYBERjournal (http://www.oc-j.com/dec00/risks.htm) and the American Academy of Pediatric Dentistry Guidelines on Informed Consent (AAPD 2011–12b)

L. Comprehensive Treatment Plan
- Comprehensive orthodontic care to include two-phase treatment consisting of protraction headgear in phase one and comprehensive bracketing in phase two

M. Post-Operative Intra-oral Photographs
- N/A

N. Prognosis and Discussion
- The prognosis is guarded and the need for orthognathic surgery cannot be ruled out

O. Complications and Alternative Treatment Plan
- Complications to this patient's care include the possibility of poor compliance or lack of protraction headgear treatment response, even with good compliance
- Alternative treatment could include waiting until growth is complete and addressing the skeletal discrepancy surgically

Self-study Questions

1. *What are the three basic components of a comprehensive orthodontic assessment for a patient?*

2. *Is it true that diagnostic records for orthodontic patients must include a cephalometric evaluation?*

3. *What new imaging technique may influence substantial changes in the way comprehensive orthodontic assessments have been done in the past?*

4. *Name the four broad areas of treatment that need to be covered during the process of informed consent*

5. *What are the most common specific areas covered when reviewing orthodontic informed consent with a patient?*

Answers are located at the end of the case.

Bibliography

American Academy of Pediatric Dentistry. 2011–2012a. Guidelines on management of the developing dentition, Reference Manual. *Pediatric Dentistry* 33(6), pp. 229–41.

American Academy of Pediatric Dentistry. 2011–2012b. Guideline on Informed Consent, Reference Manual. *Pediatric Dentistry* 33(6), pp. 285–7.

Proffit WR, Sarver DM, Ackerman JL. 2007. Orthodontic diagnosis: The development of a problem list. In: *Contemporary Orthodontics*, 4th edition. Proffit WR, Fields HW, Sarver DM (eds) Elsevier Publishing, St Louis. pp 167–233.

SELF-STUDY ANSWERS

1. Patient questionnaire, examination (oral health, function, and facial proportions), and diagnostic records

2. No, this is not true. Depending on the severity of the patient's problem, certain orthodontic records may not be necessary

3. Cone beam computer tomography (CBCT) may eliminate the need to make separate dental study models, intra-oral radiographs, and cephalometric radiographs because all three of these items can be captured in the 3-dimensional CBCT image

4. Type of treatment to be rendered, the risks, the benefits, and the alternatives to this treatment

5. Risk for caries, root resorption, periodontal disease, necrotic pulp, discomfort, trauma, temporomandibular joint disorder (TMD), impacted teeth, length of treatment, prognosis, and relapse

Case 2

Space Management: Premature Loss of Primary Second Molar in Preschool Child

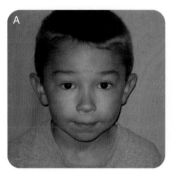
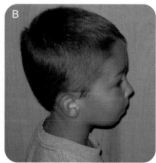

Figure 6.2.1a–b. Facial photographs

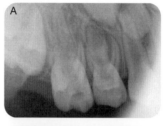
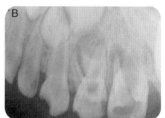
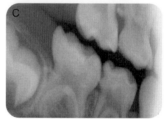
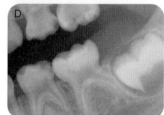
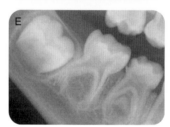
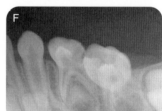

Figure 6.2.2a–f. Pre-op radiographs

A. Presenting Patient
- 3-year-, 10-month-old Caucasian male

B. Chief Complaint
- Mother states, "My son has a bunch of cavities and pain in an upper left tooth"

C. Social History
- Patient is in preschool daycare
- Parents are divorced, no siblings
- Mother is the primary caregiver and works a full-time job
- Socio-economic status is low

D. Medical History
- Non-contributory

E. Medical Consult
- Not necessary at this time

F. Dental History
- Optimal water fluoridation levels (city water)
- Highly cariogenic diet
- Unsupervised brushing

G. Extra-oral Exam
- Normal facial symmetry with convex facial profile

H. Intra-oral Exam
- Primary dentition with distal step primary molar terminal plane
- 6-mm-deep overbite with 2-mm overjet, adequate dental spacing and arch circumference
- Soft tissue within normal limits
- Moderate plaque accumulation
- Extensive severe dental decay, including sensitivity to percussion on several teeth

I. Diagnostic Tools
- Pre-op radiographs: Four periapicals and two bitewings

FUNDAMENTAL POINT 1
History for Space Management

- Obtain a thorough medical history to determine if a patient can tolerate intra-tissue metal extensions (distal shoe) in the oral cavity. For example, is there a history of a congenital heart defect, heart surgery or bleeding disorder?
- Obtain a thorough dental history to manage all oral health problems, including restorative, preventive, educational, in conjunction with the space maintenance care
- Consider occlusal relationships and options for management of the early loss of the second primary molars. Which treatment will provide the most benefit with the least drawbacks?

Durward (2000) Terlaje and Donly (2001)

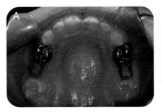
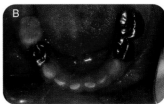

Figure 6.2.3a–b. Intra-oral photos showing space maintenance appliances in maxillary arch

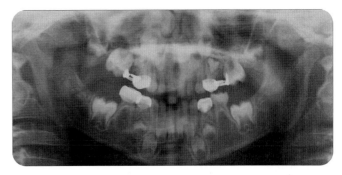

Figure 6.2.4. Post-op panoramic radiograph at age 5 yrs 5 mo

- Severe dental decay noted
- Periapical pathology noted with maxillary second molars

J. Differential Diagnosis
- N/A

K. Diagnosis and Problem List
Diagnosis
- Early childhood caries
- Poor diet
- Poor oral hygiene

Problem List
- High caries risk due to poor diet and oral hygiene
- Premature loss of the maxillary second primary molars

L. Comprehensive Treatment Plan
- A detailed informed consent should be obtained for this care. The patient will receive posterior stainless steel crowns, extraction of the maxillary right and left second primary molars, and placement of two distal shoe space maintainers to guide the eruption of the maxillary right and left first permanent molars
- Establish a dental home and aggressive preventive care to include caries risk assessment, parent education, adequate oral hygiene, fluoride varnish, and special maintenance intervals tailored to the responsiveness of the parent and child to the preventive care
- Prevent malocclusion with use of distal step primary molar terminal plane
- Maintain distal shoe space maintainer and eventually follow up with replacement bilateral maxillary lingual arch (Nance appliance)

M. Post-operative Intra-oral Photographs
- Post-op photos and panoramic radiograph were obtained at age 5 years, 5 months, showing stainless steel crowns and distal shoe space maintainers all in good repair

N. Prognosis and Discussion
- Prognosis for caries is now good secondary to compliance with the aggressive preventive plan that was implemented
- Prognosis for preventive occlusion management (space maintainers) is good secondary to success to date with the bilateral distal shoes and initial eruption of the first permanent molars. It will be essential that the patient continue regular dental visits to have the distal shoes removed and a bilateral maxillary lingual arch (Nance appliance) placed, once the first permanent molars are erupted far enough for banding

O. Complications and Alternative Treatment Plan

- Complications to this patient's care could include premature loss of the distal shoes, mismanagement of the distal shoes (particularly if the first permanent molars erupted under the most gingival aspect of the distal shoe blades), and lack of adequate follow-up by the mother

---

BACKGROUND INFORMATION 1

Distal Shoes and Alternatives

- The second primary molar is essential to the proper eruption and positioning of the first permanent molar, which is an essential tooth in establishing a normal permanent dentition occlusion
- Early loss of the second primary molar can lead to multiple occlusal problems such as space loss and altered eruption; however, these problems can be prevented with proper space maintenance
- While there are a few ways to address premature loss of this primary tooth, maintenance of its space minimizes orthodontic correction problems
- Distal shoe space maintainers or acrylic pressure (free-end) appliances are useful in guiding the eruption of the first permanent molar, but require some careful management and close follow-up

Barberia (2006), Brill (2002)

Self-study Questions

1. **What alternative management plans related to the maxillary second primary molars were available for this patient at the initiation of care?**

2. **What alternatives to bilateral distal shoes could be considered as this patient matures?**

3. **What angulation is usually built into the distal shoe blades from an occlusal to gingival direction and why?**

4. **What about this patient's occlusal relationships presents a positive prognosis regarding the need for future orthodontic care?**

5. **What about this patient's occlusal relationships presents a negative prognosis regarding the need for future orthodontic care?**

Answers are located at the end of the case.

Bibliography

Barberia E, Lucayechi T, Cardenas D, Maroto M. 2006. Free-end space maintainers: design, utilization and advantages. *J Clin Pediatr Dent* 31(1):5–8.

Brill WA. 2002. The distal shoe space maintainer chairside fabrication and clinical performance. *Pediatr Dent* 24(6): 561–5.

Durward CS. 2001. Space maintenance in the primary and mixed dentition. *Ann R Austral Coll Dent Surg* 15:203–5.

Terlaje RD, Donly KJ. 2001. Treatment planning for space maintenance in the primary and mixed dentition. *J Dent Child* 68(2):109–14.

SELF-STUDY ANSWERS

1. Aggressive pulpectomies of the second primary molars, although given the clinical signs and symptoms and the periapical radiographic appearance, particularly the maxillary left second primary molar, the prognosis is questionable

2. Either no space management at this time, permitting the permanent molars to drift mesially and impacting the second premolars, or the use of a removable acrylic pressure appliance that would guide the first permanent molars via pressure and without penetrating the alveolar mucosa

3. Angled mesially to help prevent the first permanent molar from getting impacted under the distal shoe blade

4. Adequate primary dentition spacing needed for the transition into the full permanent dentition

5. Deep overbite, distal step primary molar terminal plane and convex facial profile that would most likely lead to a class II deep overbite relationship in the permanent dentition

Case 3

Bilateral Space Management in the Mixed Dentition

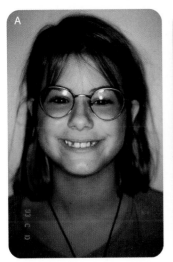
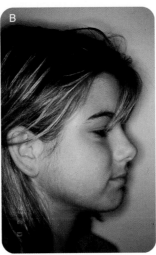

Figure 6.3.1a–b. Facial photographs

A. Presenting Patient
- 12-year-old Caucasian female

B. Chief Complaint
- Mom states, "My child has crooked and missing teeth"

C. Social History
- Patient is a happy, well developed adolescent
- Lives with mother and father
- Middle class socio-economic status
- One younger brother

D. Medical History
- Non-contributory

E. Medical Consult
- Not necessary at this time

F. Dental History
- Regular dental maintenance visits
- Optimal water fluoridation levels (city water)

- Fairly healthy diet with low caries risk
- Supervised brushing

G. Extra-oral Exam
- Normal facial symmetry with slightly convex facial profile

H. Intra-oral Exam
- Healthy mixed dentition with lower lingual arch in place (Figure 6.3.2)
- 4-mm overbite with 1 mm-overjet
- Soft tissue within normal limits
- Mild plaque accumulation
- Good oral hygiene
- Caries free with sound pit and fissure sealants on the first permanent molars

I. Diagnostic Tools
- Panoramic radiograph reveals congenitally missing and ectopically erupting teeth (Figure 6.3.3)

J. Differential Diagnosis
- N/A

K. Diagnosis and Problem List
Diagnosis
- Class I mixed dentition malocclusion

Problem List
- Congenitally missing teeth numbers 4 and 7
- Ectopic teeth numbers 6 and 11
- Peg lateral incisor number 10
- Moderate lower incisor irregularity

L. Comprehensive Treatment Plan
- Maintain current caries prevention program with routine maintenance appointments and effective home oral hygiene
- Placement of lower lingual arch to maintain the leeway space until complete eruption of the second permanent molars

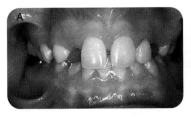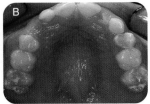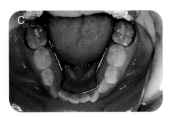

Figure 6.3.2a–c. Intra-oral photos showing bilateral space maintenance appliance

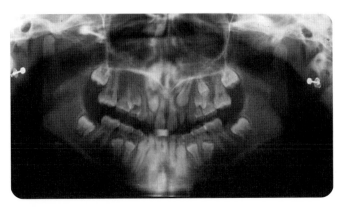

Figure 6.3.3. Panoramic radiograph

FUNDAMENTAL POINT 1
Space Maintenance

- Posterior space maintenance is indicated when there is premature loss of primary molars. Failure to hold the space for the premolars often leads to significant ectopic eruption or impaction of these teeth. Management in the mixed dentition can include (Dean et al. 2004):
  - For unilateral loss: Band and loop spacer
  - For bilateral loss prior to eruption of the permanent incisors: Bilateral band and loop spacers (concerns about the anterior portion of the lower lingual arch wire precludes consideration of this appliance until the incisors erupt)
  - For bilateral loss after eruption of the permanent incisors: Lower lingual arch or acrylic partial denture
- See American Academy of Pediatric Dentistry management of the developing dentition guidelines at: http://aapd.org/media/Policies_Guidelines/G_DevelopDentition.pdf

BACKGROUND INFORMATION 1
Mixed Dentition Space Analysis

- The mixed dentition primary molars and canines are typically larger in width, mesial to distally, than the permanent dentition premolars and canines. This extra space is called the leeway space, and keeping the permanent molars from shifting mesially after the second primary molars exfoliate can be beneficial in patients with crowding issues. Space analysis methods have been developed to aid in determining how much leeway space might be available. One simple method is the Tanaka and Johnston Analysis (Tanaka and Johnston 1974):

1. Divide the width of the lower permanent incisors in half

2. To this number, add 10.5 mm for the lower buccal segment; add 11 mm for the upper buccal segment

3. Subtract the number calculated above from the combined widths of the primary molars and canine for the buccal segment in question to get the leeway space for that area

- Once the permanent dentition is fully erupted, initiate comprehensive orthodontics and prosthetic treatment

M. Post-operative Intra-oral Photographs

- Note the significant amount of space that has developed in the mandibular premolar area by holding the permanent molars in place with the lower lingual arch. This should allow the canines and incisors to drift distally somewhat to alleviate the anterior crowding (Figure 6.3.4)

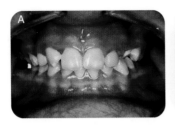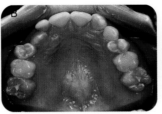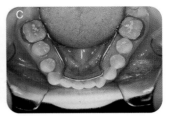

Figure 6.3.4a–c. Post-op intra-oral photos showing space in the mandibular arch

---

FUNDAMENTAL POINT 2

Space Analysis

- Mixed dentition space analysis is an important adjunct in diagnosing and managing developing dentitions

- Lower anterior crowding can be managed in a number of different ways, depending on the amount of crowding, dental development, and type of malocclusion. General options in the mixed dentition based on the amount of crowding include:

  - Space redundancy: Wait until the permanent dentition has erupted to close the space, do bonding, or consider tooth replacement

  - No crowding: Even with no crowding, long-term alignment cannot be guaranteed in some

patients. Development of alignment problems later on in life may benefit from retention

- Mild crowding (1 to 4 mm): Use of a lower lingual arch to hold the leeway space, disking of select primary teeth

- Moderate crowding (5 to 9 mm): Flaring of anterior teeth, distalization of permanent first molars, or arch expansion with appliances such as a lip bumper or limited orthodontic with bands on the molars, brackets on the incisors ("2 × 4") and open coil springs

- Severe crowding (10 mm or more): Serial extraction, or wait until the permanent dentition and consider extraction, followed by full orthodontics

Brennan and Gianelly (2000)

N. Prognosis and Discussion

- As long as the lingual arch appliance is left in place until the second permanent molars fully erupt, the prognosis is good. However, the congenitally missing and ectopic teeth in this patient's maxillary arch significantly complicate her care

O. Complications and Alternative Treatment Plan

- Long-term retention is necessary to maintain the lower anterior alignment for this type of patient

- An alternative treatment plan would have been to wait until eruption of the permanent dentition to initiate orthodontic treatment; however, regaining the space after mesial movement of the permanent molars would have made this difficult. The simple use of a lower lingual arch has significant advantages in this type of case

Self-study Questions

1. **What is the major treatment effect of placing a lower lingual arch in the case of multiple missing primary molars or lower anterior crowding?**
2. **Why should lower lingual arches not be placed prior to eruption of the permanent lower incisors?**
3. **Will lingual arches resolve crowding issues in cases with more than 5 mm of crowding?**

4. **What is the name of the extra space available in the transition from the primary molars and canine to the permanent premolars and canine?**
5. **Is measurement of the unerupted permanent premolars and canines off of radiographs the only way to predict how much arch space is needed for these teeth?**

Answers are located at the end of the case.

Bibliography

Brennan MM, Gianelly AA. 2000. The use of the lingual arch in the mixed dentition to resolve incisor crowding. *Am J Orthod Dentofacial Orthop*, 117(1):81–5.

Dean JA, McDonald RE, Avery DR. 2004. Management of the developing occlusion. In: *Dentistry for the Child and Adolescent*. McDonald RE, Avery DR, Dean JA (eds) Mosby: St. Louis. pp. 640–4.

Tanaka MM, Johnston LE. 1974. The prediction of the size of unerupted canines and premolars in a contemporary orthodontic population. *J Am Dent Assoc* 88:798–801.

SELF-STUDY ANSWERS

1. Prevent mesial drifting of the permanent molars causing loss of space
2. The anterior portion of the lingual wire can interfere with normal eruption of the incisors
3. Although they can contribute to the correction, lingual arches typically hold only 3 to 5 mm of space in the transition to the permanent dentition

4. Leeway space
5. No, several mixed dentition arch analyses use a standardized prediction formula to fairly accurately predict the size of these teeth by measuring already erupted permanent teeth, i.e., the lower incisors

Case 4

Interceptive Orthodontics: Habit Appliances

A. Presenting Patient
- 12-year-, 5-month-old African American female

B. Chief Complaint
- Mother states that her child has been a thumb sucker and they "don't like the space between her top and bottom teeth"

C. Social History
- Patient is an active seventh grader
- Parents are divorced
- Mother is the primary caregiver and works full time
- Middle socio-economic status
- Two older brothers

D. Medical History
- Non-contributory

E. Medical Consult
- Not necessary at this time

F. Dental History
- Maintains routine dental checkups
- Optimal water fluoridation levels (city water)
- Moderate cariogenic diet
- Unsupervised brushing

G. Extra-oral Exam
- N/A

H. Intra-oral Exam
- Class I molars and canines
- 2-mm open bite with 2-mm overjet
- Excessive arch length redundancy
- Soft tissue within normal limits
- Mild plaque accumulation
- Fair oral hygiene
- No active caries

I. Diagnostic Tools
- A full orthodontic diagnostic work-up was completed and evaluated

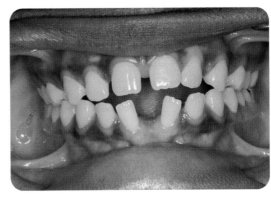

Figure 6.4.1. Intra-oral photo showing anterior open bite due to habit

---

FUNDAMENTAL POINT 1
Oral Habits

- Oral habits such as non-nutritive sucking, bruxing, and abnormal tongue swallowing and positioning can apply forces to the teeth and dentoalveolar structures that may cause deleterious effects
- Whereas mild habits many times are not of concern and the child may eventually stop on their own, habits of higher frequency, intensity, and duration can be associated with significant problems such as decreased arch width and crossbites, as well as an increased overjet and decreased overbite or open bite
- Correction involves two important concepts:
  - Often, parental anxiety and scolding about the habit increases its intensity, instead of ameliorating it
  - The child must be old enough to understand the need to stop the habit and must want to stop the habit for interventions to be helpful
- Treatment is directed toward behavior modification techniques and appliance therapy, such as a palatal crib

Dean et al. (2004)

J. Differential Diagnosis

- N/A

K. Diagnosis and Problem List

Diagnosis

- Class I permanent dentition malocclusion

Problem List

- Flaring of maxillary and mandibular incisors
- Anterior open bite secondary to thumb-sucking habit
- Excessive arch length redundancy

L. Comprehensive Treatment Plan

- The treatment plan included placement of a "Bluegrass" type habit appliance. This appliance (see Figure 6.4.2a) is comprised of a palatal wire attached to banded molars. The palatal wire has an acrylic roller bead that serves as a reminder to the patient not to suck her thumb and to encourage normal tongue positioning and swallowing. This appliance is usually effective over the course of two to three months, followed with traditional orthodontic appliances to close the space redundancy and continued use of the habit appliance

M. Post-operative Intra-oral Images

- N/A

N. Prognosis and Discussion

- Treatment with this type of habit appliance is usually successful but must be performed in patients willing to stop the habit. Thumb sucking should be significantly reduced and the patient's open bite should close down, giving her some minimal overbite
- Although the success rate of this type of treatment is high, there are patients of this age who are determined to continue the habit despite an intra-oral appliance. In these cases the patient may not truly want to stop the habit and a child

therapist should be consulted to determine if there are other psycho-social issues involved

O. Complications and Alternative Treatment Plan

- Complications for this patient could include relapse of the open bite once the appliances are removed.

BACKGROUND INFORMATION 1
Treatment Alternatives

- Once the practitioner is assured that the patient is both old enough to understand the need for cessation of the habit and is ready and willing to comply, options for treatment can be considered. Treatment alternatives fall into three main areas. A staged progression of these options or a combination of them may be best, depending on the particular needs of the patient involved

  - Behavior modification: This technique uses positive reinforcement to encourage the child's compliance. One good example is a timed rewards calendar. A short written agreement is made about goals and rewards. Then, over a period of weeks for a predetermined period of time that successively increases each week, the child does not suck his digit. A star is placed on the calendar each successful day, and at the end of each week some small reward, such as a toy or book, is given. If the parents remain dedicated to this, cessation usually occurs, if it is going to occur, within a month's time

  - Extra-oral means: Various options are available including wrapping an Ace bandage around the elbow at night to keep the child from bending her arm to place their digit in her mouth (must be careful not to cut off blood circulation), placement of bitter-tasting liquids on the digit (Kozlowski 2007), and use of a glove-like appliance that covers the thumb and straps around the wrist (Thumbusters, LLC)

  - Intra-oral appliances: Palatal appliances with cribs, loops, irritating spurs, or beads can all be helpful

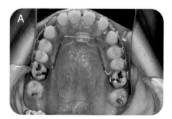 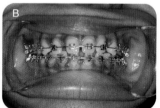

Figure 6.4.2a–b. Post-op intra-oral photos showing: A. Bluegrass appliance, B. orthodontic appliances

This could happen because of her poor swallowing pattern or thumb sucking returning

- Alternative treatment plans might include treatment with an appliance that had pointed spurs on it to irritate the tongue into a more posterior posture.

Another option is to just close the anterior spacing with bracketing and no habit appliance; however, without attempting to retrain the tongue and decrease the habit there would be a high risk of relapse

Self-study Questions

1. **What is the main difference between non-nutritive sucking habits that are benign and those that have deleterious oral effects?**

2. **In managing a patient's sucking habit, what is the most critical component to consider for success?**

3. **What intra-oral appliance types are available to aid in habit correction?**

4. **What types of extra-oral techniques can be used to reduce nonnutritive sucking habits?**

5. **Deleterious effects on the teeth and supporting structures are minimized if children will stop their digit sucking habits by approximately what age?**

Answers are located at the end of the case.

Bibliography

Dean JA, McDonald RE, Avery DR. 2004. Management of the developing occlusion. In: *Dentistry for the Child and Adolescent*, 8th edition. McDonald RE, Avery DR, Dean JA (eds) Mosby: St. Louis. pp. 625–83.

Kozlowski JT. 2007. A non-invasive method for ending thumb- and fingersucking habits. *J Clin Orthod* Oct;41(10):636.

SELF-STUDY ANSWERS

1. Patients with habits of minimal frequency, duration, or intensity have no or milder deleterious effects

2. The patient must be old enough to understand the need and must want to discontinue the habit

3. The Bluegrass or bead-type appliances and palatal spur or loop appliances

4. Commercially available foul tasting liquids painted on the digits, methods to isolate the digit from being inserted into the mouth such as a sock taped over the hand or a commercial strap wrapped around the thumb

5. Before age 6; that is, before eruption of the permanent teeth

Case 5

Interceptive Orthodontics—Anterior Crossbite in a Child in the Mixed Dentition

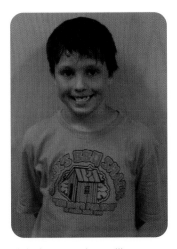

Figure 6.5.1. Facial photograph, smiling

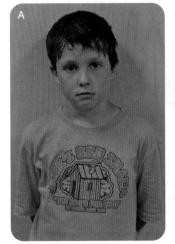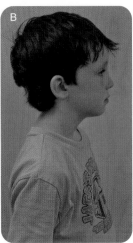

Figure 6.5.2a–b. Frontal and profile photos

A. Presenting Patient
- 8-year-, 1-month-old Caucasian male

B. Chief Complaint
- Mom states, "His teeth are very crooked"

C. Social History
- Non-contributory

D. Medical History
- Non-contributory

E. Medical Consult
- Not necessary at this time

F. Dental History
- The patient is seen for regular dental care and preventive measures. He has had minor restorative care
- Optimal water fluoridation levels (city water), with healthy diet, but has poor oral hygiene practices

G. Extra-oral Exam
- Mesofacial pattern with normal facial symmetry and slightly convex facial profile

H. Intra-oral Exam
- Dental class I relationship in the mixed dentition (Figure 6.5.3)
- 4-mm deep overbite with -5-mm overjet
- Anterior crossbite with no mandibular protrusive shift into maximum intercuspation
- Soft tissue normal, other than mild localized gingivitis
- Moderate plaque accumulation

I. Diagnostic Tools
- Panoramic and cepahalometric radiographs showed no significant skeletal discrepancies

J. Differential Diagnosis
- N/A

K. Diagnosis and Problem List
Diagnosis
- Dental and skeletal class I mixed dentition malocclusion

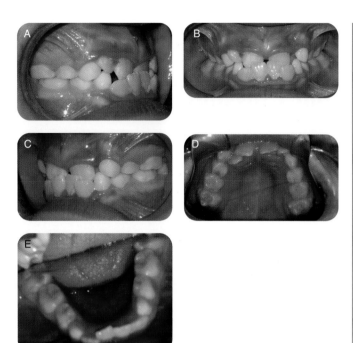

Figure 6.5.3a–e. Pre-op photos showing anterior crossbite

Problem List

- Anterior crossbite without anterior functional shift
- Moderate anterior crowding
- Need for improved oral hygiene

L. Comprehensive Treatment Plan

- Some single tooth anterior crossbites can be corrected with straightforward techniques such as finger springs. However, because of the amount of crowding and the fact that multiple teeth were involved in the crossbite, it was decided to treat this problem with maxillary orthodontic bands and brackets, as well as a lower lingual arch. The parents were cautioned that a second phase of orthodontic treatment would be needed in the permanent dentition

M. Peri-operative Intra-oral Photographs
Intra-operatively (Figure 6.5.4)

- This patient's sequence of treatment included:

1. Banding of second primary molars (since treatment alignment of first permanent molars

FUNDAMENTAL POINT 1
Diagnosis and Rationale for Treatment

- When considering treatment for crossbites, either anterior or posterior, it is important to evaluate the shifts of the mandible during closure, from the point of initial contact to maximum intercuspation. In either case, the clinician is evaluating the extent to which the crossbite etiology is dental inclination, skeletal positioning problems, or some combination of the two. As a general rule, dental inclinations are more easily managed than skeletal discrepancies. While many patients with crossbites will receive some benefit from correction, those with mandibular shifts, either protrusive or excursive, may benefit the most. The longer a patient with a shift retains that shift, the more long-term skeletal asymmetries will develop. Having these crossbites with shifts are like wearing a full-time functional appliance; however, unlike the appliances, the effect is not beneficial.

Anterior Crossbite Shifts

- Typically, an individual with an anterior crossbite will tend to shift the mandible in a protrusive direction. If there is a significant amount of protrusive shift and the maxillary incisors are very upright, the crossbite is usually more *dental* in nature and may be managed by flaring the maxillary incisors labially. If there is little to no protrusive

shift and the maxillary incisors are not necessarily upright, the patient should be evaluated cephalometrically for a class III *skeletal* problem. Usually, this can be accomplished by comparing the anterior portion of the maxilla (point A) with the anterior portion of the mandible (point B); that is, the "ANB" angle. It is also beneficial to evaluate the incisal inclination on the cephalometric radiograph. Class III skeletal problems may benefit from protraction headgear or some other skeletal correction, particularly in growing patients

Posterior Crossbite Shifts

- A mandibular shift from initial contact into maximum intercuspation and a crossbite indicates a bilateral posterior crossbite which can be from a maxillary skeletal constriction or dental buccal segment tipping. Bilateral crossbite patients will exhibit a shift of the dental midlines during closure, too, whereas those with unilateral crossbites will not. Interestingly, many appliances (W-arch, Hyrax, Quad helix, Expansion Plate, etc.) to varying extents, will effectively correct bilateral crossbites, both dental and skeletal. However, true unilateral crossbites benefit from an appliance design that only addresses the maxillary arch side that is causing the crossbite

Malandris and Mahoney (2004), Ngan et al. (1997)

was not problematic) and bracketing of remaining anterior teeth. A small amount of resin was added to the lower second primary molars to temporarily open the bite to prevent shearing off of the anterior brackets

2. After initial leveling and aligning, an open coil spring was placed to develop room for the lingually displaced tooth number 10. Once space was made, the tooth was brought into position

3. In an attempt to improve the lower alignment without bracketing and to maintain the class I permanent molar relationship during the transition into the full permanent dentition, the mesial surfaces of teeth M and R were disked and a lower lingual arch was placed

4. After maxillary debanding, a Hawley retainer was delivered

Post-operatively (Figure 6.5.5)

- Although tooth number 23 is still displaced labially, no additional treatment was planned until after leeway space utilization and transition into the permanent dentition had occurred

N. Prognosis and Discussion

- Correction of the crossbite should be retained well with little chance of relapse

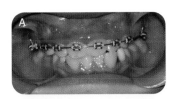
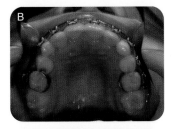
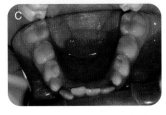

Figure 6.5.4a–c. Intra-operative intra-oral photos

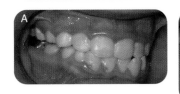
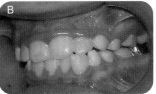
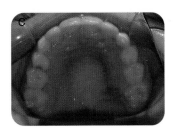
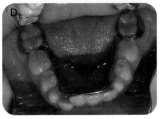

Figure 6.5.5a–d. Post-operative intra-oral photos showing correction of the crossbite and the lower lingual arch

O. Complications and Alternative Treatment Plan

• Expected complications are minimal. Due to the position of tooth number 23 after treatment,

bracketing of the lower anterior teeth or additional disking of teeth M and R might be necessary

---

Self-study Questions

1. *When correcting anterior and posterior crossbites, is it important to disclude or "open the bite" so that the treatment mechanics can move the affected teeth past the point of the crossbite?*

2. *An obtuse interincisal angle, "upright incisors," is a sign of which type of problem associated with an anterior crossbite, dental or skeletal?*

3. *Are coincident dental midlines upon maximum intercuspation a sign of a unilateral or bilateral posterior crossbite?*

4. *Is it true that a distinct advantage of early orthodontic treatment is that mandibular skeletal length can have clinically significant increases with early functional type appliances?*

5. *Name three reasons why a practitioner may decide to provide early orthodontic treatment.*

Answers are located at the end of the case.

Bibliography

Kluemper GT, Seeman CS, Hicks EP. 2000. Early orthodontic treatment: what are the imperatives? *J Am Dent Assoc* 131:613–20.

Malandris M, Mahoney EK. 2004. Aetiology, diagnosis and treatment of posterior cross-bites in the primary dentition. *Inter J Paed Dent* 14:155–66.

Ngan P, Hu AM, Fields Jr HW. 1997. Treatment of class III problems begins with differential diagnosis of anterior crossbites. *Pediat Dent* 19:386–95.

Tulloch JF, Proffit WR, Phillips C. 2004. Outcomes in a 2-phase randomized clinical trial of early Class II treatment. *Am J Orthod Dentofacial Orthop* 125(6):657–67.

SELF-STUDY ANSWERS

1. An often misunderstood concept is that occlusal acrylic pads or other bite opening technique is needed to correct crossbites. In fact, this is generally not necessary. The main reasons for doing so would be if the crossbite itself interferes with the appliance to be used or if there is pathology associated with the affected teeth

2. Upright incisors are an indication of a dental etiology

3. Unilateral crossbite, because there is no mandibular shift as the teeth occlude straight into the crossbite

4. No, research has shown that typical initial significant improvements in mandibular length do not maintain themselves when patients are re-examined at the end of normal growth

5. (a) Pathology exists, such as with traumatic occlusion; (b) failure to correct the malocclusion will result in skeletal asymmetries, such as with a bilateral posterior crossbite; (c) the patient/parent understands some of the inherent inefficiencies, but requests early correction for esthetic reasons

Case 6

Patient with Craniofacial Anomaly

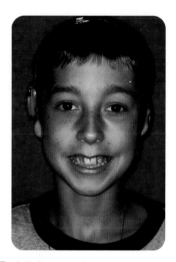

Figure 6.6.1. Facial photograph

A. Presenting Patient
- 13-year-old Caucasian male

B. Chief Complaint
- Mom states, "My child has a cleft, jaw problems, a hearing problem, and dental problems"

C. Social History
- Patient is a happy, well developed adolescent
- Parents are married and living with children
- Middle income socioeconomic status
- One younger brother

D. Medical History
- Bilateral otomandibular dysostosis
- Cleft palate
- Congenital bilateral aural atresia (development failure of the external ear canal)

E. Medical Consult
- Patient is followed by a children's hospital craniofacial anomalies team, which includes multispecialty providers

---

FUNDAMENTAL POINT 1
Craniofacial Team Management

- Craniofacial team management is extremely important for patients with craniofacial anomalies. Multispecialty collaboration in a unified team clinic setting allows for ready communication and well coordinated care. Team members typically include pediatricians, otolaryngologists, audiologists, speech pathologists, plastic surgeons, oral surgeons, pediatric dentists, orthodontists, nurses, feeding specialists, and others. Of particular importance are established treatment guidelines established by various groups, including the American Cleft Palate Craniofacial Association: http://www.acpa-cpf.org/teamcare/Parameters04rev.pdf. Also see FACES: The National Craniofacial Association: http://www.faces-cranio.org/

Jones et al. (2004)

F. Dental History
- The child has had regular dental maintenance visits
- Optimal water fluoridation levels (city water)
- High-carbohydrate diet with extremely poor oral hygiene habits

G. Extra-oral Exam
- Dolichofacial pattern with significant mandibular retrognathia and significant dysplasia of his right ear with the external portion of his audient bone conduction hearing device visible in his pre-op photos (Figure 6.6.2.)

H. Intra-oral Exam
- Permanent dentition with generalized white spot and multiple cavitated carious lesions (Figure 6.6.3.)

- Moderate to severe generalized gingivitis and missing teeth number 3 and 19.
- 1-mm overbite with 5-mm overjet
- Mild to moderate plaque accumulation
- Very poor oral hygiene

I. Diagnostic Tools

- Patient's initial panoramic radiograph reveals periapical pathology on teeth number 3 and 30, unerupted third molars (Figure 6.6.4.)
- Short-term follow-up panoramic radiograph after initiation of caries management program (Figure 6.6.5.)
- The lateral cephalogram demonstrates long lower facial height and severe mandibular retrognathia and steep mandibular plane angle (Figure 6.6.6.)

J. Differential Diagnosis

- N/A

K. Diagnosis and Problem List

Diagnosis

- Class II skeletal and dental malocclusion
- Multiple carious lesions
- Severe gingivitis

Problem List

- High caries risk (Stec-Slonicz, Szczepanska, and Hirschfelder 2007)

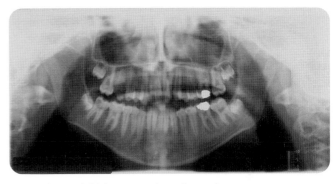

Figure 6.6.4. Initial panoramic radiograph

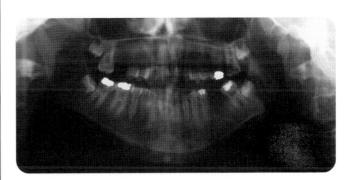

Figure 6.6.5. Pre-op panoramic radiograph showing restorations

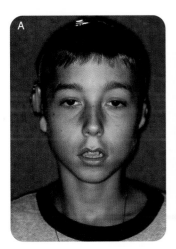
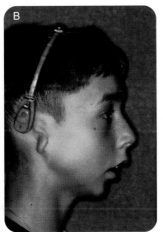

Figure 6.6.2a–b. Pre-op extra-oral photos

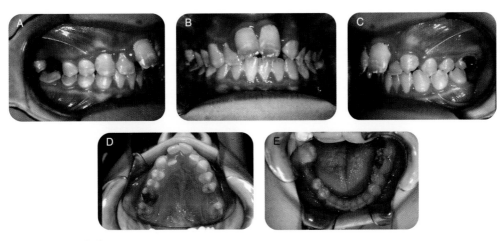

Figure 6.6.3a–e. Pre-op intra-oral photos

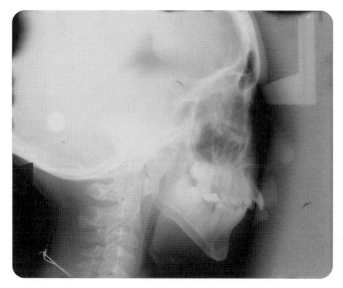

Figure 6.6.6. Pre-op lateral cephalometric radiograph

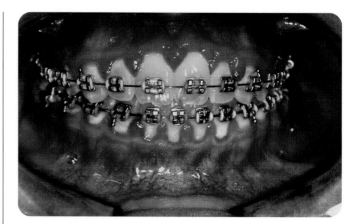

Figure 6.6.7. Pre-surgical intra-oral photo

BACKGROUND INFORMATION 1
Orthognathic Surgery Basic Overview

- Maxilla-Le Fort I osteotomy: Involves a transverse sectioning of the maxilla to accomplish various repositionings of the bone for proper three-dimensional alignment with the base of the skull and mandible

- Mandible-bilateral split sagittal osteotomy: Involves a vertical sectioning of the mandible in the mandibular ramus, distal to the dentition for the most part to allow either forward or backward repositioning of the anterior segment of the mandible

- Chin button-genioplasty: This procedure involving the bony portion of the chin allows realignment or recontouring of the chin to enhance its position relative to the face

- For a more complete discussion of orthognathic surgery with extensive diagrams and clinical photos, see eMedicine from WebMD (http://www.emedicine.com/plastic/topic177.htm)

Chigurupati (2005)

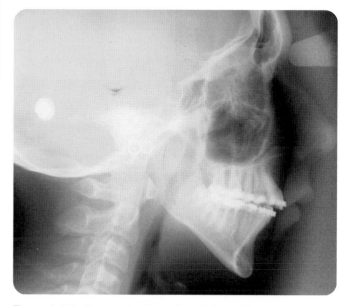

Figure 6.6.8. Pre-surgical lateral cephalometric radiograph

- Poor oral hygiene contributing to gingivitis
- Extracted teeth numbers 3 and 19
- Mandibular retrognathia
- Steep mandibular plane angle
- Long lower facial height

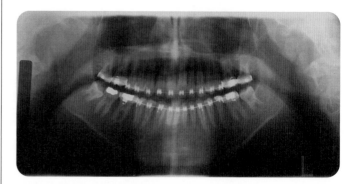

Figure 6.6.9. Pre-surgical panoramic radiograph

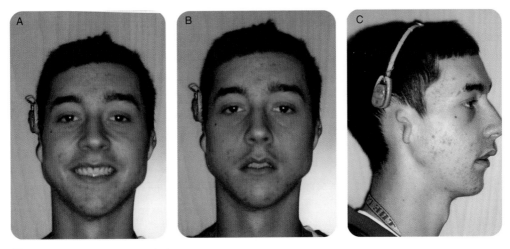

Figure 6.6.10a–c. Two-year post-op extra-oral photos

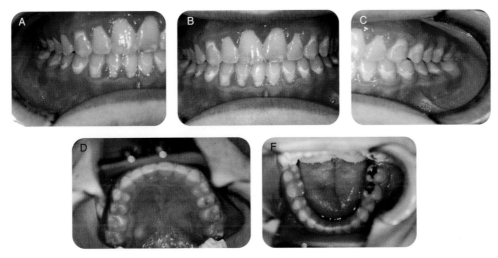

Figure 6.6.11a–e. Two-year post-op intra-oral photos

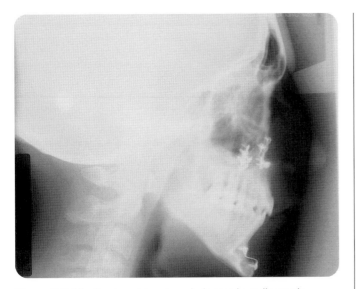

Figure 6.6.12. Post-op lateral cephalometric radiograph

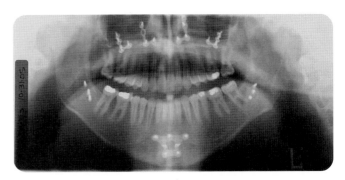

Figure 6.6.13. Post-op panoramic radiograph

L. Comprehensive Treatment Plan

- The patient's caries management program was initiated, including appropriate oral hygiene instruction, diet counseling, fluoride analysis and therapy, and dental restorations and extractions
- Coordinated case conference and treatment plan with pediatric dentist, orthodontist, oral surgeon, and plastic surgeon
- Plan included caries management, pre- and post-surgical orthodontics, orthognathic surgery to include Le Fort I maxillary osteotomy impaction and bilateral sagittal split ramus osteotomy for mandibular advancement, genioplasty, and eventual ear reconstruction

M. Immediate Pre-surgical Images

- Note the generally acceptable alignment and space closure secondary to presurgical orthodontics (Figures 6.6.7, 6.6.8, and 6.6.9.)

N. Post-operative Images

- Two years after surgery (Figures 6.6.10, 6.6.11, 6.6.12, and 6.6.13.)

- Note that malocclusion is corrected but, due to poor oral hygiene, multiple areas of caries and demineralization exist

O. Prognosis and Discussion

- The overall result and prognosis for this patient is good. The dental alignment was excellent; however, he still presents with a significant convex facial profile and lengthened lower facile height

P. Complications and Alternative Treatment Plan

- As in many cases with significant dental and skeletal changes, long-term stability for this case is a concern. However, more than two years after his surgery, his result has suffered little relapse
- Despite attempts to manage his caries and gingivitis, the patient's poor compliance resulted in significant demineralization of the facial surfaces of multiple teeth. Although multiple avenues for remedy (bleaching, enamel microabrasion, bonding, etc.) were recommended, the patient has not pursued any additional dental care

Self-study Questions

1. *Hemifacial microsomia includes what constellation of problems?*
2. *What are the timing considerations when considering extraction of badly carious first permanent molar to be substituted by the second permanent molar?*
3. *List some advantages of team management of craniofacial patients*

4. *What are the names of three common orthognathic surgical procedures?*
5. *What are some common procedures to manage high-caries-risk patients during orthodontic treatment?*

Answers are located at the end of the case.

Bibliography

Chigurupati R. 2005. Orthognathic surgery for secondary cleft and craniofacial deformities. *Oral Maxillofac Surg Clin North Am* 17(3):503–17.

Jones JE, Sadove AM, Dean JA, Huebener DV. 2004. Multidisciplinary team approach to cleft lip and palate

management. In: *Dentistry for the Child and Adolescent.* McDonald RE, Avery DR, Dean JA (eds) Mosby: St. Louis. pp. 684–711.

Stec-Slonicz M, Szczepanska J, Hirschfelder U. 2007. Comparison of caries prevalence in two populations of cleft patients. *Cleft Palate Craniofac J* 44(5):532–7.

SELF-STUDY ANSWERS

1. Underdevelopment on one side of the mandible, which involves problems with the ear and hearing

2. If possible, it is advantageous to extract the first permanent molar months prior to eruption of the second permanent molar (by age 10) to facilitate mesial drift, molar substitution, and uprighting

3. Increased coordination and communication between specialty providers, development of management protocols for efficiency and effectiveness, team cooperation and consultation for increased quality of care, and reduced patient/parent absence from school/work because appointments are simultaneous and coordinated

4. Maxillary Le Fort I osteotomy, mandibular bilateral split sagittal osteotomy, genioplasty

5. Do not start treatment until caries risk is considered to be low. Increase oral hygiene (brushing, flossing, high frequency toothbrushes, parental involvement in hands-on oral hygiene procedures), at-home fluoride mouth rinses, in-office fluoride varnish administration, fluoride-releasing orthodontic elastic ties, use of remineralizing products containing amorphous calcium phosphate (ACP)

7

Behavior Management and Medical Emergencies

Michael D. Webb, Diane L. Howell, and Amr M. Moursi

Clinical Cases in Pediatric Dentistry, First Edition. Edited by Amr M. Moursi.
© 2012 Blackwell Publishing Ltd. Pubished 2012 by Blackwell Publishing Ltd.

Case 1

Non-pharmacological Behavior Management

A. Presenting Patient
- 5-year-, 10-month-old Hispanic female

B. Chief Complaint
- Mom states, "My daughter needs a check up"

C. Social History
- Parents are married
- Mother is the primary caregiver and does not work outside the home, father is a construction worker
- Lower socio-economic status
- One brother, age 4
- The child does not participate in activities outside the home

D. Medical History
- Review of systems is negative
- No allergies to medication, mild seasonal allergies
- No routine medications
- No previous hospitalizations or surgeries; no emergency room visits

E. Medical Consult
- Not necessary at this time

F. Dental History
- This is the patient's first comprehensive dental visit. She has been examined at a dental screening in a nearby community center. Patient was uncooperative for exam but mother was told the patient had no decay
- Patient lives in a fluoridated community and uses city water
- Brushes unsupervised twice daily with fluoridated toothpaste. Patient "does not allow" mother to assist with brushing
- Highly cariogenic diet with frequent snacks and juice
- No previous dental treatments

- No history of dental trauma or habits
- Parents and siblings have not had any dental care in "several years"
- Patient clings to the parent as they are escorted to the operatory. Patient barely speaks to members of the dental team

G. Extra-oral Exam
- Head and neck: Within normal limits
- Weight and height, BMI: Within normal limits
- Exposed extremities (bruising, etc.): Within normal limits

H. Intra-oral Exam
Soft Tissues
- Within normal limits

Hard Tissues
- Occlusal caries on teeth S and L, good spacing with no interproximal caries noted

---

BACKGROUND INFORMATION 1
Functional Inquiry

- The functional inquiry consists of the following questions:
  - How do you think your child has reacted to past medical procedures?
  - How would you rate your own anxiety (fear, nervousness) at this moment?
  - Does your child think there is anything wrong with his or her teeth, such as a chipped tooth, decayed tooth, gum boil?
  - How do you expect your child to react in the dental chair?

Wright and Stigers (2010)

Dentition
- Full primary dentition

Occlusion
- Mesial step with normal overjet and overbite

I. Diagnostic Tools
- No additional diagnostics were obtained

J. Differential Diagnosis
- N/A

K. Diagnosis and Problem List
Diagnosis
- Early childhood caries

Problem List
- Fearful patient

FUNDAMENTAL POINT 1

Communication Techniques for Anxious Patients

- Child should be welcomed in to a child friendly environment
- There is a triangular relationship between the dentist, the child and the family
- Functional inquiry should be part of the history form: negative response to more than one question increases the chance of encountering a behavior problem
- Consider the communication advantages of having the parent in the operatory:
  - Parent can see firsthand how the child behaves
  - Parent may be able to facilitate communication, especially with a special needs child or when language is an issue
  - Very young children may not separate easily from the parent
- Consider the communication disadvantages of having the parent in the operatory:
  - Parent can interfere with communication between the dentist and the child
  - The child may divide her attention between the dentist and the parent
  - The child may be less willing to cooperate with the dentist when the parent is present

Wright and Stigers (2010)

- Poorly compliant parent
- Poor diet
- Poor oral hygiene
- No dental home

L. Comprehensive Treatment Plan
- Establish dental home
- Establish aggressive caries prevention plan
- Restore decay on teeth S and L using appropriate behavior management
- Recall on three-month interval

M. Prognosis and Discussion
- The child is apprehensive during the examination but will sit in the chair by herself with the mother sitting nearby. The patient follows instructions to open and close mouth but with apprehension and some crying. The tell-show-do method should be effective in this situation

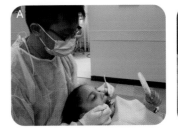
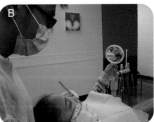

Figure 7.1.1a–b. Tell-show-do. A mirror is used while telling the patient what to expect

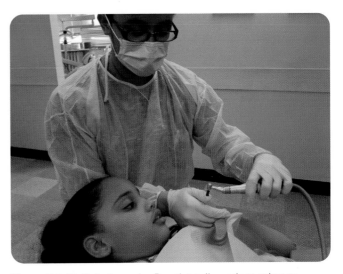

Figure 7.1.2. Tell-show-do. Dentist tells patient what to expect

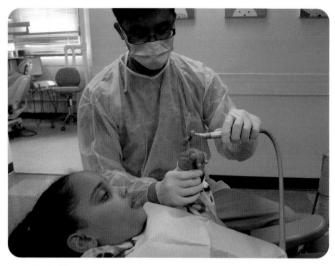

Figure 7.1.3. Tell-show-do. Dentist shows patient what to expect

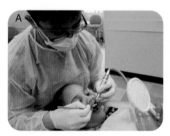 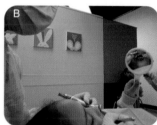

Figure 7.1.4a–b. Tell-show-do. Dentist does what patient expects while patient watches in mirror. Note anxious sibling in background

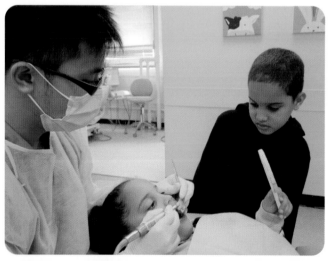

Figure 7.1.5. Modeling. Dentist demonstrates while sibling watches

N. Common Complications and Alternative Treatment Plans

- Despite her initial cooperation, the patient could became uncooperative and combative later on. If this occurs, then other forms of behavior management may need to be considered

BACKGROUND INFORMATION 2
Non-pharmacologic Behavior Management Techniques
Tell-Show-Do

- See Figures 7.1.1 through 7.1.4
- Tell the patient what to expect using phrases that are appropriate to the developmental level
- Show the procedure or instrument in a non-threatening manner
- Perform the procedure without deviating from the explanation and reminding the patient of the previous explanations and demonstrations

Voice Control

- Use controlled modulation of voice volume to direct the patient's behavior. This technique should be described to parents unfamiliar with its use

Positive Reinforcement

- Reward positive behavior through social (voice tone) and non-social (tokens, prizes) reinforcement

Distraction

- Divert the patient's attention from what may be perceived as an unpleasant experience. This can be visual (watching a movie) or auditory (listening to music or a story)

AAPD (2011–12)

Self-study Questions

1. *What are the important questions to ask to assess the possible behavior of the patient?*
2. *How do you accomplish tell-show-do?*
3. *What are the advantages and disadvantages of having a parent in the operatory?*

4. *Should the dental team be trained in behavior management skills? Why?*
5. *What are the options available for behavior management if communication methods fail?*

Answers are located at the end of the case.

Bibliography

American Academy of Pediatric Dentistry. 2011–2012. Reference Manual, *Guideline on Behavior Guidance for the Pediatric Dental Patient*, 33(6):161–73.

Wright GZ, Stigers J. 2010. Non-pharmacolgical management of children's behavior. In *Dentistry for the Child and Adolescent*, 9th Edition. McDonald R, Avery D, Dean J (eds) Mosby: Maryland Heights, MO.

SELF-STUDY ANSWERS

1. It is important to ask questions in the functional inquiry about behavior at previous medical or dental visits, parental anxiety about dentistry, the child's perception of her oral health, and how the parents expect the child to behave. It is also helpful to ask about child development status, behavior in daycare or preschool, and previous dental experiences of parents and siblings

2. First tell the patient what is going to be done, then demonstrate the action, and then perform the procedure and simultaneously explain it

3. The advantages of having a parent in the operatory are that the parent can see firsthand how the child behaves, the parent may be able to facilitate communication—especially with a disabled child—and very young children may not separate from the parent. The disadvantages are that the parent can interfere with communication between the pediatric dentist and the child, the child may divide her attention between the dentist and the parent, and the dentist may divide his attention between the child and the parent. Sometimes the child may not be as willing to cooperate with the dentist's instructions when the parent is present

4. The dental team should be trained in behavior management techniques because the staff is an extension of the dentist. This allows the dental team to work together to communicate with the child

5. If communication methods fail, protective stabilization or pharmacological methods can be considered

Case 2

Pharmacological Behavior Management

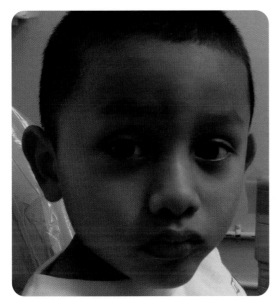

Figure 7.2.1. Facial photograph

A. Presenting Patient
- 4-year-, 10-month-old Hispanic male

B. Chief Complaint
- Mom states, "My son is here to have his cavities fixed with sedation"

C. Social History
- Mother is the primary caregiver
- Patient lives with parents and one brother, age 10
- Mother works full-time outside the home; father is unemployed
- Lower socio-economic status
- Patient does not participate in any sports

D. Medical History
- Review of systems is negative
- No known allergies to any foods or medications
- No medications

FUNDAMENTAL POINT 1
Patient Assessment

- When reviewing the patient's medical history and performing an assessment of the patient's general health on the day of sedation, keep in mind that the American Society of Anesthesiologists (ASA) uses a physical status classification system which serves as a risk assessment

- A careful pre-sedation evaluation for underlying health conditions that would place the patient at an increased risk for complications during sedation must be completed

- Only patients who are ASA I are routinely accepted as appropriate candidates for in-office moderate sedation

- Patients who are ASA II or III require consultation with the patient's primary care provider to identify any concerns regarding the administration of sedation medications

- Patients who are ASA III typically are treated in the hospital setting with anesthesiologists to manage potential complications

ASA Physical Status Classification System

- Class I: Normal healthy patient
- Class II: Patient with mild systemic disease
- Class III: Patient with severe systemic disease
- Class IV: Patient with a severe systemic disease that is a constant threat to life
- Class V: Moribund patient who is not expected to survive without the operation

See http://www.asahq.org/clinical/physicalstatus.htm for the complete ASA classification system

- Hospitalization at age 3 for dental treatment under general anesthesia
- American Society of Anesthesiologists (ASA) class I

E. Medical Consult
- Not necessary at this time

F. Dental History
- Highly cariogenic diet with frequent sugared soft drinks and snacks
- Patient lives in a fluoridated community using city water, and mom states the child brushes his teeth once every day with fluoridated toothpaste without supervision; does not floss
- Patient was treated for full mouth dental rehabilitation under general anesthesia in the ambulatory care center at age 3. Treatment also included surgical repair of a left mandibular abscess that had resulted in left facial cellulitis
- After the initial post-operative follow-up appointment the patient did not return for recall visits
- No history of trauma
- Patient is uncooperative and extremely anxious, clinging to his mother

G. Extra-oral Exam
- Head and neck: Within normal limits
- Weight and height, BMI: Within normal limits
- Exposed extremities: Within normal limits, negative for bruising
- Other: Heart sounds normal, breath sounds clear with no evidence of upper respiratory infection
- Patient has not taken any food or liquid by mouth (NPO) since midnight

H. Intra-oral Exam
Soft Tissues
- Within normal limits, Brodsky scale 2

Hard Tissues
- Multiple severe carious lesions

Dentition
- Primary dentition

Occlusion
- Crossbite on right

FUNDAMENTAL POINT 2
Goals of Pharmacological Behavior Management

- As stated by the American Academy of Pediatric Dentistry, the goals of sedation for children undergoing diagnostic and therapeutic procedures include:
  - Ensure the patient's safety and welfare
  - Minimize discomfort and pain
  - Control anxiety and minimize psychological trauma
  - Maximize amnesia
  - Control behavior or patient movement so the procedure can be completed safely
  - Return the patient to the pre-sedation level to allow for safe discharge from medical supervision
- The provider shall obtain and document appropriate informed consent according to local, state, and institutional requirements

§ For further information see the American Academy of Pediatric Dentistry *Clinical Guideline on Monitoring and Management of Pediatric Patients During and After Sedation for Diagnostic and Therapeutic Procedures*

http://www.aapd.org/media/policies.asp

I. Diagnostic Tools
- Bitewing radiographs

J. Differential Diagnosis
- N/A

K. Diagnosis and Problem List
Diagnosis
- Recurrent early childhood caries

Problem List
- No dental home
- Poor oral hygiene and diet
- Uncooperative and exhibits situational anxiety

L. Comprehensive Treatment Plan
- Establish dental home

FUNDAMENTAL POINT 3
Patient Assessment: Brodsky Scale

- To help minimize the potential for airway obstruction in children receiving oral sedation medications, an airway assessment must be completed prior to sedation to check for airway abnormalities or large tonsils

- The Brodsky scale indicates how much space the tonsillar tissue occupies in the pharyngeal area

- Patients with a Brodsky of +3 (meaning the tonsillar tissue takes up more than 50% of the pharyngeal space) are at an increased risk of developing airway obstruction (see example in Figure 7.2.2)

- Patients with a Brodsky of +3 or greater should be considered for alternative pharmacologic management, i.e., general anesthesia or no sedation to maintain a patent airway

McDonald et al. (2004)

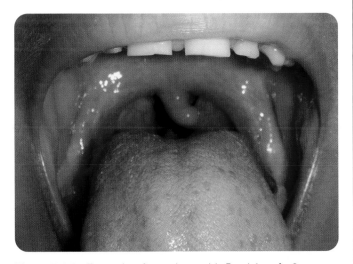

Figure 7.2.2. Example of a patient with Brodsky of +3

- Implement aggressive caries prevention plan
- Due to anxiety and the extent of the restorations, treatment will require the use of oral sedative medications in conjunction with nitrous oxide to assure the patient's comfort level and tolerance of the procedure

Post-op Care

- Minimize vigorous activity for the patient
- Pay attention to lip numbing while the patient attempts to eat
- Maintain a bland and soft diet for the day
- Follow-up visit in two weeks

M. Prognosis and Discussion

- Based on the history, this child has a high likelihood of caries recurrence
- Patient has already required a general anesthesia appointment and sedation to treat caries
- An aggressive prevention plan should be implemented
- The parent should be advised that routine recall visits of at least three months interval are necessary to maintain the patient's oral health and monitor home care. These less invasive visits will provide an opportunity to reduce anxiety about dental visits

N. Common Complications and Alternative Treatment Plans

- What are your options if the oral sedative medications fail to adequately control the patient's anxiety and movement during the case?
- What is the appropriate intervention if the patient becomes apneic?

FUNDAMENTAL POINT 4
American Academy of Pediatric Dentistry Guidelines for Monitoring

- Continuous monitoring of oxygen saturation and heart rate, and intermittent recording of respiratory rate and blood pressure that should be recorded on a time-based record

- Frequent checking of restraint devices to prevent airway obstruction or chest restriction

- Frequent checking of the patient's head position to ensure airway patency

- Presence of a functioning suction apparatus

- Monitoring requirements depend on the level of sedation. Minimal, moderate, and deep sedation all have different monitoring guidelines

FUNDAMENTAL POINT 5
Selecting Sedative Medications

- To achieve the goals of sedation in children while minimizing adverse events, the lowest dose of a drug with the highest chance of success for the procedure should be chosen
- For painful procedures, include an analgesic such as an opiod like Meperidine
- For non-painful procedures, a sedative can be used, such as a benzodiazepine like Midazolam (Versed®). A sedative hypnotic also can be used, such as Chloral Hydrate

- For procedures that require both sedation and analgesia, choose either single agents with both sedative/analgesic properties, or combination drug therapy
- Anxiolysis and amnesia are also considered when choosing drug regimens
- The more drugs that are mixed, the greater the chance of adverse events such hypoventilation, apnea, or airway obstruction

McDonald, et al. (2004), AAPD (2011–12)

BACKGROUND INFORMATION 1
Pharmacology of Benzodiazepines

- Benzodiazepines are commonly used as amnestics in the outpatient sedation of children
- Benzodiazepines enhance the binding of GABA, the primary inhibitory neurotransmitter of the central nervous system
- Benzodiazepines produce sedation, anxiolysis, amnesia, and suppression of seizure activity
- At moderate doses, patients who have received benzodiazepines will be conscious, yet sedate, and will not remember the procedure

- At high doses, benzodiazepines will result in unconsciousness and loss of protective airway reflexes
- Common benzodiazepines include Midazolam (Versed®) and Diazepam (Valium®)
- When combined with narcotics, the respiratory depressant effects are synergistic
- Benzodiazepines produce little direct cardiovascular effects

Coté et al. (2001), Duke and Rosenburg (1996)

BACKGROUND INFORMATION 2
Pharmacology of Opioids

- The main opioid receptors are Mu_1 and Mu_2
  - Analgesia occurs through Mu_1 receptors
  - Respiratory depression, bradycardia, and euphoria occur through Mu_2
- Meperidine is commonly used in the outpatient sedation of children, usually in combination with Versed® or Chloral Hydrate
  - There tends to be less respiratory depression with meperidine than morphine in children, but each child responds differently, so monitoring is essential

Duke and Rosenburg (1996), Katzung (1998)

BACKGROUND INFORMATION 3
Pharmacology of Chloral Hydrate

- Chloral hydrate is considered an older sedative hypnotic, an alcohol by structure
- Commonly used, inexpensive, and well absorbed by mouth (PO), it has minimal effects on respiration, with sedation in about 30 to 45 minutes
- It is NOT an analgesic
- Sedation can result in airway obstruction, especially in the presence of large tonsils
- Chloral Hydrate tastes bad and can cause nausea and vomiting

Duke and Rosenburg (1996), Katzung (1998)

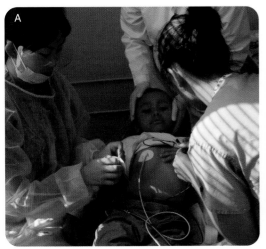
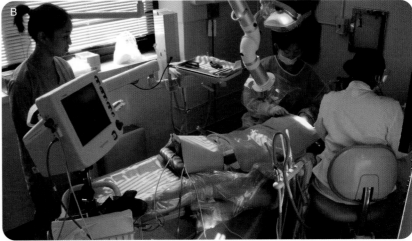

Figure 7.2.3a–b. Patient with monitors and protective stabilization during sedation

---

FUNDAMENTAL POINT 6
Discharge Criteria

- Children should be monitored as they recover from sedation. Do not be fooled by thinking that just because the dentistry is done, the child is recovered. With the loss of surgical stimuli, the child may actually become more sedated

- Children are ready to be discharged if at least the following criteria are met:
  - Pre-sedation level of consciousness is attained
  - Respiratory rate and rhythm, heart rate, and oxygen saturation are within normal limits
  - Pre-sedation level of ambulation is attained

- Patient can swallow oral fluids; demonstrates return of gag reflex or cough
- Patient has no nausea, vomiting, dizziness
- Medications with a longer half life may require longer periods of supervised recovery due to the possibility of resedation
- Patients who have received reversal agents also require a longer period of supervised recovery because the sedative medication tends to last longer than the reversal agent, posing a potential for resedation

Coté et al. (2001), AAPD (2011–12)

Self-study Questions

1. **What important history and physical observations are required before administering sedative medications to a patient?**

2. **To minimize risk to the pediatric dental patient receiving sedation, what are the requirements of a safe environment for in-office administration of sedation?**

3. **What are some of the potential complications of sedation in the office that the provider should be prepared to handle?**

4. **What are the different types of sedation available to patients, provided the dentist has the proper educational qualifications?**

Answers are located at the end of the case.

Bibliography

American Academy of Pediatric Dentistry. 2011–2012. *Clinical Guideline for Monitoring and Management of Pediatric Patients During and After Sedation for Diagnostic and Therapeutic Procedures*. Reference manual. Pediatr Dent 33(6):185–201.

Coté CJ, Ryan J, Todres ID, Goudsouzian NG. 2001. *A Practice of Anesthesia for Infants and Children*, 3rd edition. W.B. Saunders Company: Philadelphia.

Duke J, Rosenburg SG. 1996. *Anesthesia Secrets*. Hanley and Belfus, Inc.: Philadelphia.

Katzung BG. 1998. *Basic and Clinical Pharmacology*, 7th edition. Appleton and Lange: Stamford.

McDonald RE, Avery DR, Dean JA. 2004. *Dentistry for the Child and Adolescent*, 8th edition. Mosby: St. Louis.

SELF-STUDY ANSWERS

1. The pre-sedation history and physical should include information regarding allergies to foods or medicines, current prescription or over-the-counter medications, medical disease processes, previous hospitalizations and surgeries, review of body systems, weight in kilograms, history of anesthesia or sedation and any complications, vital signs, airway evaluation, ASA class, and NPO status

2. Requirements for a safe environment for in-office administration of sedative agents include appropriate educational training, support personnel trained in monitoring the patient, and adequate rescue equipment and personnel who know how to use it. Everyone should be competent in basic life support techniques, and the primary provider should be trained in pediatric advanced airway skills

3. Common complications of sedation include hypoventilation, airway obstruction, allergic reactions, apnea, laryngospasm, aspiration, and cardiopulmonary impairment. Personnel involved in the sedation of pediatric patients must be trained in airway rescue techniques that support ventilation and oxygenation, as well have portable oxygen sources and bag-valve-mask apparatus available for use

4. The American Academy of Pediatric Dentistry defines and characterizes three types of sedation: minimal, moderate, and deep. The other type of sedation available is general anesthesia, which, with the right educational requirements, can be in office or in a hospital setting.

Case 3

Intraoperative Pain Management

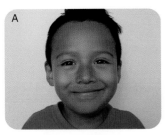 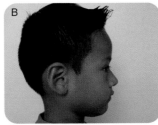

Figure 7.3.1a–b. Facial photographs

A. Presenting Patient
- 6-year-, 2-month-old male

B. Chief Complaint
- Mom states, "My son is here to get his teeth fixed"

C. Social History
- Parents are married
- Mother is the primary caregiver and does not work outside the home
- Patient lives with both parents and a younger brother, age 3
- Socio-economic status is middle class
- Patient is in first grade

D. Medical History
- Review of systems is negative
- No allergies
- No routine medications
- No previous hospitalizations or surgeries
- One emergency room visit for trauma to patient's arm when he fell off a swing set at age 5

E. Medical Consult
- Not necessary at this time

F. Dental History
- This is the patient's third dental visit.
- He was previously seen for a new patient examination then had restorative care

- The patient lives in a fluoridated community and uses city water
- Mother brushes the child's teeth once a day with a fluoridated toothpaste
- Cariogenic diet
- No history of dental trauma
- The patient is cooperative and gets up in the dental chair by himself

G. Extra-oral Exam
- Head and neck: Within normal limits
- Weight and height, BMI: Within normal limits
- Exposed extremities (bruising, etc.): Within normal limits

H. Intra-oral Exam
Soft Tissues
- Within normal limits

Hard Tissues
- Dental decay on teeth J and K requiring intracoronal restorations. Occlusal restorations present in teeth A and T

Dentition
- Full primary dentition

Occlusion
- Flush terminal plane with normal overjet and overbite

I. Diagnostic Tools
- Bitewing radiographs show normally developing dentition with no evidence of interproximal decay

J. Differential Diagnosis
- N/A

K. Diagnosis and Problem List
Diagnosis
- Dental caries

Problem List

- No dental home
- Poor oral hygiene and diet
- Caries risk assessment is high

L. Comprehensive Treatment Plan

- Patient is cooperative for dental treatment
- Dental caries requiring restoration using local anesthesia
- Implement aggressive prevention plan
- Recall visits at least every six months

M. Prognosis and Discussion

- The patient has a guarded prognosis for future dental caries due to poor oral hygiene and diet and the lack of a dental home

---

BACKGROUND INFORMATION 1

Local Anesthesia Administration

- Discomfort of local anesthesia administration can be lessened by:

  - Use of topical anesthetics: Available in gels and sprays

  - Counter irritation: Application of vibratory stimulation or moderate pressure at the site of injection (Figure 7.3.3.)

  - Distraction: Maintain constant communication to keep attention away from syringe

  - Slow rate of administration: Administration of a cartridge of anesthetic should take at least one minute

Pinkam et al. (2005)

FUNDAMENTAL POINT 1

Maximum Doses of Local Anesthetics in Children

- Articaine: 7.0 mg/kg, 3.2 mg/lb, 500 mg total
- Lidocaine: 4.4 mg/kg, 2 mg/lb, 300 mg total
- Mepivicaine: 4.4 mg/kg, 2 mg/lb, 300 mg total
- Prilocaine: 6 mg/kg, 2.7 mg/lb, 400 mg total
- Bupivicaine: 2 mg/kg, 0.9 mg/lb, 90 mg total
- Etidocaine: 8 mg/kg, 3.6 mg/lb, 400 mg total

Vargas (2011)

- Establishment of a dental home and compliance with a rigorous prevention plan would improve the prognosis and caries risk assessment
- It is important to give very clear post-operative instructions to the patient and parents. They must be instructed to avoid any manipulation (chewing, scratching, etc.) of the anesthetized tissue to avoid self-inflicted trauma

N. Common Complications and Alternative Treatment Plans

- What should you do if you reach the maximum recommended amount of local anesthetic and the child is still complaining of pain?

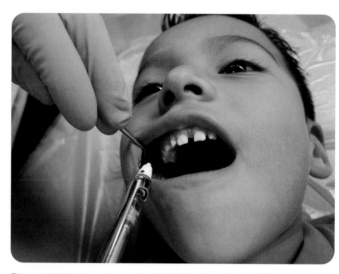

Figure 7.3.2. Local anesthetic infiltration in maxillary vestibule

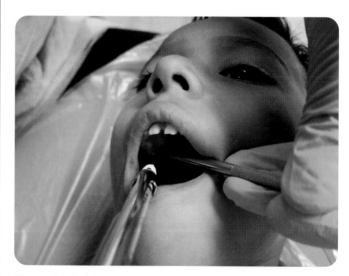

Figure 7.3.3. Local anesthetic palatal infiltration. Mirror handle is used as counter irritation.

- What should you do if the child bites his lip or tongue after receiving local anesthesia?
- What other types of local anesthetics could be used?

- What are some behavior management techniques that could be used to help with the administration of local anesthesia?
- What are the subjective signs of local anesthesia?

BACKGROUND INFORMATION 2

Local Anesthesia Complications

Paresthesia From Local Anesthesia

- Defined as persistent anesthesia beyond the expected duration
- Caused by trauma to the nerve or "electric shock" on injection
- Risk is 1:1,200,000 for 0.5%, 2%, and 3% local anesthetics
- Risk is 1:500,000 for 4% local anesthetics
- Most cases resolve in eight weeks

Soft Tissue Trauma

- Caused by chewing or biting soft tissue while numb
- Bilateral mandibular block does not increase the risk of soft tissue trauma when compared to unilateral mandibular block

- Use local anesthetics that minimize the residual soft tissue anesthesia
- Advise caregivers of the amount of time that the soft tissue will be numb
- If possible, have the child bite on cotton rolls until the soft tissue anesthesia has worn off

Signs of Local Anesthetic Toxicity (Overdose)

- Early signs: Dizziness, anxiety, confusion, tachycardia, increased blood pressure
- Later signs: Seizure activity, bradycardia, cardiac arrest

AAPD (2011–12)

Self-study Questions

1. **What is the maximum mg/kg and total dose of: (a) lidocaine, (b) mepivicaine, and (c) articaine?**
2. **What is the total amount of lidocaine that can be given to this child if he weighs 52 pounds?**
3. **What is an anatomical difference between children and adults with respect to**

administration of the inferior alveolar nerve block?

4. **What is the mechanism of action of local anesthetics?**
5. **What are the signs of local anesthetic toxicity?**

Answers are located at the end of the case.

Bibliography

American Academy of Pediatric Dentistry. 2011–2012. Guideline on Use of Local Anesthesia for Pediatric Dental Patients, Reference Manual. *Pediatr Dent* 33(6):174–80.

Vargas KG. 2011. Pain Control. In: The Handbook of Pediatric Dentistry, 4th Edition. Nowak AJ, Casamassimo PS (eds). American Academy of Pediatric Dentistry, pp. 168–72.

Pinkam P, Casamassimo PS, Fields HW, McTigue DJ, Nowak AJ. 2005. *Pediatric Dentistry: Infancy Through Adolescence*, 4th Edition. Mosby: St. Louis.

SELF-STUDY ANSWERS

1. The maximum mg/kg and total doses of commonly used local anesthetics in pediatric dentistry are: (a) lidocaine: 4.4 mg/kg (2 mg/lb), 300 mg total; (b) mepivicaine 4.4 mg/kg (2 mg/lb) 300 mg total; (c) articaine 7 mg/kg (3.2 mg/lb) 500 mg total

2. A 52-pound child could receive a total of 104 mg of lidocaine

3. The mandibular foramen is lower than the occlusal plane in children, so the injection should be made lower and slightly more posterior in children

4. Local anesthetics act by interfering with the entry of sodium ions in sodium channels of the nerve cell membrane

5. The signs of local anesthetic toxicity are a central nervous system excitatory phase (dizziness, anxiety, confusion, tachycardia, increased blood pressure) followed by depression of the central nervous system (seizure activity, bradycardia, cardiac arrest)

Case 4

General Anesthesia

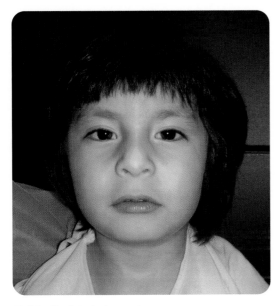

Figure 7.4.1. Facial photograph

A. Presenting Patient
- 3-year-, 7-month-old Hispanic female

B. Chief Complaint
- Mother states, "My daughter has some bad teeth and she would not let the other dentist treat her"

C. Social History
- Parents are divorced
- Mother is the primary caregiver and works outside the home on a part-time basis
- Child lives with mother, grandmother, and two siblings, ages 2 and 7
- Lower socio-economic status

D. Medical History
- Review of systems is positive for sickle cell trait
- Allergy to penicillin; mother reports the child developed a rash with amoxicillin
- No routine medications

- No previous hospitalizations or surgeries
- No emergency room visits

E. Medical Consult
- Request medical consult by pediatrician to update status of sickle cell trait and allergies

F. Dental History
- This is the patient's third dental visit
- She was previously seen for a new patient examination and an attempt at restorative treatment with nitrous oxide and local anesthesia
- The patient lives in a fluoridated community and uses city water
- Mother brushes the child's teeth once daily with a fluoridated toothpaste but does not floss
- Highly cariogenic diet
- No history of dental trauma

G. Extra-oral Exam
- The patient appears hesitant as she and her mother are escorted to the operatory
- Head and neck: Within normal limits
- Weight and height, BMI: Within normal limits
- Exposed extremities (bruising, etc.): Within normal limits

H. Intra-oral Exam
Soft Tissues
- Within normal limits

Hard Tissues
- Extensive dental decay involving all four quadrants and the maxillary anterior teeth

Dentition
- Full primary dentition

Occlusion
- Mesial step with normal overjet and overbite

I. Diagnostic Tools

- Bitewing radiographs from previous office confirm extensive interproximal decay

J. Differential Diagnosis

- N/A

K. Diagnosis and Problem List

Diagnosis

- Severe early childhood caries

Problem List

- Extremely apprehensive patient
- No dental home
- Poor diet
- Poor oral hygiene

L. Comprehensive Treatment Plan

- Patient is apprehensive and keeps asking, "Are you going to stick me with a needle like the other dentist did?" Due to anxiety and the extent of the restorations, treatment will require the use of general anesthesia

Post-op Instructions

- Minimize vigorous activity for the patient
- Pay attention to lip numbing while the patient attempts to eat
- Maintain a bland and soft diet for the day
- Follow up with a visit in two weeks
- Establish a dental home
- Implement an aggressive caries prevention plan
- Recall visits at least every six months

M. Prognosis and Discussion

- Treatment under general anesthesia has a high prognosis for success because no patient cooperation is necessary.
- The parent should be presented the option of having the general anesthesia performed in a hospital or an in-office setting.

N. Common Complications and Alternative Treatment Plans

- The most common obstacles to general anesthesia treatment are pre-operative complications such as illness or poor compliance with no-food-by-mouth (NPO) instructions

---

FUNDAMENTAL POINT 1

Indications for General Anesthesia in Pediatric Dentistry

- Certain physical, mental, or medically compromising conditions
- Ineffective local anesthesia due to acute infection, anatomic variations, or allergy
- Extremely uncooperative, fearful, anxious, physically resistant, or uncommunicative child or adolescent in whom there is no expectation that the behavior will soon improve
- Extensive orofacial/dental trauma
- Patients with immediate needs who would not otherwise receive comprehensive care
- Patients in whom use of general anesthesia may protect the developing psyche or reduce medical risks

Contraindications for General Anesthesia

- Unsuitable general anesthesia risk
- Respiratory infection
- Active systemic disease with elevated temperature
- No-food-by-mouth (NPO) guidelines violated
- Healthy cooperative patient with minimal dental needs

Weddell and Jones (2010), Post and Turner (2012)

- In the post-op period there is a risk of nausea and vomiting, and sore throat from the endotracheal tube
- If the parent did not want to use sedative agents or general anesthesia, attempts could be made to place interim restorations while trying to reduce the patient's anxiety with short, easy visits

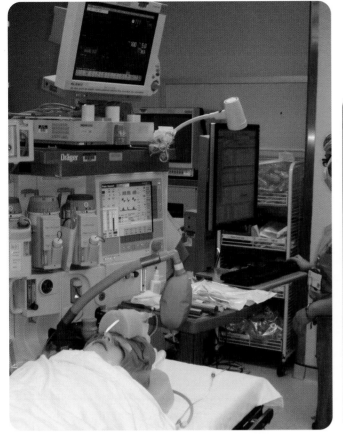 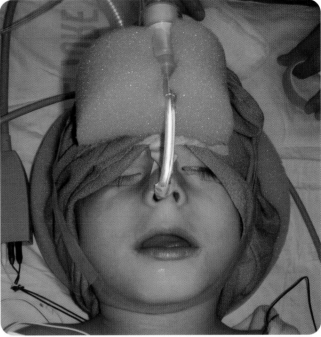

Figure 7.4.2a–b. Intubated patient in operating room

BACKGROUND INFORMATION 1

Pre-anesthetic Feeding Guidelines for General Anesthesia

- Clear liquids up to two hours prior to the procedure
- Breast milk up to four hours prior to the procedure

- Infant formula and non-human milk up to six hours prior to the procedure
- Light meal up to six hours prior to the procedure

AAPD (2011–2012), American Society of Anesthesiologists Task Force on Preoperative Fasting (1999)

Self-study Questions

1. **What children are candidates for anesthesia on an outpatient basis?**

2. **What information do you need to have prior to scheduling a patient for general anesthesia?**

3. **What are the advantages and disadvantages that general anesthesia provide in dental care to children?**

4. **What type of training is needed for a dentist to treat children under general anesthesia?**

Answers are located at the end of the case.

Bibliography

American Academy of Pediatric Dentistry. 2011–2012. Guideline for monitoring and management of pediatric patients during and after sedation. Reference Manual. *Pediatric Dentistry* Vol. 33(6), pp. 185–201.

American Society of Anesthesiologists Task Force on Preoperative Fasting. 1999. Practice Guidelines for Preoperative Fasting and the Use of Pharmacologic Agents to Reduce the Risk of Pulmonary Aspiration: Application to Healthy Patients Undergoing Elective Procedures. *Anesthesiology* March 1999, Vol.90, Issue 3. pp. 896–905.

Post C, Turner E. 2011. Hospital dentistry and general anesthesia. In: *The Handbook of Pediatric Dentistry*, 4th Edition. Nowak AJ, Casamassimo PS (eds). *American Academy of Pediatric Dentistry*, pp. 173–84.

Weddell JA, Jones JE. 2010. Hospital dental services for children and the use of general anesthesia. In: *McDonald and Avery Dentistry for the Child and Adolescent*, 9th ed. McDonald R (eds) Mosby: St. Louis.

SELF-STUDY ANSWERS

1. Children who have no significant medical, mental, or physical compromise are usually good candidates for anesthesia on an outpatient basis

2. Prior to scheduling a child for general anesthesia there should be a pre-anesthetic assessment of the medical history, an explanation of the procedure along with the risks/benefits and options for alternative treatment, and informed consent should be obtained from the parent or legal guardian

3. The advantages of general anesthesia are that all of the child's dental needs can be met in one visit, quality care can be provided, and the child's developing psyche is protected. The disadvantages include higher cost, the risk of a general anesthetic, and the inability for the opportunity for the child to learn coping skills

4. A dentist who treats children under general anesthesia should be trained in hospital protocol, operating room procedures, pre-operative assessment, and management of post-operative complications

Case 5

Airway Management

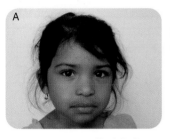 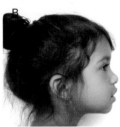

Figure 7.5.1a–b. Facial photographs

A. Presenting Patient
- 3-year-, 5-month-old female

B. Chief Complaint
- Patient referred from family dentist for full mouth dental rehabilitation under general anesthesia

C. Social History
- Mother is primary caregiver
- Patient lives with both parents and one sister, age 2
- Mother is unemployed, father works full-time in construction
- Lower socio-economic status
- Spanish is primary language

D. Medical History
- Review of systems is negative, American Society of Anesthesiologists (ASA) class I
- No known allergies to any foods or medications
- No routine prescription or over-the-counter medications
- No previous hospitalizations or surgeries
- No emergency room visits

E. Medical Consult
- Healthy patient, consult not necessary for initial visit

F. Dental History
- The patient's first dental visit was a new patient exam at the family's dentist three weeks ago
- Mother reports that the child brushes her teeth every morning with fluoridated toothpaste; mother does not routinely supervise brushing
- Does not floss
- Fluoride in their community water unknown
- Highly cariogenic diet
- No trauma history
- Behavior assessment: uncooperative with previous dentist and pediatrician, with age-appropriate anxiety

G. Extra-oral Exam
- Head and neck: Within normal limits
- Exposed extremities: Mild eczema patches
- Other: Lung sounds clear, heart sounds within normal limits, no evidence of an upper respiratory infection

H. Intra-oral Exam
Soft Tissues
- Within normal limits, Brodsky scale 2, Mallampati 1

Hard Tissues
- Multiple caries on all primary teeth in varying stages of cavitation

Dentition
- Primary

Occlusion
- Within normal limits

I. Diagnostic Tools
- Radiographs will be completed under general anesthesia

BACKGROUND INFORMATION 1
Airway Assessment

- Airway assessment is critical pre-operatively in an effort to anticipate and prepare for any airway difficulties during mask ventilation or during tracheal intubation

- The Mallampati score assesses the degree to which the practitioner can visualize the uvula during voluntary tongue protrusion. It is sometimes difficult to obtain on an uncooperative child

- The Brodsky Scale is used to evaluate the size of the tonsils and the degree to which they may obstruct the airway

- Airway assessment also includes looking for any loose or already chipped/damaged teeth, crowns, bridges, or dentures

- Prominent labial inclination of the maxillary incisors can make laryngoscopy difficult without damaging the incisors

- Other indicators of a potentially difficult mask ventilation or laryngoscopy and intubation include:
  - Micrognathia
  - Large tongue
  - Short neck
  - Limited cervical spine or temporomandibular jaw (TMJ) mobility

- Children with a high BMI or obesity can have a difficult airway, upper airway obstruction in the post-anesthesia care unit. They may also require longer post-operative recovery times and need more antiemetics

- Children with craniofacial abnormalities require a thorough pre-op airway evaluation and tools for a difficult airway should be immediately available

Nafiu et al. (2007), Morgan, Mikhail, and Murray (2005)

J. Differential Diagnosis
- N/A

K. Diagnosis and Problem List
Diagnosis
- Severe early childhood caries
- Severe situational anxiety

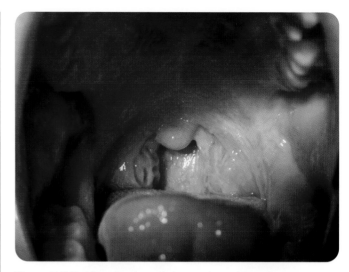

Figure 7.5.2. Visualization of the uvula and tonsils to determine the Mallampati score and Brodsky scale

Problem List
- English is not primary language, needs a competent translator (not a family member)
- Poor diet and oral hygiene
- No dental home

L. Comprehensive Treatment Plan
- Comprehensive assessment of the airway
- Obtain medical clearance from primary care provider
- Full mouth dental rehabilitation under general anesthesia due to the extensive treatment plan and patient's severe anxiety

Follow-up Care
- Supervised recovery period after extubation
- Instructions for parental monitoring of patient's status at home on the surgical day
- Post-op phone call at 24 to 48 hours
- Follow up visit in two weeks, then three-month recall visits
- Space management as needed due to multiple extractions
- Implement aggressive prevention plan

M. Prognosis and Discussion
- Full mouth dental rehabilitation with multiple extractions has a good prognosis for short-term success
- Unless significant changes occur in diet, oral hygiene, home care, and a dental home, there is a strong possibility that the patient will continue to develop dental caries and may require additional

FUNDAMENTAL POINT 1
Oxygen Therapy

- A child with respiratory insufficiency for any reason requires the administration of supplemental oxygen

- When a patient requires supplemental oxygen in an acute situation, the practitioner also must be ready to assist or provide ventilation

- Oxygen can be delivered in any of the following ways:
  - Nasal cannula
  - Face mask
  - Blow-by or face tent
  - An invasive, secured airway such as an endotracheal tube

- The least invasive yet maximally effective route should be chosen first to minimize increasing the child's anxiety, which will only serve to increase oxygen demand

- Oxygen masks require spontaneous respirations
  - Low-flow, simple mask delivers 35% to 60% oxygen
  - Partial rebreathing mask delivers 50% to 60% oxygen
  - Nonrebreathing mask delivers 95% to 100% oxygen
  - High-flow, Venturi mask delivers 25% to 60% oxygen

- Nasal cannulas also require spontaneous ventilation, and only provide up to approximately 32% oxygen

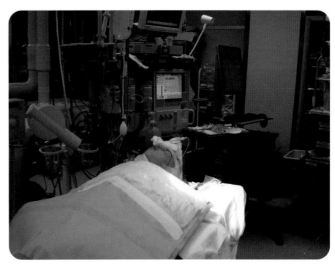

Figure 7.5.3. Intubated patient in the operating room

treatment in the operating room under general anesthesia

- One of the major benefits of treatment under general anesthesia is airway support and protection. This is difficult to obtain in an unsedated child of this age, especially with the extent of restorative and extraction treatment necessary

- Airway problems are one of the most common complications to care under nitrous oxide/oxygen, conscious sedation, or general anesthesia. Upper airway congestion, infections of the airway or lungs, enlarged tonsils, and anatomical variations can all pose difficulties pre-, intra-, or post-operatively

FUNDAMENTAL POINT 2
Use of a Bag-Valve-Mask

- The bag-valve-mask technique is a basic life support skill that allows the practitioner to provide effective ventilation and oxygenation to the pediatric patient

- The mask must be sized appropriately, fitting over the bridge of the nose (avoiding pressure on the eyes) and around the mouth

- It is important not to compress the soft tissue of the young patient's airway with remaining fingers while creating a seal between the face and the mask (Figure 7.5.4.)

- Holding the mask with the left hand, gently deliver a tidal volume with your right hand squeezing the bag; watch for chest rise. Don't overinflate!

- Gentle repositioning of the head and neck may be required to find the best position for ventilation

- Make sure the apparatus is properly connected to an oxygen source

- Healthcare providers serving children should have, at a minimum, basic life support skills in airway management and use of the bag-valve-mask device

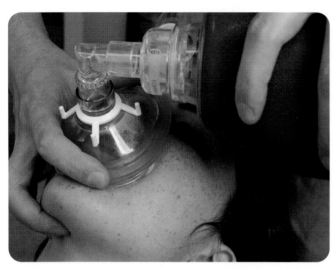

Figure 7.5.4. Use of bag and mask for ventilation

N. Common Complications and Alternative Treatment Plans

- The child with spontaneous respirations but signs and symptoms of a partial airway obstruction requires the gentle application of approximately 5 to 10 cm of continuous positive airway pressure (CPAP). This is generally accomplished by obtaining and maintaining a good seal with the face mask and a breathing circuit that will allow CPAP to be provided
- During assisted or controlled ventilation with a face mask, insufflation of the stomach can occur, especially if the practitioner is attempting to ventilate around a partial obstruction. This is a common complication that could result in aspiration or regurgitation of gastric contents

---

BACKGROUND INFORMATION 2

Differences Between the Child and Adult Airways

- It is important to understand the differences between a child's airway and an adult's airway to minimize airway obstruction and prevent hypoxemia
- The tongue is the most common cause of obstruction in the unconscious or sedated pediatric patient
  - In the child, the tongue is bigger in relation to the oral cavity
  - The larger occiput of the child tends to flex the child's neck, contributing more to obstruction
  - To manage this type of obstruction, use the head-tilt-chin-lift maneuver

- Children have soft tissue that can easily be compressed by the rescuer's incorrect finger placement under the chin; be sure your fingers are on the bony part of the jaw, not the soft tissue, because this will exacerbate any airway obstruction
- The cricoid is the narrowest part of a child's airway, unlike the glottic opening in adults, which necessitates the use of uncuffed endotracheal tubes in children

American Heart Association (2006), Morgan, Mikhail, and Murray (2005)

Self-study Questions

1. *In an unconscious pediatric patient with no spontaneous respirations, what is the best airway adjunct choice for initial airway management to provide ventilation and oxygenation?*

2. *In a conscious pediatric patient exhibiting signs of respiratory distress, what is the first airway adjunct that should be attempted?*

3. *Is an oral airway an appropriate airway adjunct to use in an awake child exhibiting signs of respiratory distress?*

4. *How much oxygen can a non-rebreather mask be expected to deliver if connected appropriately to an oxygen delivery source?*

5. *How is a child with a partial airway obstruction managed?*

Answers are located at the end of the case.

Bibliography

American Heart Association. 2006. Management of respiratory distress and failure. *The Pediatric Advanced Life Support Manual*, pp. 45–58.

Morgan GE, Mikhail MS, Murray MJ. 2005. *Clinical Anesthesiology*, 4th Edition. McGraw-Hill Medical: New York.

Nafiu OO, Reynolds PI, Bamgbade OA, Tremper KK, Welch K, Kasa-Vubu JZ. 2007. Childhood body mass index and perioperative complications. *Paediatr Anaesth* May;17(5):426–30.

SELF-STUDY ANSWERS

1. The bag-valve-mask device, connected to oxygen, used by either one or two rescuers

2. The least invasive yet maximally effective adjunct should be chosen first to minimize increasing the child's anxiety. Start with an oxygen cannula or simple face mask, call 911, and continually assess the child's respiratory pattern to determine the need for more invasive airway support requirements

3. No, an oral airway in any awake patient will only stimulate the gag reflex and possibly cause laryngospasm

4. A non-rebreather mask will deliver nearly 100% oxygen if connected correctly to an oxygen source delivering 10 to 15 LPM of oxygen to a patient who is breathing spontaneously

5. To manage a child with a partial airway obstruction, first make sure the airway is positioned correctly. Obtain a good seal with the face mask by pulling the child's face into the mask, and creating a seal with the index finger and thumb (review the E-C technique from the *Pediatric Advanced Life Support Manual,* American Heart Association). Be sure to stay off the soft tissue under the mandible, and provide supplemental oxygen. Do not use an oral airway in a child who is conscious

Case 6

Allergic Reactions

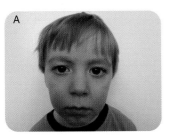 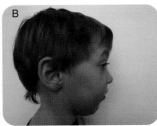

Figure 7.6.1.a–b. Facial photographs

A. Presenting Patient
- 3-year, 2-month-old Caucasian male

B. Chief Complaint
- Mother states, "My son needs his teeth cleaned and has one loose tooth"

C. Social History
- Parents are separated
- Mother is the primary caregiver and works full-time
- Patient has two healthy siblings, ages 8 and 11, with some environmental allergies
- Middle class socio-economic status

D. Medical History
- Review of systems is negative
- Allergic to bananas and mangoes; no allergies to medications
- No routine over-the-counter or prescription medications
- No previous hospitalizations or surgeries
- No emergency room visits

E. Medical Consult
- Consultation with primary care provider to test for sensitivity to latex

F. Dental History
- Has had regular dental visits since age 2
- Positive behavior for all recalls

FUNDAMENTAL POINT 1
Latex Allergy
- Food allergies that should alert the practitioner to a possible latex allergy include bananas, mangos, avocado, kiwi, and passion fruit
- Symptoms upon exposure to latex should be gathered in the medical history. In children, lip swelling or itching upon exposure to balloons can be an indication of latex sensitivity
- Latex anaphylaxis in children has an estimated incidence of 1 in 10,000
- Chronic exposure to latex and a history of atopy (an immediate reaction) increases the risk of sensitization; children who have a history of multiple surgeries or frequent exposure to urinary catheters are possibly at risk for latex allergy
- Latex allergies range in severity from mild dermatitis to life-threatening anaphylactic reactions
- Most serious latex reactions involve a direct immunoglobulin E-mediated response to the polypeptides found in natural latex

Morgan, Mikhail, and Murray (2005)

- Optimal water fluoridation
- Healthy, low-cariogenic diet
- Brushes once or twice a day, usually unsupervised

G. Extra-oral Exam
- Head and neck: Within normal limits
- No significant findings

H. Intra-oral Exam
Soft Tissues
- Mild plaque accumulation, mild gingivitis

FUNDAMENTAL POINT 2
Causes of Allergic Reactions

- Allergic reactions are exaggerated immunological responses to allergens

- Exposure can occur via the nose, eyes, skin, lungs, gastrointestinal tract, or intravenously/intramuscularly

- There are four types of hypersensitivity reactions (Background Information 1: Physiology of Allergic Reactions)

- Common causes of allergies include certain foods, medications, animals, insect venom, cosmetics, perfumes, and latex

Morgan, Mikhail, and Murray (2005)

BACKGROUND INFORMATION 1
Physiology of Allergic Reactions

- Type I, or immediate, hypersensitivity reactions involve antigens cross-linking with immunoglobulin E antibodies. This cross-link triggers mast cells to release inflammatory mediators. Severe allergic reactions, or anaphylaxis, can result

- Type II, or cytotoxic, hypersensitivity reactions involve Immunoglobulin G (IgG) antibodies, which bind with antigens on cell surfaces. This IgG binding causes cell lysis, i.e., hemolytic transfusion reactions

- Type III, or immune complex, hypersensitivity reactions occur when antigen-antibody complexes are deposited into tissues. After the complex is deposited, neutrophils are activated and cause tissue injury from the release of lysosomal enzymes and other toxic products

- Type IV, or delayed/cell-mediated, hypersensitivity reactions are mediated by T lymphocytes that have been exposed to the antigen before. Re-exposure to the antigen causes the production of lymphokines that activate inflammatory cells over about 48 to 72 hours, i.e., contact dermatitis

Morgan, Mikhail, and Murray (2005)

Hard Tissues

- Full primary dentition, no cavities

Occlusion

- Within normal limits

I. Diagnostic Tools

- Bitewing and occlusal radiographs show no cavities

J. Differential Diagnosis

- N/A

K. Diagnosis and Problem List

Diagnosis

- Good oral health

Problem List

- Food allergies
- Poor oral hygiene

L. Comprehensive Treatment Plan

- Improve oral hygiene
- Must rule out latex allergy

FUNDAMENTAL POINT 3
Recognizing Allergic Reactions

- Symptoms of allergic reactions can range from mild to severe

- Mild symptoms include watery, itchy eyes with a rash and possibly nose and/or chest congestion

- Moderate reactions can include the above symptoms, but also display itchiness and/or difficulty breathing

- Severe allergic reactions, or anaphylaxis, result in differing degrees of angioedema (swelling) that can make it difficult for the patient to swallow or breathe. Other symptoms include:

  - Abdominal pain, vomiting
  - Cramps, diarrhea
  - Mental confusion and/or dizziness

- Other clinical signs and symptoms of allergic reactions include:

  - Tachycardia, hypotension, arrhythmias
  - Cough, bronchospasm, laryngeal edema, hypoxia
  - Facial edema, pruritus, generalized itching

AAPD (2011–12), Morgan, Mikhail, and Murray (2005)

FUNDAMENTAL POINT 4

Anaphylaxis

- IgE-mediated allergic reactions: The body produces antibodies to a substance on first exposure. On second exposure, the body releases the antibodies and huge amounts of histamine. This can be potentially life threatening without immediate intervention. Symptoms appear quickly and can include increased heart rate, extreme shortness of breath, sudden weakness, a drop in blood pressure, shock, unconsciousness, and death.

AAPD (2011–12), Morgan, Mikhail, and Murray (2005)

- Continue six-month recalls

M. Prognosis and Discussion

- This cavity-free child is in good oral health but needs to improve his oral hygiene practices by increasing brushing more and with parental assistance and supervision. If latex sensitivity is found to be positive, then proper precautions should be taken to avoid latex exposure

N. Common Complications and Alternative Treatment Plans

- What complications should you be prepared for in a patient with known allergies to mangoes and bananas?
- What preparations should you make for this patient's visit?

FUNDAMENTAL POINT 5

Treatment of Allergic Reactions

- If an allergic reaction is suspected due to drug administration, discontinue the medication
- Discontinue all sources of the allergy-causing substance
- Administer diphenhydramine:
  - Children: 1 mg/kg PO qid, 0.5 to 1 mg/kg IV
  - Adults: 25 to 50 mg PO qid
- For anaphylactic reactions, recognize a true medical emergency:

- Call 911
- Administer epinephrine (IM or sq), 0.01 mg/kg q 5 minutes
- Administer supplemental oxygen
- Monitor vital signs
- Provide airway support as required
- Consult the American Academy of Pediatric Dentistry guidelines on the management of medical emergencies

AAPD (2011–12)

Self-study Questions

1. *Besides food and drug allergies that the patient has, what are some common sources of potential allergic reactions in your office?*

2. *Type I, or immediate, hypersensitivity reactions are modulated by which immunoglobulin?*

3. *Anaphylactic reactions occur after the second exposure to an allergen (antigen), upon which the body releases which substance?*

4. *State the common signs and symptoms of an allergic reaction.*

5. *State the common food allergies that would make you suspicious that your patient has a latex allergy.*

Answers are located at the end of the case.

Bibliography

American Academy of Pediatric Dentistry. 2011–12. *Management of Medical Emergencies*, Reference manual. *Pediatric Dentistry* 33(6):345–6.

Morgan GE, Mikhail MS, Murray MJ. 2005. *Clinical Anesthesiology*, 4th Edition. McGraw-Hill Medical: New York.

SELF-STUDY ANSWERS

1. Common sources of allergies in the office setting include anything containing latex (gloves, the powder inside gloves, rubber dams, tourniquets), medications (especially antibiotics), some local anesthetics (rare allergies)

2. Type I, or immediate, hypersensitivity reactions are modulated by IgE

3. Anaphylactic reactions occur after the body has been sensitized to the antigen upon first exposure. The second and all subsequent exposures cause the body to release massive amounts of histamine, resulting in shortness of breath, tachycardia, and rapidly declining cardiovascular function

4. The common signs and symptoms of an allergic reaction include watery, itchy eyes with a rash and possibly nose and/or chest congestion; generalized itchiness and/or difficulty breathing; and tachycardia, hypotension, arrhythmias, cough, bronchospasm, laryngeal edema, hypoxia, and facial edema

5. The common food allergies that should alert the practitioner to a potential latex allergy include mangoes, bananas, avocados, passionfruit, and kiwi

Case 7

Asthma

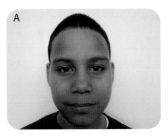 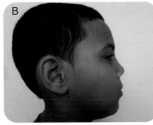

Figure 7.7.1.a–b. Facial photographs

A. Presenting Patient
- 8-year, 1-month old Hispanic male

B. Chief Complaint
- Mother states, "He is here for his six-month check-up"

C. Social History
- Parents are married
- Patient has three healthy siblings, age 15, 11, and 10
- Both parents work full time outside the home
- Upper middle class socio-economic status

D. Medical History
- Patient has moderate persistent asthma
- Patient has required two trips in the last 12 months to the emergency department for exacerbation of his asthma symptoms; has never been hospitalized overnight
- Current medications include Pulmicort inhaled nebulizer treatments BID; Singulair chewable tabs, 4 mg QD; and Nasonex AQ nasal spray, one spray to each nostril QD
- PRN medications include Albuterol (Ventolin) nebulizer treatments, which he requires once or twice per month, depending on the season
- Parents note that they occasionally miss doses of his medications

---

FUNDAMENTAL POINT 1
Asthma History
- Complete a thorough inquiry into the extent of the disease, how well it is controlled, and what exacerbates symptoms is required
- Ask how frequent the attacks are, what typically causes the attacks, and what is required to relieve them
- Ask about recent emergency department visits, and what treatment was required
- Ask if the patient has any activity restrictions
- See Chapter 1 Case 7, Asthma

McDonald, Avery, and Dean (2004)

- No known allergies to any foods or medications
- No surgeries

E. Medical Consult
- Consultation with primary care provider is advised in order to have a through understanding of the patient's medical history and the state of asthma control

F. Dental History
- Routine six-month check-ups since age 14 months
- Very uncooperative, with extreme anxiety
- Optimal water fluoridation levels
- Healthy, low-cariogenic diet (occasional sweets)
- Brushes twice a day with supervision
- Uses fluoridated toothpaste; does not floss

G. Extra-oral Exam
- Head and neck: Within normal limits
- No other significant findings

BACKGROUND INFORMATION 1
Types of Asthma
Mild Intermittent Asthma

- Symptoms twice/week or less with nighttime symptoms twice/month or less
- Brief exacerbations of varying intensity

Mild Persistent Asthma

- Symptoms more than twice/week but less than once/day
- Nighttime symptoms more than twice/month
- Exacerbations may affect activity

Moderate Persistent Asthma

- Daily symptoms with daily use of inhaled β-2 agonists
- Exacerbations affect activity and occur twice/week or more
- Nighttime symptoms more than once/week
- Exacerbations could last for days

Severe Persistent Asthma

- Continual symptoms with frequent exacerbations and nighttime symptoms
- Limited physical activity

Rollant, Hamlin, and Piotrowski (2001), Behrman, Kliegman, and Jenson (2001)

BACKGROUND INFORMATION 2
Pathophysiology of Asthma

- Chronic airway disease characterized by bronchial constriction
  - Inflammation and edema of the mucous membranes
  - Production of copious and tenacious secretions
  - Smooth muscle spasms of the bronchi and bronchioles
- Chronic disease with acute exacerbations of varying severity
- Attacks can be triggered by:
  - Environmental irritants (dust, smoke, pollen)
  - Strenuous exercise or increased stress
  - Weather (cold air or increased humidity)
  - Upper respiratory infections
- Oral Findings
  - Xerostomia
  - Increased levels of gingivitis

Rollant, Hamlin, and Piotrowski (2001), Behrman, Kliegman, and Jenson (2001), McDonald, Avery, and Dean (2004)

H. Intra-oral Exam
Soft Tissues

- Moderate gingivitis, xerostomia

Hard Tissues

- Within normal limits, no caries

Dentition

- Primary dentition

Occlusion

- Within normal limits

I. Diagnostic Tools

- Bitewing and occlusal radiographs show no cavities

J. Differential Diagnosis

- N/A

K. Diagnosis and Problem List
Diagnosis

- Moderate persistent asthma
- Moderate gingivitis

Problem List

- Xerostomia
- Poorly compliant parents

L. Comprehensive Treatment Plan

- Obtain medical consult
- Consider water-based chlorhexidine to reduce gingivitis
- Discuss with parents options for reducing dry mouth

M. Prognosis and Discussion

- The patient is at risk for an asthma attack during the dental visit due to possibly poor compliance with medications and the stress of the dental visit. Caution should be taken to complete a through assessment and be prepared to manage an acute asthmatic attack
- The patient may be at increased risk for caries due to the xerostomia caused by the medications. Fortunately, the patient has a well-developed oral hygiene routine with the help and support of both parents. The parents should be advised to try to

keep the mouth moist with sugarless candies and beverages. Rinsing several times a day with a solution of salt and baking soda can help buffer the acidic oral environment

N. Common Complications and Alternative Treatment Plans

- If this patient presents with a slight upper respiratory infection, the stress of the dental visit could exacerbate his asthma symptoms. How do you recognize the symptoms of an asthma attack?

FUNDAMENTAL POINT 2
Recognition of an Asthma Attack

- Audible expiratory wheezing with restlessness and apprehension
- Hacking, non-productive cough
- Dyspnea
- Nasal flaring and intercostal retraction
- Cyanosis; look around the lips and the nailbeds
- Coarse rhonchi
- Tachycardia
- In an acute asthma attack, the loss of the wheezing sound is a BAD sign: the airways are totally collapsed and a respiratory arrest is likely

Rollant, Hamlin, and Piotrowski (2001), Behrman, Kliegman, and Jenson (2001)

FUNDAMENTAL POINT 3
Treatment of an Asthma Attack

- Call 911 if it is an in-office emergency
- Help patient into a position of comfort, usually sitting
- Give airway support as needed
  - Supplemental oxygen and ventilation support as needed with a bag-valve-mask
  - Only people with advanced airway training should attempt an intubation

Administer Appropriate Medication if Adequately Trained

- β-2 agonists
  - Inhaled medications such as Albuterol inhalers or nebulized breathing treatments
  - Subcutaneous injections of epinephrine or terbutaline
- Anticholinergics
  - Inhaled Atrovent
- Corticosteroids
  - Oral prednisone

AAPD (2011–12)

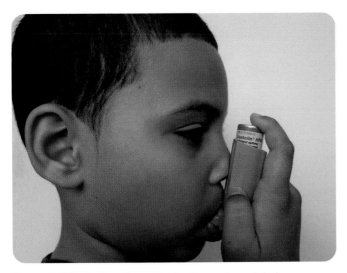

Figure 7.7.2. Asthmatic patient using asthma inhaler

Self-study Questions

1. *What are the important questions to ask regarding the child's asthma history?*
2. *What are the different classifications of asthma?*
3. *What determines the classification of asthma?*
4. *What are the common signs of an acute asthma attack?*
5. *What are the common triggers for asthma exacerbation?*

Answers are located at the end of the case.

Bibliography

American Academy of Pediatric Dentistry. 2011–2012. *Management of Medical Emergencies*, Reference manual *Pediatr Dent* 33(6):345–6.

Behrman RE, Kliegman RM, Jenson HB. 2001. *Textbook of Pediatrics*, 16th ed. W.B. Saunders: Philadelphia.

McDonald RE, Avery DR, Dean JA. 2004. *Dentistry for the Child and Adolescent*, 8th ed. Mosby: St. Louis.

Rollant PD, Hamlin JJ, Piotrowski KA. 2001. *Maternal-Child Nursing*, 2nd ed. Mosby: St. Louis.

SELF-STUDY ANSWERS

1. The questions to be reviewed with the parents include the following: Frequency and severity of symptoms, daily and rescue medications, how frequently the child requires rescue meds, what brings on an attack in the child, history regarding hospitalization and emergency room visits due to asthma exacerbations

2. The different classifications of asthma are: Mild intermittent, mild persistent moderate persistent, severe persistent

3. Asthma is classified according to: Frequency of symptoms in a week's time, frequency of nighttime symptoms, frequency of exacerbations and their impact on activity, medications required to manage asthma, peak expiratory flow, and forced expiratory volume

4. The common signs of an acute asthma attack (can occur in any order) are: Dyspnea, nasal flaring, intercostal retractions; restlessness, apprehension, diaphoresis; expiratory and/or inspiratory wheezing; prolonged expiration; cyanosis around the lips or in the nailbeds; coarse rhonchi

5. The common triggers for an asthma exacerbation include: Allergens: dust, smoke, pollen, food; cold weather; increased humidity; strenuous exercise; stress; viral infections

8

Special Needs Patients

Nancy Dougherty

Clinical Cases in Pediatric Dentistry, First Edition. Edited by Amr M. Moursi.
© 2012 Blackwell Publishing Ltd. Pubished 2012 by Blackwell Publishing Ltd.

Case 1

Trisomy 21 (Down Syndrome)/New Patient

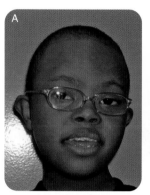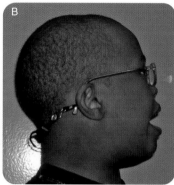

Figure 8.1.1a–b. Facial photographs

A. Presenting Patient
- 6-year-, 6-month-old, African-American male
- Diagnosed with Trisomy 21 (Down syndrome) (see Background Information 1)
- New patient visit

B. Chief Complaint
- Mother states, "My son has been to other dentists, but they were not able to take care of him"

C. Social History
- Patient attends school; in class for children with special educational needs
- Mother is primary caregiver
- Lower mid-level socio-economic status
- Patient has two sisters, ages 8 and 11

D. Medical History
- Cardiac: Ebstein's anomaly (congenital defect of tricuspid valve). Patient's defect is mild and has not required surgical repair. He is not currently on any medications and is followed by pediatric cardiology on an outpatient basis (see Fundamental Point 1).

BACKGROUND INFORMATION 1
Trisomy 21
- Trisomy 21 consists of a characteristic group of cognitive and physical findings that result from having an extra copy of chromosome 21.
- Most individuals with Trisomy 21 function in the range of mild to moderate intellectual disability.
- Craniofacial characteristics include:
  - Hypoplastic midface and maxilla
  - Mild microcephaly
  - Upslanting palpebral fissures
  - Short neck
- Health conditions frequently seen in individuals with Trisomy 21 include:
  - Congenital heart disease
  - Hypotonia
  - Compromised immune function
  - Hearing problems
  - Thyroid dysfunction
  - Skeletal abnormalities
  - Eye problems, especially cataracts
  - Increased risk for development of leukemia
  - Early development of senile dementia

National Institute of Child Health and Human Development (2007)

- History of frequent otitis media and upper respiratory infections.
- Patient was hospitalized at age 3 for myringotomy and placement of tympanostomy tubes. Due to post-operative complications, patient was

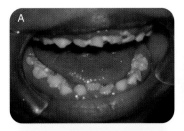
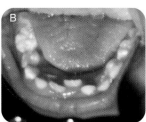
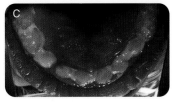

Figure 8.1.2a–c. Intra-oral photos showing generalized marginal gingival inflammation.

required to stay in the hospital for three days post-operatively.

E. Medical Consult

- Cardiology consult requested. Patient cleared for routine dental treatment. Antibiotic prophylaxis not required.

F. Dental History

- Mother has taken patient to three other dentists, but she was dissatisfied with care provided.
- Patient's behavior was uncooperative for previous dental examinations.
- Optimal water fluoridation levels
- Patient is not a frequent snack eater, but does drink large amounts of sugary beverages.
- Patient does not brush teeth himself. Allows mother to brush his teeth under duress.

G. Extra-oral Exam (Figures 8.1.1 a–b)

- Patient has characteristic facies of Trisomy 21, as discussed in the background information.
- No other significant findings

H. Intra-oral Exam (Figures 8.1.2 a–c and Fundamental Point 2)

- Early mixed dentition
- Erupting mandibular central incisors
- Poor oral hygiene
- Generalized marginal gingival inflammation
- Caries-free dentition

- Occlusion: class III skeletal relationship, mesial step primary molars

I. Diagnostic Tools

- Radiographs were not obtained for the following reasons:
  - Patient was unable to cooperate for radiographic exam
  - No caries were noted
  - It was determined that the patient would require sedation for radiographic exam; due to absence of caries and the patient's past history

of post-anesthesia complications, the practitioner did not feel sedation presented an appropriate risk/benefit balance for this patient at this time (see Fundamental Point 3).

FUNDAMENTAL POINT 3
Sedation Considerations

- Individuals with Trisomy 21 show an increased incidence of the following anatomic variations/ medical conditions, which may place them at an increased risk for complications associated with sedation and general anesthesia:
  - Congenital heart defects
  - Small naso-pharyngeal complex
  - Increased incidence of airway anomalies, including laryngomalacia, tracheomalacia, bronchomalacia
  - Increased incidence of cervical spine instability
  - Obesity
  - Hypotonia
  - Obstructive apnea
- A careful risk/benefit analysis should be conducted for each child with Trisomy 21 who is being considered for treatment under sedation or general anesthesia.

J. Differential Diagnosis

- N/A

K. Diagnosis and Problem List

Diagnosis

- Trisomy 21
- Congenital heart defect (triscuspid valve prolapse)
- Frequent otitis media
- Gingivitis
- Poor oral hygiene
- Malocclusion

Problem List

- High caries risk due to special needs status, high intake of sugared beverages, and poor oral hygiene
- Lack of a dental home
- Increased risk for periodontal disease due to poor oral hygiene and compromised immunity
- Increased risk for ectopic eruption or impaction of teeth, especially in maxillary arch (due to maxillary hypoplasia)

FUNDAMENTAL POINT 4
Trisomy 21 Oral Health

- Caries risk: Use the American Academy of Pediatric Dentistry Caries Assessment Tool (CAT) in assigning a patient's risk category AAPD (2011–2012)
- Periodontal disease: Onset of periodontal disease in individuals with Trisomy 21 is frequently seen by the late teen years. Incidence in some adult populations has been reported to be over 90%. This is probably due to the reduced immune response in these people. Early, aggressive therapy, including frequent cleanings and possible systemic antibiotic therapy, should be considered.
- Malocclusion, ectopic eruption, impactions:
  - The class III malocclusion seen in Trisomy 21 involves midface hypoplasia, and would, in most cases, require extensive surgical procedures to correct.
  - Patients should be monitored for dental crowding, ectopia, and impactions. These problems may be correctable with orthodontic and minor oral surgical treatment.

Pilcher (1998)

L. Comprehensive Treatment Plan (see Fundamental Point 4)

- Establish a dental home
- Dental prophylaxis and topical fluoride
- Encourage parent to reduce sugared beverage intake
- Encourage improved oral hygiene, (in this case, with parent) focusing on brushing and flossing
- Three-month recall
  - Re-evaluate caries risk
  - Re-evaluate oral hygiene status
  - Monitor eruption of permanent dentition
  - Re-evaluate patient's ability to cooperate for radiographic exam. If cooperative, take radiographs to evaluate for interproximal caries and development of permanent dentition.

M. Prognosis and Discussion

- There have been reports that individuals with Trisomy 21 have a lower incidence of dental caries than the general population. However, they do experience caries and this patient's high intake of sugary beverages and poor oral hygiene increases his risk for caries. Dietary modifications and increased recall visits including topical fluoride treatments should reduce this patient's caries risk.

- This patient is at high risk for development of periodontal disease due to a combination of compromised immune response and poor oral hygiene. Improved oral hygiene and increased recall visits, including prophylaxis and monitoring for periodontal problems, may help improve this patient's periodontal prognosis.

- Behavioral capabilities, both in the dental setting and at home, are always a consideration when treating children with intellectual disabilities. There is a wide range of behaviors in children with Trisomy 21, and many of them are treatable for routine dental care with little or no modifications in care necessary. Diagnostic exams for this particular patient were compromised by the fact that he has, up to now, been uncooperative for radiographs. An oral examination, prophylaxis, and fluoride varnish treatment were made possible with the mother's assistance, holding her child in the dental chair. Tell-show-do was used with limited effectiveness.

As per the mother's report, the child's behavior also makes it difficult for her to accomplish adequate oral hygiene at home. An attempt was made to keep the dental visit as atraumatic as possible, and it is possible that, in the future, the child may become more cooperative. As discussed earlier, these children are at an increased risk for complications related to sedation and general anesthesia, and careful consideration must be made for each individual as to whether or not an anesthetic procedure is warranted for routine diagnostic and dental procedures.

N. Complications and Alternative Treatment Plan

- If this patient had clinically detectable caries, would the behavior management techniques previously used be adequate to accomplish needed treatment?

- If this child had cervical spine (atlanto-axial) instability, how might the practitioner need to modify the way in which dental care was delivered?

- Would there be any differences in this child's orthodontic care at this age if his behavior was cooperative?

Self-study Questions

1. **What are some systemic findings in children with Trisomy 21 that could significantly impact longevity and/or quality of life?**

2. **List four characteristic craniofacial features of individuals with Trisomy 21.**

3. **Name common intra-oral findings in individuals with Trisomy 21.**

4. **List features of Trisomy 21 that make these patients poor candidates for outpatient sedation procedures.**

5. **What is the probable explanation for the increased incidence of early, aggressive periodontal disease in many individuals with Trisomy 21?**

Answers are located at the end of the case.

Bibliography

American Academy of Pediatric Dentistry. 2011–2012. Guideline on Caries-risk Assessment and Management for Infants, Children, and Adolescents, Reference Manual. *Pediatr Dent* 33(6):110–15.

Freeman SB. et al. 1998. Population-based study of congenital heart defects in Down syndrome. *Am J of Medical Genetics* 16;80(3):213–17.

Mitchell RB, Call E, Kelly J. 2003. Ear, nose and throat disorders in children with Down syndrome. *Laryngoscope* 113(2):259–63.

National Institute of Child Health and Human Development. www.nichd.nih.gov/health/topics/Down_Syndrome.cfm.

Pilcher, ES. 1998. Dental care for the patient with Down syndrome. *Down Syndrome Research and Practice* 5(3):111–16.

Shaw L, Saxby MS. 1986. Periodontal destruction in Down's syndrome and in juvenile periodontitis; how close a similarity? *J of Periodontology* 57:709–13.

Yavuzyilmaz E. et al. 1993. Neutrophil chemotaxis and periodontal status in Down syndrome patients. *J of Nihon University School of Dentistry* 35:91–5.

SELF-STUDY ANSWERS

1. Congenital heart defects, cognitive impairment, compromised immune response, thyroid disorders, cervical spine instability, increased risk for development of leukemia, increased incidence of early development of senile dementia

2. Hypoplastic midface, mild microcephaly, upslanted palpebral fissures, short neck

3. Hypodontia, microdontia, delayed dental eruption, ectopic dental eruption, dental impactions, crowding of maxillary dentition, relative macroglossia, class III malocclusion

4. Increased incidence of airway anomalies, small naso-pharyngeal complex, hypotonia, obesity, increased incidence of congenital heart defects, increased incidence of spinal deformities and instability

5. Individuals with Trisomy 21 have a compromised immune response, which places them at increased susceptibility for chronic infectious processes. This is the probable explanation for their relatively high incidence of periodontal disease.

Case 2

Cerebral Palsy, Bronchopulmonary Dysplasia

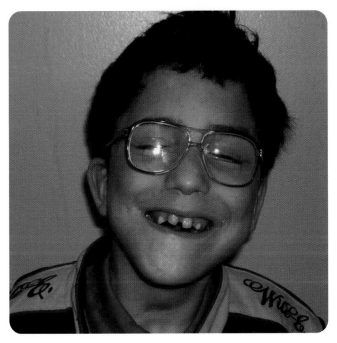

Figure 8.2.1. Facial photograph

A. Presenting Patient

- 8-year-, 2-month-old Caucasian male
- Diagnosed with cerebral palsy, bronchopulmonary dysplasia, asthma, and mild intellectual disability

B. Chief Complaint

- Patient presenting for recall appointment; last dental visit was 18 months ago

C. Social History

- Patient attends school; is in a class for children with special educational needs
- Child lives at home with mother, father, and 3 older siblings
- Father works full time; mother is a full-time homemaker
- Socio-economic status is lower middle class

BACKGROUND INFORMATION 1
Cerebral Palsy

- Cerebral palsy can be described as "A group of disorders of the development of movement and posture causing activity limitations that are attributed to non-progressive disturbances that occurred in the developing fetal or infant brain. The motor disturbances of cerebral palsy are often accompanied by disturbances of sensation, cognition, communication, perception, and/or behavior and/or a seizure disorder." (Bax et al. 2005)
- Bronchopulmonary dysplasia (BPD) is a common complication of preterm birth. It is seen most frequently in infants born prior to 30 weeks gestational age and weighing <1,200g at birth. It is related to the need for positive-pressure ventilation (PPV) in neonates with poorly developed pulmonary systems. PPV can result in injury to the pulmonary microvasculature and alveolar structures. Neonates with BPD are at increased risk for abnormal pulmonary function into late childhood and possibly adulthood (Blayney et al. 1991, Jobe and Bancalari 2001).

D. Medical History (see Background Information 1)

- Premature birth (child was born at 26 weeks gestational age, birth weight = 978 g) (see Fundamental Point 1)
- Cerebral palsy, mixed type (spastic and dyskinetic)
- Status post bronchopulmonary dysplasia secondary to long neonatal course of positive pressure ventilation
- Hospitalization for aspiration pneumonia at age 2

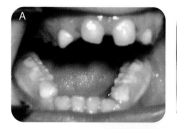
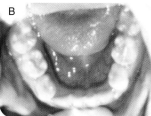
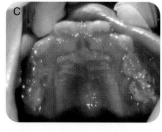

Figure 8.2.2a–c. Intra-oral photos showing generalized marginal gingivitis and mandibular crowding

- Mild/moderate asthma, currently managed with Flovent (fluticasone) and albuterol inhalers used on a daily basis
- Mild intellectual disability

E. Medical Consult

- Consulted with primary care physician to ascertain patient's current respiratory status, which is stable

F. Dental History

- Has been managed at the same dental clinic since 3 years of age
- Attendance at clinic has been sporadic (last visit 18 months ago)
- Positive behavior for brief procedures, but very active in dental chair: Try to keep appointments short
- Not a frequent snacker, eats mostly at meal time
- Optimal water fluoridation levels
- Brushes without supervision (once or twice per day)

G. Extra-oral Exam (Figure 8.2.1)

- No significant findings

H. Intra-oral Exam (see Figures 8.2.2a–c and Fundamental Point 2)

- Early mixed dentition (slightly delayed for age)

Occlusion

- 9-mm overjet, anterior open bite
- Moderate crowding of the lower arch
- Mesial step primary molars, class I canines

Poor Oral Hygiene

- Generalized marginal gingivitis
- Clinical exam suggests caries-free dentition

I. Diagnostic Tools

- Radiographs (bitewings and a panoramic film) were attempted, but were of poor diagnostic quality due to patient's difficulty staying still

J. Differential Diagnosis

- N/A

K. Diagnosis and Problem List

Diagnosis

- Cerebral palsy
- Cognitive impairment (mild)
- Status post bronchopulmonary dysplasia with current mild/moderate asthma

Problem List

- Irregular use of a dental home
- Gingival inflammation due to poor oral hygiene
- High caries risk due to poor oral hygiene and asthma medications
- Unknown caries status of interproximal surfaces
- Large overjet increases risk of traumatic dental injury
- Moderate mandibular crowding

FUNDAMENTAL POINT 2

Oral Considerations in Cerebral Palsy

- Possible intra- and extra-oral concerns in patients with cerebral palsy (CP) (Ortega et al. 2007):
  - Hypotonia of the tongue and perioral musculature can result in anterior open bites and constricted palates. (This particular patient does not have a constricted palate).
  - Immature swallow pattern, with characteristic tongue thrust, can also contribute to anterior open bite.
- A poor swallow reflex, seen in some patients with CP, can result in persistent drooling, which can irritate skin in the peri-oral region.
- Patients who use inhaled medication for control of asthma may show the following oral findings (McDonald, Avery, and Dean 2011):
  - Increased caries risk (due to reduced salivary flow)
  - Gingivitis
  - Throat irritation
  - Candidiasis

FUNDAMENTAL POINT 3

Maintaining Oral Health with Cerebral Palsy

- Caries risk: Use the American Academy of Pediatric Dentistry Caries Assessment Tool (CAT) in assigning a patient's risk category AAPD (2011–2012a)
  - Provide dietary counseling to the parent AAPD (2011–2012a and b)
- Gingival inflammation
  - Stress to parent the importance of daily oral home care. Instruct the parent to help with child's oral hygiene.
  - Schedule recall visits at more regular intervals to assess home care, perform prophylaxis, and monitor gingival inflammation (AAPD 2011–2012c)
- Malocclusion: Conduct orthodontic evaluation in early mixed dentition
  - Assess tooth size, shape, position
  - Conduct space analysis (AAPD 2011–2012d)

L. Comprehensive Treatment Plan

- Dental prophylaxis (sedation may be necessary)
- Fluoride treatment
- Review of oral hygiene and diet (with parent and child)
- Orthodontic consultation
  - Space analysis to evaluate arch length
  - Evaluate patient's behavior regarding his ability to cooperate for orthodontic treatment (if treatment is indicated at this time).
- Three-month recall
  - Re-evaluate caries risk
  - Re-evaluate oral hygiene and soft tissue status

M. Intra-Oral and Post-operative Images

- N/A

N. Prognosis and Discussion

- Although the patient is in a high risk category for dental caries due to poor oral hygiene, he has never had a carious lesion. The prognosis for continued periodontal pathology is high due to poor

hygiene, but could improve with better daily oral hygiene. Even performing a thorough prophylaxis may be difficult and sedation may be considered (see Fundamental Point 4).

- The prognosis for malocclusion is poor. Although the patient is fairly cooperative for oral examinations and prophylaxis, it is not clear what his level of cooperation would be for lengthier or more complicated treatments. This must be evaluated and taken into consideration before a decision is made to begin orthodontic treatment.

O. Complications and Alternative Treatment Plan

- If the patient had dental caries present, would the behavior management techniques previously used be adequate to accomplish the needed treatment?
- Is this child an appropriate candidate for in-office sedation, or would he be better managed in a hospital operating room setting, if treatment needs dictated?
- Would there be any difference in this child's orthodontic treatment at this age, if behavior was not a consideration?

FUNDAMENTAL POINT 4
Sedation Considerations

- This patient's history of bronchopulmonary dysplasia, aspiration pneumonia, and mild/moderate asthma puts him at risk for respiratory complications during sedation. According to the American Society of Anesthesiologists (ASA) physical status classification system, the patient would be ASA class II (mild systemic disease). If the patient required dental procedures that could not be completed without sedation and/or general anesthesia, his respiratory history should be taken into consideration when deciding the most appropriate setting (i.e., outpatient clinic or hospital OR) and type of anesthesia. (AAPD 2011–2012e)

Self-study Questions

1. **What are some common complications of extreme low birth weight that can have long-term sequelae?**

2. **Name three oral/perioral complications sometimes seen in patients with cerebral palsy.**

3. **What is the etiology for the complications mentioned in question 2?**

4. **True or False: Cerebral palsy is a progressive neurologic disorder.**

5. **In what category of neonates does bronchopulmonary dysplasia most frequently develop?**

Answers are located at the end of the case.

Bibliography

American Academy of Pediatric Dentistry. 2011–2012a. Guideline on Caries-risk Assessment and Management for Infants, Children, and Adolescents, Reference Manual. *Pediatr Dent* 33(6):110–15.

American Academy of Pediatric Dentistry. 2011–2012b. Policy on Dietary Recommendations, Reference Manual. *Pediatr Dent* 33(6):53–4.

American Academy of Pediatric Dentistry. 2011–2012c. Periodicity of Examination, Reference Manual. *Pediatr Dent* 33(6):102–9.

American Academy of Pediatric Dentistry. 2011–2012d. Management of the Developing Dentition, Reference Manual. *Pediatr Dent* 33(6):229–41.

American Academy of Pediatric Dentistry. 2011–2012e. Guideline for Monitoring and Management of Pediatric Patients During and After Sedation for Diagnostic and Therapeutic Procedures, Reference Manual. *Pediatr Dent* 33(6):185–201.

Bax M, Goldstein M, Rosenbaum P, et al. 2005. Proposed definition and classification of cerebral palsy. *Dev Med Child Neurol* Aug; 47(8):571–6.

Blayney M, Kerem E, Whyte H, O'Brodovich H. 1991. Bronchopulmonary dysplasea: improvement in lung function between 7 and 10 years of age. *J Pediatrics* Feb; 118(2):201–6.

Hack M, Taylor HG, Drotar D, et al. 2005. Chronic conditions, functional limitations, and special health care needs of school-aged children born with extremely low-birth-weight in the 1990s. *JAMA* Jul 20;294(3):318–25.

Jobe AH, Bancalari D. 2001. Bronchoplmonary dysplasia. *Am J Respir Crit Care Med* June;163(7):1723–9.

McDonald RE, Avery DR, Dean JA. 2011. *Dentistry for the Child and Adolescent*, 9th edition. Mosby: St. Louis. 479.

Ortega AOL, Guimaraes SS, Ciamponi ALL, Mari, SKN. 2007. Frequency of parafunctional oral habits in patients with cerebral palsy. *J of Oral Rehab* 34;323–8.

SELF-STUDY ANSWERS

1. Cerebral palsy, respiratory disorders, intellectual disability, visual impairment, hearing impairment, congenital heart defects

2. Anterior open bite, narrow palate, persistent drooling

3. Hypotonia (low muscle tone) of the perioral musculature

4. False. Cerebral palsy (CP) is sometimes termed a "static encephalopathy." The original lesion in the brain does not progress or result in further deterioration to the central nervous system (CNS). Be aware, however, that the clinical presentation of CP, especially muscle function, can change as an individual matures and ages.

5. Bronchopulmonary dysplasia develops most frequently in infants born with extremely low birth weights (<1,000 grams) and/or prior to 30 weeks gestation.

Case 3

Congenital Adrenal Hyperplasia, Hearing Loss, Intellectual Disability

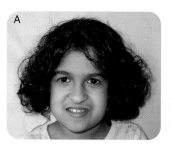 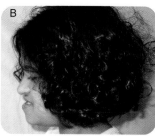

Figure 8.3.1a–b. Facial photographs

BACKGROUND INFORMATION 1
Congenital Adrenal Hyperplasia

- Congenital adrenal hyperplasia (CAH) is a term used for several autosomal recessive disorders, all of which exhibit defects in aldosterone synthesis, cortisol synthesis, or both.

- The resulting cortisol and/or aldosterone deficiencies can result in different clinical findings in females and males:

  - Females: Virilization, with ambiguous genitalia at birth, accelerated skeletal maturity, hirsutism, oligomenorrhea, infertility, inability to maintain sodium balance ("salt-wasting"), hypertension

  - Males: Often not diagnosed as a neonate because of the normal appearance of the genitalia. May present at several months of age due to failure to thrive, vomiting, dehydration, hypotension, hyponatremia, hyperkalemia. Later in childhood, these males may exhibit precocious puberty and accelerated skeletal maturity.

Wilson (2006), Robertson and Shilkofski (2005), Gorlin, Cohen, and Levin (1990)

A. Presenting Patient
- 9-year-, 10-month-old Arab-American female
- New patient visit

B. Chief Complaint
- Routine examination and evaluation for orthodontic treatment

C. Social History
- Patient lives at home with both parents and three brothers. All siblings are healthy.
- Patient attends special education class at public school; receives speech therapy and extra help with academic coursework.

D. Medical History
- Primary diagnosis: 21-hydroxylase deficiency type of congenital adrenal hyperplasia (CAH), also sometimes called simple virilizing adrenal hyperplasia. Another characteristic of this form of CAH is salt-wasting, in which the body is unable to maintain proper sodium balance. This patient's condition was diagnosed at birth, due to virilization of the genital organs (see Background Information 1).
- Patient is currently followed by a pediatric endocrinologist; routine visits every three months
- Hearing loss; cochlear implant was placed at age 3
- Cognitive impairment (mild-moderate range)
- Status post surgical correction of genital organs
- Current medications:
  - Hydrocortisone: 2.5 mg in a.m. and at noon, 5 mg in p.m.
  - Florinef (fludrocortisone acetate): 0.1 mg in a.m., 0.05 mg in p.m. to maintain mineralocorticoid levels
  - Gluco- and mineralocorticoid levels are checked every three months. Medication dosages may be altered based on laboratory findings.

FUNDAMENTAL POINT 1
Corticosteroid therapy

- A consideration for patients who have been on long-term corticosteroid therapy is that they many be unable to produce endogenous steroids adequate to cope with stressful situations (such as a surgical or dental procedure). It is advisable to consult with the patient's physician to determine current dosages of corticosteroids, explain the planned treatment to the physician, and determine if steroid supplementation is advisable prior to and after any procedures.

- Dehydration can be a precipitating factor in adrenal crisis. Therefore, it is important to ensure that these patients are adequately hydrated prior to dental treatment.

- Symptoms of adrenal crisis include:
  - Headache
  - Weakness
  - Nausea, vomiting
  - Confusion
  - Rapid heart rate
  - Sweaty face, palms of hands
  - Low blood pressure
- Treatment of adrenal crisis
  - IV or IM injection of hydrocortisone
  - Supportive treatment of low blood pressure with IV fluids
  - Lack of timely treatment may result in shock

Hurd (2006), Lockhart (2004)

E. Medical Consult (see Fundamental Point 1)

- Consult with the patient's endocrinologist resulted in the following recommendations:
  - For diagnostic procedures and cleaning, no supplementation of corticosteroids needed.
  - For procedures requiring local anesthetic, double corticosteroid dosages for 24 hours, starting the morning of the procedure.
  - The endocrinologist also felt that if general anesthetic (GA) was indicated for treatment, the patient should be admitted to the hospital one day prior to the procedure for management by pediatric endocrine service.

F. Dental History

- Patient had been to previous dentist and had cleanings performed. Previous dentist had been unable to take radiographs due to uncooperative behavior. Patient has never required any restorative treatment.
- Optimal water fluoridation levels
- Healthy, low-cariogenic diet
- Brushes without supervision once per day. Mother is aware that child does a poor job of brushing, and has tried to help. However, child is resistant to having another person help with brushing.

G. Extra-oral Exam

- Patient has an underdeveloped midface region, with relative prognathism of the jaw (see Figure 8.3.1b).

H. Intra-oral Exam (Figures 8.3.2 a–e)

- Anterior and bilateral posterior crossbites
- Class III malocclusion
- Anterior open bite (approximately 5 mm)
- Moderate crowding of maxillary arch with ectopic eruption of maxillary canines
- Plaque and calculus deposits throughout mouth
- Marginal gingivitis secondary to poor oral hygiene
- No caries noted

I. Diagnostic Tools (see Fundamental Point 2)

- Two bitewings (poor diagnostic quality in maxillary arch due to crowding and patient's inability to cooperate fully for radiographic exam). Radiographs were obtained with the assistance of the patient's mother. She helped to steady patient's head and keep film holder in patient's mouth. No interproximal caries noted.
- Panoramic film was attempted, but due to patient's inability to stand still for radiograph, no exposure was made.

J. Differential Diagnosis

- N/A

K. Diagnosis and Problem List
Diagnosis

- Congenital adrenal hyperplasia
- Hearing loss (status post placement of cochlear implant)
- Intellectual disability
- Malocclusion
- Poor oral hygiene

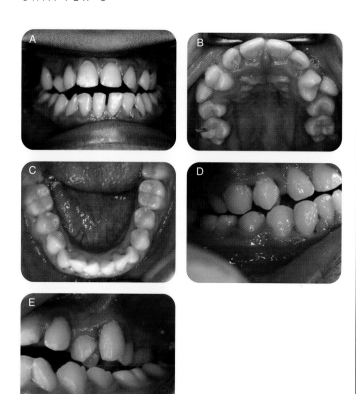

Figure 8.3.2a–e. Intra-oral photos showing malocclusion and gingivitis

Problem List

- High caries risk due to poor oral hygiene (see Fundamental Point 3)
- Gingival inflammation due to poor oral hygiene
- Class III malocclusion, mandibular prognathism
- Anterior open bite
- Moderate maxillary crowding; ectopic eruption of maxillary canines
- Patient was resistant to treatment

L. Comprehensive Treatment Plan

- Establish dental home
- Dental prophylaxis
- Fluoride treatment
- Review of oral hygiene; work with mother to establish techniques that may allow her to assist with daily oral hygiene regimen
- Orthodontic consultation
- Three-month recall
    - Re-evaluate oral hygiene and gingival status

M. Prognosis and Discussion

- Patient is unable to provide adequate oral hygiene for herself at this point, although with instruction

---

FUNDAMENTAL POINT 2
Radiographic Examination

- The American Dental Association (ADA) recommends that a new patient with permanent dentition receive a baseline radiographic examination consisting of posterior bitewings and a panoramic film, or posterior bitewings and selected periapical images. The American Academy of Pediatric Dentistry (AAPD) goes on to clarify that in cases in which diagnostic-quality radiographs are unobtainable, the risks of behavior management techniques, such as sedation, must be weighed against the possible benefits to the patient in obtaining these radiographs.

- In this patient, because she was currently caries-free on clinical examination and did not have a history of caries, the decision was made not to pursue additional behavioral management techniques to obtain radiographs.

- When a family member is asked to help with a radiographic exam, that person must be appropriately shielded to minimize radiation exposure. Placement of the film in the patient's mouth should be done by the oral health provider, with the family member being shown carefully how to maintain that placement.

http://www.ada.org/sections/professionalResources/pdfs/topics_radiography_examinations.pdf

AAPD (2011–2012a)

---

and reinforcement, her abilities in this area may improve in the future. The prognosis for improvement of gingival inflammation is poor unless mother (and/or other family members) can be trained to help provide oral hygiene on a daily basis.

- Patient has extensive orthodontic and, possibly, orthognathic treatment needs. A key consideration for a positive outcome in this area is the patient's ability to cooperate for treatment. Based on initial evaluation, the patient currently has limited ability to tolerate oral procedures. Further behavioral evaluation will be made when the patient returns for prophylaxis and fluoride treatment.

N. Complications and Alternative Treatment Plan

- If patient had clinically visible caries, what behavioral management techniques could be

considered to allow completion of the radiographic examination and restorative treatment?

FUNDAMENTAL POINT 3
Oral Considerations

- Caries risk: Use the American Academy of Pediatric Dentistry Caries Assessment Tool (CAT) in assigning a patient's risk category (AAPD 2011–2012b)

- Malocclusion: Patient referred to orthodontist for evaluation for treatment. A critical factor in making orthodontic treatment decisions will be the patient's ability to cooperate for lengthy, sometimes uncomfortable procedures, and her ability to improve and maintain oral hygiene.

Self-study Questions

1. **What class of medications is used to manage the clinical manifestations of congenital adrenal hyperplasia (CAH)?**
2. **What is the pattern of genetic inheritance associated with CAH? What is the chance that two parents with this defective gene will have a child with CAH?**

3. **What are two precipitating factors that can lead to adrenal crisis in patients with adrenal insufficiency?**
4. **Name four clinical signs of adrenal crisis.**
5. **Provide one important reason why outpatient oral sedation is not an appropriate management option for this patient.**

Answers are located at the end of the case.

Bibliography

American Academy of Pediatric Dentistry. 2011–2012a. Prescribing Dental Radiographs Reference Manual. *Pediatr Dent* 33(6):289–91.
American Academy of Pediatric Dentistry. 2011–2012b. Guideline on Caries-risk Assessment and Management for Infants, Children, and Adolescents, Reference Manual. *Pediatr Dent* 33(6):110–15.
Gorlin R, Cohen MM, Levin LS. 1990. *Syndromes of the Head and Neck*, 3rd edition. Oxford University Press: New York. 1617–22.

Hurd R. 2006. Medline Plus, U.S. National Library of Medicine, National Institute of Health, www.nlm.nih.gov/medlineplus/ency/article/000357.htm.
Lockhart PB. 2004. *Dental Care of the Medically Complex Patient*, 5th edition. Elsevier/Wright: Edinburgh. 102, 108–9.
Robertson J, Shilkofski N (eds). 2005. *The Harriet Lane Handbook*, 17th edition. Elsevier/Mosby: Philadelphia. 256.
Wilson TA. 2005. *Congenital Adrenal Hyperplasia*, www.emedicine.com/ped/topic48.htm.

SELF-STUDY ANSWERS

1. Corticosteroids, both glucocorticoids and mineralocorticoids

2. CAH is associated with an autosomal recessive inheritance pattern. If two parents are carriers of the defective gene responsible for this disorder, they have a 1:4 chance of having a child with the disorder.

3. Stress and dehydration can both lead to adrenal crisis in patients with adrenal insufficiency.

4. The following may be signs of adrenal crisis: headache, nausea, vomiting, rapid heartbeat, low blood pressure, excessive sweating, confusion, weakness.

5. Children receiving oral sedative medications are generally kept NPO for a number of hours prior to the procedure. This could result in dehydration, which can be a precipitating factor for adrenal crisis.

Case 4

Seizure Disorder, Intellectual Disability

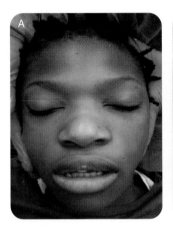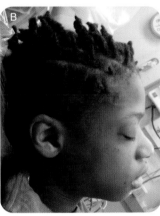

Figure 8.4.1a–b. Facial photographs

A. Presenting Patient

- 13-year-, 10-month-old African-American female
- Seizure disorder (epilepsy), cognitive impairment (severe)
- Visit for treatment under IV sedation

B. Chief Complaint

- Patient had maxillary anterior tooth avulsed due to trauma during a seizure. Patient's mother would like this tooth to be replaced.

C. Social History

- Patient lives at home with mother, grandmother, and one younger sister.
- Patient attends special education classes in public school system.

D. Medical History

- Patient was born full-term in Antigua.
- Patient has history of generalized seizures, tonic/clonic type. According to mother's report, patient had her first seizure at 4 months of age.
- Patient's last seizure was 1 1/2 years ago.

- Patient did not walk independently until 2 1/2 years of age.
- Patient has never developed age-appropriate verbal skills; makes needs and wants known primarily through body gestures.
- According to her neurodevelopmental report, patient functions at a level of severe intellectual disability.
- Current medication: Valproic acid (anti-epileptic)

E. Medical Consult

- Patient's primary care physician was consulted prior to scheduling for IV sedation. According to the physician, the patient's seizures are currently well controlled. No other systemic conditions exist to contraindicate sedation. Since the patient's seizures have been well controlled for more than a year, she is considered to have either an ASA II or III status, according to the American Society of Anesthesiologists (see Fundamental Point 1).

F. Dental History

- Patient has been treated in current clinic for 10 years, with annual visits.
- Patient has always been extremely resistant to dental treatment, although she allows her mother to brush her teeth twice daily.
- Due to behavioral resistance, all treatment other than cursory examination has been accomplished under IV sedation.
- Patient first avulsed her maxillary left central incisor four years ago. It was reimplanted within an hour of avulsion and subsequently required endodontic treatment. The tooth was re-avulsed 1 1/2 years ago, while the patient was at summer camp, and the tooth was not reimplanted at that time.
- A removable appliance (similar to a Hawley) to replace the missing tooth was fabricated a year ago, but the patient refused to wear the appliance.

BACKGROUND INFORMATION 1

Seizure Disorders

Definitions

- Seizure: Synchronized discharges from a population of cortical neurons resulting in a clinically evident alteration of function or behavior.

- Epilepsy: Two or more seizures not precipitated by a known cause (i.e., idiopathic seizure activity).

- 70% to 75% of seizure disorders are idiopathic.

Non-idiopathic Seizure Etiologies

- Fevers, particularly in children under 2 years old

- Inborn errors of metabolism

- Congenital brain malformation

- Acquired cortical defect (neoplasm, infection, trauma)

- Neurodegenerative disease

- Neurocutaneous disorders

- Electrolyte imbalances

- Toxins/drugs

Classification of Seizures

- Generalized (involve both cerebral hemispheres)
  - Involves loss of consciousness

- Partial (limited to a discrete segment of the cerebral cortex)
  - No loss of consciousness; may have altered consciousness

- Status epilepticus: Prolonged, non-self-limiting seizure activity; can be life threatening

- Generalized and partial seizures are sub-classified depending on clinical manifestations

Lockhart (2004), Robertson and Shilkofski, (2005), Turner and Glickman (2005)

- Optimal water fluoridation levels
- Healthy, low-cariogenic diet

G. Extra-oral Exam (Figures 8.4.1 a–b)

- No significant findings

H. Intra-oral Exam (Figures 8.4.2 a–e)

- Permanent dentition
- Maxillary left central incisor missing secondary to trauma

FUNDAMENTAL POINT 1

Obtaining a History for Seizure Disorder

- When evaluating a patient with a seizure disorder, it is important to know if the seizures are currently well-controlled or if the patient continues to have seizures despite anti-seizure treatment. The following information should be elicited, either through parental report or from medical consult (Lockhart 2004):
  - Type of seizures
  - Frequency of seizures
  - Date of last seizure
  - Anti-epileptic medications being taken
  - Precipitating factors (if known)

- The classification of physical status provided by the American Society of Anesthesiologists (ASA) is the most commonly used pre-operative risk evaluation system used in the U.S. (American Society of Anesthesiologists 2007):
  - An ASA II patient has mild systemic disease
  - An ASA III patient has severe systemic disease

- Intact amalgam restorations in teeth number 2, 3, 30, and 31
- Occlusion: Class I molar and canine relationships, 70% overbite, 1 mm overjet
- Soft tissue within normal limits
- Good oral hygiene
- No active caries noted

I. Diagnostic Tools (Figure 8.4.3)

- Four bitewing radiographs taken while patient was sedated show no signs of interproximal caries. A maxillary anterior periapical radiograph was taken six months prior to this visit (not shown).

J. Differential Diagnosis

- N/A

K. Diagnosis and Problem List

Diagnosis

- Seizure disorder (see Fundamental Point 2)
- Severe cognitive impairment

Problem List

- Maxillary left central incisor missing secondary to trauma
- Extremely resistant to dental treatment

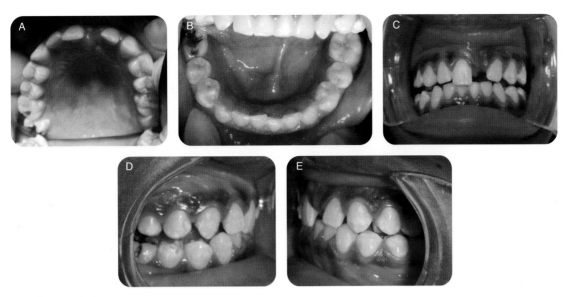

Figure 8.4.2a–e. Intra-oral photos

FUNDAMENTAL POINT 2
Complications of Seizure Disorders

- Patients who experience seizures that involve loss of consciousness and/or loss of motor control are at higher risk for dental trauma and oral soft tissue trauma than the general population.

- Gingival hypertrophy is often associated with use of the anti-epileptic drug (AED) Dilantin (phenytoin). Oral side effects are not commonly reported with other AEDs.

- Valproic acid can cause decreased platelet count. Although thrombocytopenia is not usually severe, planning for significant elective surgery should include laboratory evaluation of bleeding parameters.

Aragon and Burneo (2007)

L. Comprehensive Treatment Plan

- Patient scheduled for two treatment sessions under IV sedation
- At the first session, the following treatment was completed:
  - Thorough oral examination
  - Radiographic examination
  - Prophylaxis, topical fluoride treatment
  - Impressions of the upper and lower arches were taken so the laboratory can fabricate an appliance to replace tooth number 9.

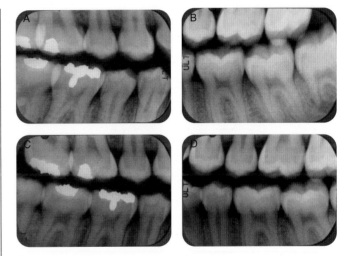

Figure 8.4.3. Pre-op bitewing radiographs

- At the second IV session, the appliance will be cemented in place.
- Unless the patient has problems with the appliance (or other dental problems), she will be seen under IV sedation for an annual examination.

M. Prognosis and Discussion

- The prognosis for the appliance to replace tooth number 9 is questionable, even though it is considered a temporary solution until the patient is old enough for an implant. Although her seizures seem to be well controlled at this point, there is greater concern about how the patient will tolerate the appliance. The patient has already shown that she will not tolerate a removable appliance, so it remains to be seen if she will tolerate the cemented one.

- Patient has a mother who is extremely conscientious about oral care, and motivated to keep her daughter's mouth clean. Therefore, her oral hygiene at this time is excellent. If a time comes when the mother is no longer the primary caregiver, the prognosis for continued good oral health is questionable. The patient's behavior is difficult, and maintaining her dentition and periodontium in optimal health will require a dedicated caregiver.

N. Complications and Alternative Treatment Plan

- Be aware of the risk for future trauma when planning treatment in patients who have sustained dental trauma during a seizure. In this case, it was already known that the patient would not tolerate a removable appliance. The use of a removable appliance in a patient with uncontrollable seizures is not advised, because it could become dislodged during the seizure and cause intra-oral soft tissue trauma, or possibly block the airway. Likewise, a Maryland bridge was not considered, because of the possibility of dislodgement and aspiration during a seizure. A fixed 3- (or 4-) unit bridge was not thought to be appropriate for this patient for several reasons. First, the remaining maxillary incisors were in excellent condition, so there was a reluctance to prepare them for crowns. Second, placing a fixed bridge in this area would make the abutment teeth more vulnerable, as a group, to trauma during a future seizure. After careful consideration, it was decided that an implant was the most appropriate treatment to replace tooth number 9, with the temporary banded, cemented appliance shown as an interim restoration.

FUNDAMENTAL POINT 3
Emergency Management of Seizures

- If a patient has a seizure in the dental office:
  - Remove all instruments from patient's mouth and away from dental chair
  - Place dental chair in a supine position as close to the floor as possible
  - Place patient on his side, if possible
  - Do not attempt to restrain patient
  - Time the seizure
  - Call 911 if the seizure lasts longer than three minutes or if the patient becomes cyanotic at any time
  - Administer oxygen at a rate of 6 to 8 L/minute

- After seizure, try to evaluate patient's level of consciousness
- Do not allow the patient to leave the office if his/her level of awareness has not returned to baseline (this may be difficult to determine in a patient who has significant cognitive impairment)
- Do a brief oral examination to determine if any oral injuries were sustained during seizure
- Depending on patient's post-ictal status, either discharge to home with responsible adult or transfer to emergency room for further monitoring and evaluation

Aragon and Burneo (2007)

Self-study Questions

1. *What are the two main classifications for seizure disorders?*
2. *What is the definition of epilepsy?*
3. *What are important questions that need to be asked before treating a patient with a history of seizures?*
4. *The American Society of Anesthesiologists (ASA) has developed a pre-anesthesia scale that attempts to measure what?*
5. *Do most anti-epileptic medications cause gingival hyperplasia?*

Answers are located at the end of the case.

Bibliography

American Society of Anesthesiologists (ASA). 2007. Physical Status Classification System, www.asahq.org/clinical/physicalstatus.htm.

Aragon CE, Burneo JG. 2007. Understanding the patient with epilepsy and seizures in the dental practice. *J of the Canadian Dent Assoc* 73:1, 71–6.

Lockhart PB. 2004. *Dental Care of the Medically Complex Patient*, 5th edition. Elsevier/Wright: Edinburgh. 90–2.

Robertson, J, Shilkofski N. 2005. *The Harriet Lane Handbook*, 17th Edition, Mosby: Philadelphia. 513–20.

Turner MD, Glickman RS. 2005. Epilepsy in the oral and maxillofacial patient: current therapy. *J Oral Maxillofacial Surg* 63:996–1005.

SELF-STUDY ANSWERS

1. Generalized (abnormal electrical activity involves both cerebral hemispheres) and partial (seizure activity is limited to discrete section of cerebral cortex).

2. The diagnosis of epilepsy is based on a history of at least two *unprovoked* (idiopathic in nature) seizures.

3. What type of seizures does the patient experience? When was the last seizure? What is the frequency of seizures? Is the patient on anti-epileptic medication, and if yes, what medication? Are there any specific precipitating factors associated with the patient's seizures?.

4. The ASA system classifies patient physical status with the aim of evaluating pre-operative risk.

5. No. Dilantin (phenytoin) causes gingival hyperplasia in approximately 50% of the patients who take it. Gingival hyperplasia is not a reported side-effect of other anti-epileptic drugs.

Case 5

Asperger's Syndrome

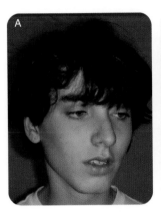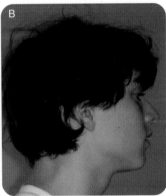

Figure 8.5.1a–b. Facial photographs

A. Presenting Patient
- 14-year-, 2-month-old Caucasian male
- Recall visit

B. Chief Complaint
- Patient presenting for a recall exam; however, according to mother, child has bleeding gums.

C. Social History
- Patient lives at home with both parents and 11-year-old brother
- Patient attends private school
- Both parents work full time
- Upper middle class socio-economic status

D. Medical History
- Patient has been diagnosed with Asperger's Syndrome (see Background Information 1)
- Patient has history of asthma in early childhood. According to mother, has not had an asthmatic attack for at least three years; is not currently on any medication for asthma.
- Patient is followed on an annual basis by a pediatric urologist for hydronephrosis (distention of the

kidney due obstructed urine flow), which was discovered on a prenatal ultrasound (family history of kidney disorder). Kidney function has always been within normal limits.
- Patient is generally in good health, and is not currently on any medications.

E. Medical Consult
- Not necessary at this time

F. Dental History
- Patient has been treated in the same clinic since 3 years of age. Comes regularly at six-month intervals.
- Lives in area without water fluoridation. Took vitamins with fluoride supplementation from 1 year of age until about 8 years of age.
- Resistant to oral examinations and treatment as a young child, but behavior has improved as he has grown older. Level of cooperation is much higher when he is allowed to distract himself with a hand-held video game (see Fundamental Point 1).
- Brushes without supervision (will not allow anyone to assist with oral care) once or twice daily. Oral hygiene is consistently poor.
- Has a fairly limited diet (due to issues with food textures, he prefers soft foods that do not require much chewing), but it has a low cariogenic potential.

G. Extra-oral Exam (Figures 8.5.1 a–b)
- No significant findings

H. Intra-oral Exam (Figures 8.5.2 a–e)
- Permanent dentition; all teeth erupted except for third molars
- Occlusion: 2-mm overjet, 50% overbite; class I molar and canine relationships
- Marginal gingivitis, most pronounced in maxillary and mandibular incisor regions
- Moderate/heavy plaque accumulation

BACKGROUND INFORMATION 1
Asperger's Syndrome

- The diagnosis of Asperger's is based on behavioral characteristics. In the *Diagnostic and Statistical Manual of Mental Disorders (DSM-IV)*, it is included in the section of autistic spectrum disorders, under the subcategory of pervasive developmental disorders.

Diagnostic Criteria

- Impairment in social interaction. Must include at least two of the following:
  - Impairment of nonverbal behaviors such as facial expression, body postures, eye-to-eye contact
  - Failure to develop age-appropriate peer relationships
  - Lack of seeking to share enjoyment, interests, or achievements with others
  - Lack of social or emotional reciprocity
- Restricted repetitive and stereotyped patterns of behavior, interests, and activities. Must include at least one of the following:
  - Preoccupation with one or more restricted pattern of interest; abnormal in intensity or focus
  - Inflexible adherence to specific routines or rituals
  - Stereotyped and repetitive motor mannerisms
  - Persistent preoccupation with parts of objects
- Clinically significant impairment in social, occupational, or other important areas of functioning.
- No clinically significant delay in language.
- No clinically significant delay in cognitive development or in the development of age-appropriate self-help skills, adaptive behavior, and curiosity about the environment.
- Criteria are not met for another specific pervasive developmental disorder or schizophrenia.

DSM-IV (1995)

FUNDAMENTAL POINT 1
Behavioral Considerations

- Ability to cooperate in the dental setting is a primary consideration when treating children with a diagnoses from the autistic spectrum disorders. These children often experience heightened reactions to sensory input such as light, touch, and auditory stimuli. It can be imagined that a routine visit to a dental office could be perceived by the child with autism as a virtual bombardment of the senses. Although children with Asperger's syndrome have good verbal and cognitive skills, they are still subject to many of the sensory issues common to other autistic spectrum disorders.
- A parent can be very helpful in providing information concerning which type of stimuli might be most disturbing to his child. The parent might also be able to inform the dentist about distraction techniques that have worked in the past to help the child through stressful situations. These may include listening to music (or some other type of auditory input) through headphones or using a hand-held game system, such as the patient discussed in this case.
- Desensitization, a technique in which a patient is taught to replace fearful or maladaptive responses with non-fearful responses, also may be useful for enabling treatment of individuals with autism. Although some dentists may be familiar with desensitization techniques, and may use these routinely with all children, true desensitization for a phobic or hypersensitive patient is a time-consuming endeavor. If the dental office is not prepared to offer desensitization, referral to a behavioral therapist who works with children with autism may be an appropriate alternative.

Grandin (2006), Friedlander et al. (2006), Connick et al. (2000)

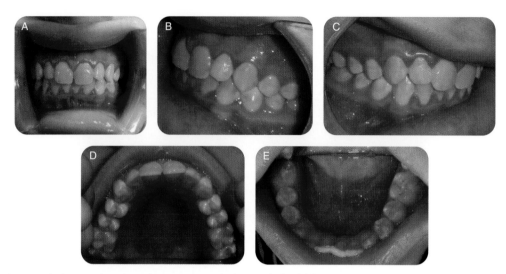

Figure 8.5.2a–e. Intra-oral photos showing plaque accumulation and gingivitis

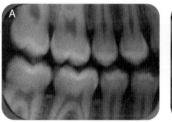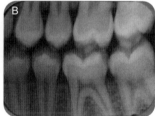

Figure 8.5.3. Bitewing radiographs

- Oral hygiene is poor
- Caries-free dentition
- Sealants present on all first molars

I. Diagnostic Tools

- Two bitewing radiographs show no interproximal caries (Figure 8.5.3)

J. Differential Diagnosis

- N/A

K. Diagnosis and Problem List

Diagnosis

- Asperger's syndrome
- Poor oral hygiene
- Marginal gingivitis

Problem List

- Increased caries and periodontal health risk due to poor oral hygiene (see Fundamental Point 2)

L. Comprehensive Treatment Plan

- Dental prophylaxis
- Fluoride treatment

FUNDAMENTAL POINT 2
Oral Considerations in Asperger's Syndrome

- Although this patient is not taking any psychotropic medications, many patients with autism take medications to mediate behaviors. Xerostomia is a common side effect of psychotropic medications. Sialorrhea is a less commonly reported but known side effect of some of these medications. Many of these may also interact with or potentiate the effects of medications that are commonly used as sedative agents by pediatric dentists.

- Many behavioral therapies employed with children with autistic spectrum disorders use food, especially candy, as a reward. This can increase caries risk.

- Use the American Academy of Pediatric Dentistry caries assessment tool (CAT) in assigning a patient's risk category.

- Periodontal health: Poor compliance with oral hygiene is not a consistent finding in children with autism spectrum disorders. Some children are very compliant, to the point of being obsessive brushers. Others, as the patient discussed here, have oral textural and taste sensitivities that interfere with adequate hygiene.

Friedlander et al. (2006), AAPD (2011–2012a and b)

- Review of oral hygiene (with parent and child)
- Placement of sealants on second molars
- Six-month recall: Re-evaluate oral hygiene status

M. Prognosis and Discussion

- The prognosis for periodontal health is poor due to consistently inadequate oral hygiene. This has been discussed with both parent and child in the past. Patient, however, has always had oral sensitivities. He states that he "doesn't like to brush his teeth because I don't like the way any toothbrushes feel and I hate the taste of all the toothpastes." We have discussed with him that use of toothpaste is not necessary if it is so distasteful. His mother has also purchased numerous different toothbrushes,

but he continues to be resistant to home care. We suggested at this visit that use of gauze wipes might be more tolerable than a toothbrush, and he has agreed to try this method.

N. Complications and Alternative Treatment Plan

- What additional management techniques might need to be considered if this patient, who has heightened oral sensitivities, requires extensive restorative procedures?
- How might this child's oral health be affected if he was taking psychotropic medications?

Self-study Questions

1. **On what bases are any of the autistic spectrum disorders (ASD) diagnosed?**
2. **Do individuals who are diagnosed with Asperger's syndrome have cognitive impairment?**
3. **Are there any specific oral findings associated with autism?**

4. **What are the factors that might put a child with autism at high risk for dental caries?**
5. **What is desensitization?**

Answers are located at the end of the case.

Bibliography

American Academy of Pediatric Dentistry. 2011–2012a. Caries-risk assessment and Management for infants, children, and adolescents. *Pediatr Dent* 33(6):110–17.

American Academy of Pediatric Dentistry. 2011–2012b. Treatment of plaque-induced gingivitis, chronic periodontitis, and other clinical conditions. *Pediatr Dent* 33(6):307–16.

Connick C, Pugliese S, Willette J, Palat M. 2000. Desensitization: Strengths and limitations of its use in dentistry for the patient with severe and profound mental retardation. *J of Dent for Children* 250–5, July-Aug.

Diagnostic and Statistical Manual of Mental Disorders. 1995. American Psychiatric Association: Washington, DC. 75–7.

Friedlander AH, Yagiela JA, Paterno VI, Mahler ME. 2006. The neuropathology, medical management and dental implications of autism. *JADA* 137, 1517–27, November.

Grandin T. 2006. *Thinking in Pictures, and Other Reports from My Life with Autism.* Vintage Books: New York.

ANSWERS

1. The diagnosis of any autistic spectrum disorder is based on behavior. There are no imaging, blood, or genetic analyses that are used to make a diagnosis of an ASD (although these tests may be used to rule out other disorders).

2. Children diagnosed with Asperger's syndrome do not display any significant delays in either language or cognitive development.

3. No, there are no specific oral findings associated with autism.

4. Factors that could put a child with autism at high risk for dental caries include: resistant behaviors that make it difficult to maintain oral hygiene on a daily basis, as well as in the dental setting; candy being used as a frequent reward for acceptable behaviors; oral sensitivities, including hypersensitivity to taste and texture; psychotropic medications that may cause xerostomia.

5. Desensitization is a behavioral therapy in which individuals with specific phobias are gradually taught to replace fearful responses with non-fearful responses.

Case 6

Sickle Cell Anemia, Intellectual Disability

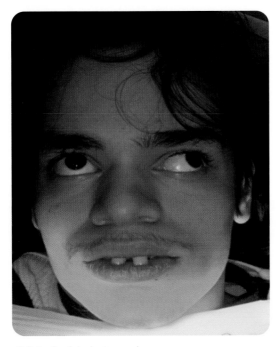

Figure 8.6.1. Facial photograph

A. Presenting Patient
- 13-year-, 2-month-old Hispanic male
- New patient visit (recent immigrant to U.S. from Dominican Republic; referred to dental clinic by pediatrician)

B. Chief Complaint
- Father states that the "doctor told us his teeth look bad, and we need to see the dentist."

C. Social History
- Patient attends public school; is in a special class for children with developmental disabilities.
- Lives with both parents and two sisters (sisters both have sickle cell trait, not full anemia)
- Father works full-time, mother is the primary caregiver

- Mother speaks only Spanish; when going for medical and dental appointments, she is accompanied by either the father or one of the daughters, who speak English.
- Socio-economic status is lower middle-class

D. Medical History
- Sickle cell anemia diagnosed in infancy (see Background Information 1 and Fundamental Point 1)
- Has been hospitalized four times for sickle cell crisis; last hospitalization was two years ago
- Hospitalization in Dominican Republic when patient was eight years old involved osteomyelitis of leg
- Severe intellectual disability
- Patient was on penicillin prophylaxis until about nine years of age; is not currently on any medication regimen

E. Medical Consult
- Hematologist stated that he does not routinely recommend antibiotic prophylaxis for his sickle cell patients who are having dental procedures
- Because of this patient's extensive treatment needs, and the plan to have treatment performed under general anesthesia (GA), the hematologist would like to have the patient admitted to the hospital one day prior to the procedure for monitoring of hemoglobin levels and possible blood transfusion. No precise guidelines exist as to what hemoglobin levels dictate the need for transfusion. The hematologist will base the decision on the patient's history and current treatment needs

F. Dental History
- According to the father, the patient was seen by a dentist only once before, many years ago, in the Dominican Republic. At that time, the patient had two primary teeth extracted
- Patient is extremely resistant to oral home care; parents feel unable to provide toothbrushing on a regular basis

BACKGROUND INFORMATION 1
Sickle Cell Anemia

- Genetic disorder that involves defect in the β-hemoglobin chain of red blood cells.
  - β-globin gene (sickle hemoglobin, HbS) is responsible
- In the most common form of sickle cell anemia, the individual is homozygous for HbS, i.e., one gene is inherited from each parent.
- If a child inherits a defective gene from only one parent, they will have the sickle cell trait, which is generally a benign condition.
  - Approximately 8% of African-Americans carry the trait; it is also found in Mediterranean, Middle Eastern, African, and Afro-Caribbean populations.
- Affected red blood cells show increased adhesion to vascular endothelium. Intravascular aggregation of cells, inflammation of microvasculature, and vasoconstriction result in the clinical symptoms of sickle cell crisis.
- Vaso-occlusive sickle cell crises can affect multiple systems in the body. Sequelae can include tissue anoxia, infarcts, necrosis, and pain. Factors that may precipitate a vaso-occlusive crisis include dehydration, hypoxia, infection, stress, and menstruation.
- Complications of sickle cell anemia are multi-systemic, each requiring its own special treatment. Psychosocial problems, related to dealing with any chronic disease state, are also frequently seen.

da Fonseca, Oueis, and Casamassimo (2007), Kelleher, Bishop, and Briggs (1996), Lockhart (2004)

FUNDAMENTAL POINT 1
Medical History for Sickle Cell Anemia

- A careful medical history must be elicited for all patients with sickle cell prior to dental treatment
  - Vaso-occlusive crises: frequency, duration, hospitalizations, date of last crisis
  - Damage to any organ systems
  - History of transfusions and any related complications
  - Current medication regimens
  - Current and past infections
  - Psychosocial issues
- Any extensive treatment needs should be discussed with hematologist prior to treatment

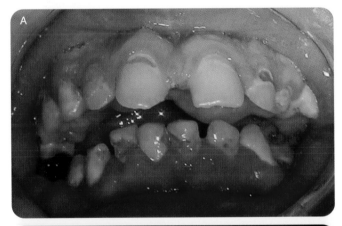

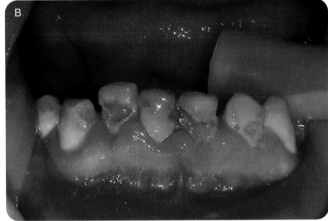

Figure 8.6.2a–b. Intra-oral photos showing severe dental decay and gingival hypertrophy

---

- Patient has a highly cariogenic diet; he frequently snacks on sweets and consumes large amounts of fruit juice

G. Extra-oral Exam (Figure 8.6.1)

- Marked strabismus
- Proclined maxillary incisors, indentations in lower lip due to pressure from incisors

H. Intra-oral Exam (see Fundamental Point 2)

- Permanent dentition with rampant cervical dental caries

FUNDAMENTAL POINT 2
Oral Consideration with Sickle Cell Anemia

- Intra-oral findings associated with sickle anemia can include:
  - Enlarged maxilla secondary to increased bone marrow activity
  - Increase in maxillary incisor proclination and interdental spacing
  - Mandibular incisor retrusion can be seen secondary to large overjet and lip pressure
  - Pallor of oral soft tissues
  - Gingival enlargement
  - Glossitis
- Radiographic findings can include:
  - Coarse trabecular ("stepladder") pattern in bone
  - Mandibular radiopaque lesions
  - Thin border of mandible
  - Granular appearance of cranial bones
  - Pulp stones
- Oral/systemic complications include:
  - Mandibular osteomyelitis
  - Mandibular nerve neuropathies
  - Pulpal necrosis in teeth without caries or history of trauma
  - Facial or dental pain secondary to vaso-occlusive crisis
  - Osteoporosis or osteopenia (patient may be taking bisphophonates)

Alves et al. (2006), da Fonseca, Oueis, and Casamassimo (2007), Kelleher, Bishop, and Briggs (1996), Licciardello, Bertuna, and Samperi (2007)

- Extremely poor oral hygiene, with generalized severe plaque accumulation (Figures 8.6.2a-b were taken after plaque deposits were removed; caries detection could not be accomplished without removal of plaque)
- Enlarged maxilla with wide interdental spacing in incisor area
- 10-mm overjet, 100% overbite
- Generalized gingival inflammation, gingival hypertrophy

I. Diagnostic Tools
- Patient's cooperation was not at a level at which intra-oral radiographs could be obtained

J. Differential Diagnosis
- N/A

K. Diagnosis and Problem List
Diagnosis
- Sickle cell anemia
- Severe intellectual disability and resistant to care
- Rampant dental caries
- Generalized gingival inflammation secondary to poor oral hygiene
- Malocclusion (large overjet, deep overbite)

Problem List
- High caries risk due to extremely poor oral hygiene, poor dietary habits (frequent consumption of fermentable carbohydrates), and behavioral resistance to treatment and home care.
- Increased risk for periodontal infection due to poor oral hygiene
- Malocclusion

L. Comprehensive Treatment Plan
- Due to extent of treatment needs and the patient's behavioral resistance, treatment was planned to be completed under general anesthesia (GA) in the operating room.
- The importance of daily oral hygiene must be discussed with the parents prior to the GA appointment. Clinic staff will work with the parents to develop techniques for an effective oral hygiene regimen that will work for the patient.
- Dietary modification (reduction of fermentable carbohydrate consumption) must also be stressed to the parents.
- A full-mouth series of radiographs will be taken once the patient is under GA. A final treatment plan will be determined at that time; some teeth may not be restorable and therefore will be extracted.
- Anterior teeth will be restored with composite resin.
- Posterior teeth will be treated with stainless steel crowns.
- Fluoride treatment will be done in the operating room.
- A dentifrice with high fluoride concentration for caries control will be prescribed.

- Following treatment, the patient is to be followed on a three-month recall schedule in the clinic to:
  - Re-evaluate oral hygiene status; discuss with parents whether they feel that the techniques taught to brush the patient's dentition have been effective.
  - Review dietary recommendations; determine whether the parents have been able to make changes.
  - Evaluate status of restorations placed in operating room.

M. Prognosis and Discussion

- Note that this patient's prognosis is complicated by his intellectual disability and behavior more than by the sickle cell anemia.
- The prognosis for continued maintenance of this patient's dentition is poor, unless the parents make a concerted effort to improve their son's daily oral hygiene and diet. There are already numerous teeth with very questionable prognoses.
- If extraction of teeth is required, the patient is not a good candidate for replacement with fixed prosthesis at this time (due to poor hygiene, soft tissue inflammation). Given the patient's resistance to intra-oral manipulations, his ability to tolerate a removable prosthesis is also questionable.
- The patient is not a candidate for orthodontic or orthognathic treatment at this time due to:
  - Poor oral hygiene
  - Resistant behavior requiring sedation or GA for any procedures other than cursory examinations and cleanings.

N. Complications and Alternative Treatment Plan

- If the patient's behavior was cooperative, would he be a good candidate for orthodontic treatment?
- How does the increased probability of osteomyelitis affect the decision to extract or restore teeth with questionable prognoses?
- What would be the primary post-operative concern in patients requiring extractions?

Self-study Questions

1. **Genetically, how does the full sickle cell genotype differ from the genotype for sickle cell trait?**
2. **Is there an ethnic prediliction for sickle cell anemia?**
3. **What are possible sequelae of a vaso-occlusive sickle cell crisis?**
4. **What is the underlying cause for the maxillary enlargement that is present in many individuals with sickle cell anemia?**
5. **Name possible precipitating factors for a vaso-occlusive crisis.**

Answers are located at the end of the case.

Bibliography

Alves PVM, Alves DKM, de Souza MMG, Torres SR. 2006. Orthodontic treatment of patients with sickle-cell anemia. *The Angle Orthodontist* 76(2):269–73.

da Fonseca MA, Oueis HS, Casamassimo PS. 2007. Sickle cell anemia: A review for the pediatric dentist. *Ped Dent* 29(2):159–69.

Kelleher M, Bishop K, Briggs P. 1996. Oral complications associated with sickle cell anemia. *Oral Med Oral Path Oral Radiol Endod* 82(2):225–8.

Licciardello V, Bertuna G, Samperi P. 2007. Craniofacial morphology in patients with sickle sell disease: a cephalometric analysis. *European J of Orthodontics* 29(3): 238–42.

Lockhart PB. 2004. *Dental Care of the Medically Complex Patient*, 5th Edition. Elsevier/Wright: Edinburgh. 116–18.

SELF-STUDY ANSWERS

1. In the most common type of sickle cell anemia in the U.S., the patients are homozygous for the HbS gene. Individuals with the sickle cell trait are heterozygous for HbS, and are asymptomatic.

2. In the U.S., sickle cell anemia is seen most frequently in African-Americans. It may also be present in individuals of Mediterranean and Middle-Eastern descent.

3. Sequelae of a vaso-occlusive crisis can include tissue anoxia, tissue necrosis, infarct, and pain. These can occur in any organ system in the body.

4. The maxillary enlargement is secondary to heightened bone marrow activity and an increase in the marrow space in the maxilla.

5. Factors that may precipitate a vaso-occlusive crisis in a patient with sickle cell anemia include hypoxia, infection, stress, dehydration, menstruation.

9

Restorative Dentistry

Kevin J. Donly

Case 1

Resin Restoration of Incipient Decay (Primary or Permanent Molar)

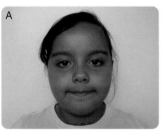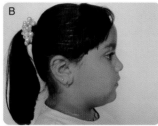

Figure 9.1.1a–b. Facial photographs

A. Presenting Patient
- 6-year-, 8-month-old Hispanic female
- Presents for a restorative visit

B. Chief Complaint
- Patient has presented previously for a comprehensive exam; this is her first restorative visit. Mother reports that "child has some small cavities"

C. Social History
- Patient is in kindergarten
- Involved in swimming and summer camps
- Parents both work as research assistants
- Socio-economic status is mid-level
- Patient is an only child

D. Medical History
- Mild intermittent asthma with symptoms related to specific allergens (see Fundamental Point 1).
- American Society of Anesthesiologists (ASA) 2
- Medications: Singulair for seasonal allergies
- Patient has never been hospitalized; has never gone to the emergency room for asthma treatments

E. Medical Consult
- Not necessary at this time

FUNDAMENTAL POINT 1
Medical History in Asthma Patients
- Obtain a thorough understanding on the severity and control of the asthma. See Chapter 1 Case 7 for a complete presentation of the clinical issues related to asthma
- Question on (Graham 2006):
  - Medications used for asthma control and frequency
  - Frequency and severity of the episodes
  - Any visits to the emergency room for the asthma
  - Symptoms experienced by the patient
  - Limitations or restrictions on any activities
- Quick relief medications, including short-acting beta agonists (e.g., albuterol) are taken as needed to promptly reverse acute airflow obstruction and relieve accompanying symptoms. Increased use of asthma medication and time of the day that the asthma medication is used could lead to xerostomia. This could be associated with increase in caries experience in the primary dentition. (Redding and Stoloff 2004, Milano et al. 2006)

F. Dental History
- Child had her first dental visit one month ago
- Positive behavior for all care given
- Optimal water fluoridation
- High cariogenic diet
- Toothbrushing with supervision twice a day

G. Extra-oral Exam (Figures 9.1.1 a–b)

- Patient is slightly overweight for height and age
- Mild deviation at opening and closing

H. Intra-oral Exam

- Early mixed dentition
- Retained primary maxillary right central incisor with slight mobility
- Occlusion: 2 mm of overjet, 5% overbite (secondary to tooth emerging in mouth); mild crowding of the lower arch; bilateral class I molars, bilateral class I canines
- Soft tissue: Within normal limits
- Moderate plaque accumulation
- Oral hygiene is poor
- Visible interproximal caries on tooth S
- Tooth T has stained occlusal groves and possible cavitation. Cavitation noted on the buccal groove.

FUNDAMENTAL POINT 2

Complications in Asthma and Obese Patients

- Possible intra- and extra-oral concerns with asthmatic patients (Steinbacher and Glick 2001):
  - Patients tend to be mouth breathers
  - Reduction in salivary flow and dry mouth may increase caries risk
  - Throat irritation
  - Dryness of mouth
  - Candidiasis
  - Gingivitis
- Overweight children can be susceptible to secondary problems including hypertension, diabetes mellitus, and increased caries rate. Appropriate diet and patient referral should be considered when necessary (Willerhausen et al. 2007)

I. Diagnostic Tools

- Two bitewing radiographs and one maxillary anterior periapical radiograph show interproximal caries, a retained primary tooth, and a radio-opaque area apical to tooth D. (Figures 9.1.3 a–c)
- No other radiographs were taken at this time due to the mother's concern for radiation exposure and no other pathology suspected
- The patient will have a panoramic film taken at a future recall and a maxillary anterior periapical radiograph as indicated to monitor emergence of tooth number 8 (see Fundamental Point 3).

J. Differential Diagnosis

- N/A

K. Diagnosis and Problem List (see Fundamental Point 2)

Diagnosis

- Mild asthma
- Overweight
- Dental caries
- Pathology apical to tooth D

Problem List

- High caries risk secondary to asthma, cariogenic diet
- Moderate plaque accumulation and lack of dental home prior to 6 years of age (determined using American Academy of Pediatric Dentistry caries assessment tool, AAPD [2011–2012b])
- Dental caries
- Over-retained tooth E with delayed eruption of tooth number 8
- Pathology apical to tooth D

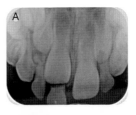
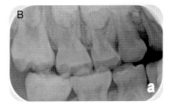
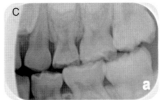

Figure 9.1.3a–c. Pre-operative radiographs

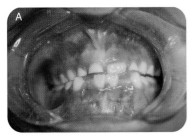
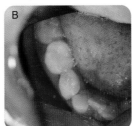

Figure 9.1.2a–b. Pre-operative intra-oral photos

L. Comprehensive Treatment Plan

- Establish a dental home
- Patient referred to oral surgeon to evaluate possible supernumerary tooth or odontoma apical to tooth D
- Preventive treatment
  - Dental prophylaxis
  - Fluoride treatment
  - Review of oral hygiene (with parent and child) at the beginning of treatment and at subsequent visits
  - Sealant on first permanent molars: numbers 3 (OL) and 14(OL)
- Restorative treatment
  - Number 19 (0) resin restoration
  - A (OL) resin restoration
  - K (MO) resin restoration
  - S (DO) resin restoration
  - T (OB) resin restoration
  - Number 30 (O) resin restoration

- Monitoring of growth and development with special attention to exfoliation of E and subsequent emergence of number 8. Consider an orthodontic consultation. Patient will have a panoramic radiograph later for monitoring growth and development
- Recall at six months and every six months thereafter

M. Treatment

- Local anesthesia: 36 mg of Lidocaine with 1:100,000 epinephrine was administered via mandibular nerve block on the right side. (Maximum recommended dosage [MR] of Lidocaine = 4.4 mg/kg. This patient weights 35.6 kg, therefore MRD = 156.64 mg Lidocaine)
- Rubber dam isolation: A W8A Ivory clamp was placed on tooth number 30 to achieve isolation for the resin restoration to be performed in tooth T (Figure 9.1.4).
- Cavity preparation: Cavity preparations for this conservative resin restoration eliminate the need for extension for prevention (see Background Information 1 and Fundamental Point 4). The cavity preparation is limited to the small areas of carious enamel or dentin. As seen in figure 9.1.5, the carious lesion was confined to three separate areas: the buccal pit and two areas in the occlusal surface. (Simonsen 1978a, Simonsen 1978b, Simonsen 2005)
- Filling of cavity preparation: Conventional etching with 37% phosphoric acid was done. Filling of the cavity preparation was performed using a hybrid composite resin. A partially filled sealant material was placed on the uncavitated areas of the tooth (Figure 9.1.6).

N. Prognosis and Discussion

- The prognosis for caries is questionable because of the patient's past experience of dental caries, as a predictor of future caries (Powell 1998)
- However, education in the form of anticipatory guidance and the establishment of a dental home could improve the patient's oral health habits and reduce her caries risk

O. Complications and Alternative Treatment Plan

- How would management differ if the patient had severe, uncontrolled asthma?
- What is the proper protocol for managing an asthmatic episode during dental treatment?
- How would management differ if the patient lived in a non-fluoridated community?

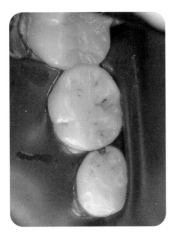

Figure 9.1.4. Tooth T, pre-operative isolation

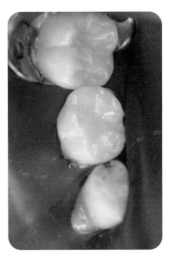

Figure 9.1.6. Tooth T, post-operative completed restoration

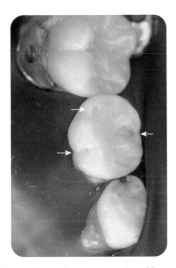

Figure 9.1.5. Tooth T, cavity preparation. Note how the cavity preparations (arrows) do not involve unaffected fissures. There is no extension for prevention

FUNDAMENTAL POINT 4

Minimally Invasive Resin Restorations

- Minimally invasive resin restorations are indicated for teeth with cavitated carious lesions in which the remaining grooves are sound but considered to be at high caries risk
- Their advantages include:
  - Conservative preparation design
  - Ability to isolate tooth
  - Sealant for prevention

Simonsen (1978a), Simonsen (1978b), Simonsen (1980), Simonsen (1982), Simonsen (2005)

BACKGROUND INFORMATION 1

Importance of Conservation of Tooth Structure

- Traditionally, amalgam was the restorative material of choice for posterior restorations. The early resin-based composites had large silica particles as fillers and they were not silinated to bond to the resin within the restorative material. These properties led to breakdown of the resin-based composite when placed in areas where significant wear occurred (Bayne et al. 1988). Although amalgam has been an effective restorative material for more than a century (Fuks 2002), extension for prevention was recommended so that all susceptible pits and fissures were included in the cavity preparation

- Minimally invasive resin restorations offer conservation of non-carious tooth structure (Donly and García-Godoy 2002). Being able to bond to dentin and enamel allows for only carious tooth structures to be removed, with bonded resin-based composite replacing tooth structure that was removed due to decay. A sealant is then placed over the entire occlusal surface, filling in any surface imperfections in the filled resin-based composite restoration that may have been created during finishing, and covering all caries-susceptible pit and fissures on the occlusal surface that were not included in the tooth cavity preparation (Simonsen 1980). The sealant provides prevention to future occlusal decay

- How would the approach to sedation change if a severely overweight patient requires moderate oral conscious sedation (Baker and Yagiela 2006)?

- Would a restoration be needed for this patient if tooth T presented with only stained grooves and no cavitation upon clinical examination?

Self-study Questions

1. **What will be helpful to identify overweight and/or obesity in children older than two years of age?**

2. **What is the purpose of the sealant placement in a preventive resin restoration (PRR)?**

3. **What is a contraindication to placing a resin restoration?**

4. **Is the wear of resin-based composite a significant concern when placing a resin restoration?**

Answers are located at the end of the case.

Bibliography

American Academy of Pediatric Dentistry. 2011–2012a. Prescribing Dental Radiographs, Reference Manual. *Pediatr Dent* 33(6):289–91.

American Academy of Pediatric Dentistry. 2011–2012b. Guideline on Caries-risk Assessment and Management for Infants, Children, and Adolescents, Reference Manual. *Pediatr Dent* 33(6):110–15.

Baker S, Yagiela JA. 2006. Obesity: a complicating factor for sedation in children. *Pediatr Dent* 28(6):487–93.

Barlow SE, Bobra SR, et al. 2007. Recognition of childhood overweight during health supervision visits: Does BMI help pediatricians? *Obesity* (Silver Spring) 15(1):225–32.

Bayne SC, Taylor DF, Roberson TM, Sturdevant JR, Wilder AD, Heymann HO, et al. 1988. Posterior composite wear factors. *Trans Acad of Dent Mater* 1:20–1.

Chinn S. 2006. Definitions of childhood obesity: current practice. *Eur J Clin Nutr* 60(10):1189–94.

Donly KJ, García-Godoy F. 2002. The use of resin-based composite in children. *Pediatr Dent* 24(5):480–8.

Fuks AB. 2002. The use of amalgam in pediatric dentistry. *Pediatr Dent* 24(5):448–55.

Graham L M. 2006. Classifying asthma. *Chest* 130(1 Suppl):13S-20S.

Milano M, Lee J Y, et al. 2006. A cross-sectional study of medication-related factors and caries experience in asthmatic children. *Pediatr Dent* 28(5):15–9.

Powell L V 1998. Caries prediction: a review of the literature. *Community Dent Oral Epidemiol* 26(6):361–71.

Redding GJ, Stoloff S W. 2004. "Changes in recommended treatments for mild and moderate asthma. *J Fam Pract* 53(9):692–700.

Simonsen RJ 1978a. Preventive resin restorations (I). *Quintessence Int Dent Dig* 9(1):69–76.

Simonsen RJ. 1978b. Preventive resin restorations (II). *Quintessence Int Dent Dig* 9(2):95–102.

Simonsen RJ. 1980. Preventive resin restorations: three-year results. *J Am Dent Assoc* 100(4):535–9.

Simonsen RJ. 1982. Preventive resin restoration. Innovative use of sealants in restorative dentistry. *Clin Prev Dent* 4(4):27–9.

Simonsen RJ. 2005. Preventive resin restorations and sealants in light of current evidence. *Dent Clin North Am* 49(4):815–23, vii.

Steinbacher DM, Glick M. 2001. The dental patient with asthma. An update and oral health considerations. *J Am Dent Assoc* 132(9):1229–39.

Willerhausen B, Blettner M, et al. 2007. Association between body mass index and dental health in 1,290 children of elementary schools in a German city. *Clin Oral Investig* 11(3):195–200.

SELF-STUDY ANSWERS

1. Body mass index (BMI) calculation (Chinn 2006, Barlow and Bobra 2007)

2. Eliminate the need to extend the preparation to prevent future decay and to fill any voids in the surface of the hybrid resin-based composite created during finishing

3. Inability to isolate the tooth; known allergy to resin-based composite material

4. No. Current materials have biomechanical properties that can reduce the risk of excessive wear

Case 2

Class II Glass Ionomer

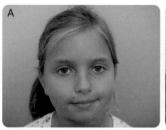
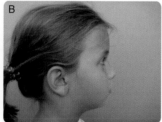

Figure 9.2.1a–b. Facial photographs

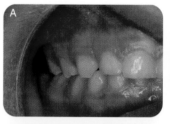
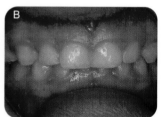
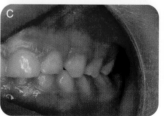
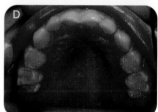
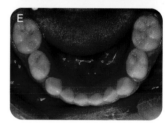

Figure 9.2.2a–e. Pre-operative photos

A. Presenting Patient
- 5-year-, 6-month-old Caucasian female
- New patient visit

B. Chief Complaint
- Mom states, "My daughter needs to see a dentist"

C. Social History
- Patient is in kindergarten
- Patient and 7-year-old brother live with mother
- Mother is the primary caregiver and has a full-time job
- Socio-economic status is lower level

D. Medical History
- Patient has no cardiovascular, pulmonary, gastro-intestinal, hepatic, renal, or genito-urinary disease or abnormality
- No medications
- No known disease or abnormality and no history of allergies (American Society of Anesthesiologists [ASA] I)

E. Medical Consult
- Not necessary at this time

F. Dental History
- Patient has never been to a dentist
- Optimal water fluoridation levels
- Moderate cariogenic diet including carbonated soda
- Toothbrushing without supervision, once daily

G. Extra-oral Exam
- No significant findings

H. Intra-oral Exam
- Primary dentition
- Occlusion: 2-mm overjet, 75% overbite; closed contacts in anterior and posterior
- Mesial step primary molars, class I canines
- Soft tissue: Within normal limits
- Moderate plaque accumulation
- Oral hygiene is poor

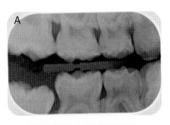

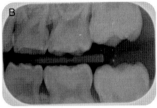

Figure 9.2.3a–b. Pre-operative bitewing radiographs

FUNDAMENTAL POINT 1
Radiographic Guidelines for Transitional Dentition

- The American Academy of Pediatric Dentistry (AAPD) recommends that a new patient with a transitional dentition should have a radiographic examination that includes posterior bitewings (if contacts between the teeth are present) and a panoramic radiograph or selective periapical radiographs. See the AAPD radiography guidelines: *http://www.aapd.org/media/ Policies_Guidelines/E_Radiographs.pdf* (AAPD 2011–2012a)

- The American Dental Association (ADA) also has radiographic guidelines similar to the AAPD. See the ADA radiography guidelines:

  http://www.ada.org/sections/professionalResources/pdfs/ topics_radiography_examinations.pdf

---

- Staining on occlusal surfaces, but no visible demineralization or cavitations

I. Diagnostic Tools

- Two bitewing radiographs show interproximal decay, B-do, I-do, J-mo, L-do (see Figures 9.2.3 a-b and Fundamental Point 1)

J. Differential Diagnosis

- N/A

K. Diagnosis and Problem List
Diagnosis

- Caries
- Need for oral hygiene improvement

FUNDAMENTAL POINT 2
Rationale for Material Selection

- The mesio-occlusal lesion in this patient was restored with a class II resin-modified glass ionomer cement restoration. Due to difficulty in isolating the tooth and the moderate caries risk status of the child, resin-modified glass ionomer cement was chosen rather than resin-based composite. Saliva contamination causes the tooth/resin interface bond to be compromised, with subsequent restoration failure with resin-based composite restorations. Glass ionomer cement can still chemically cure in the presence of minimal contamination. The fluoride release from the glass ionomer cement can aid in inhibiting tooth demineralization at restoration margins in this moderate-caries-risk patient. According to the Pediatric Restorative Dentistry Consensus Conference, primary teeth can be effectively restored with resin-modified glass ionomer cement Class II restorations (AAPD 2002)

Problem List

- Moderate caries risk due to diet, oral hygiene, and presence of decay (per American Academy of Pediatric Dentistry caries risk tool [AAPD 2011–2012b])
- Generalized plaque accumulation
- Lacks a dental home

L. Comprehensive Treatment Plan

- Establish a dental home
- Dental prophylaxis
- Fluoride treatment (5% fluoride varnish placed)
- Review of oral hygiene (with parent and child)
- Recommend use of floss
- Restore decayed teeth, B-do, I-do, J-mo, L-do
  - J-mesio-occlusal decay: To be restored with a resin-modified glass ionomer cement restoration
  - I-disto-occlusal decay: To be restored with a resin-modified glass ionomer cement restoration
- Prevention Plan
  - Three-month recall, re-evaluate oral hygiene status and caries risk
  - Prescribe a remineralizing product such as those containing amorphous calcium phosphate

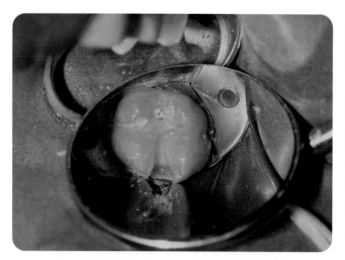

Figure 9.2.4. Isolated tooth J with mesio-occlusal preparation, including occlusal dovetail

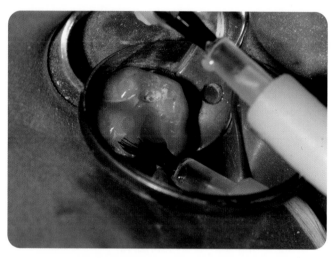

Figure 9.2.5. Primer applied

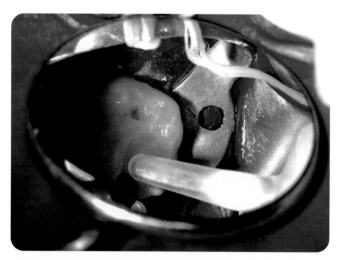

Figure 9.2.6. Resin-modified glass ionomer cement applied

BACKGROUND INFORMATION 1
Class II Resin-modified Glass Ionomer Cement Restoration

- A class II resin-modified glass ionomer cement restoration can be very effective. Caries is removed with a 330 bur, creating a rectangular box preparation with the axial wall placed in dentin as far as caries extends. The preparation buccal and lingual walls slightly converge occlusally. A dovetail is placed from the proximal box of the preparation onto the occlusal surface. This provides a bulk of glass ionomer cement which is less susceptible to fracture than just a slot preparation, in which only the proximal box is prepared and restored with restorative material. It is important to place butt cavosurface margins due to the brittleness and compressive strength of resin-modified glass ionomer cement

- A resin primer can be placed prior to the resin-modified glass ionomer cement to improve bond strength to tooth structure. Following placement of the glass ionomer cement restoration, the tooth should be isolated as best as possible so that saliva does not wash away aluminum during the acid-base chemical cure. This allows for maximum uptake of aluminum, which maximizes compressive strength

- After the restoration is finished and polished, a resin adhesive should be placed over the restoration surface. Again, this allows the aluminum that has not been uptaken into the glass ionomer setting reaction to remain at the restoration surface for uptake as the reaction continues over 24 hours

American Academy of Pediatric Dentistry (2002), Burgess et al. (2002), Donly and García-Godoy (2002), Waggoner (2005)

M. Treatment (Figures 9.2.4–9.2.7)

N. Prognosis and Discussion

- Prognosis for caries is moderate due to the patient's moderate cariogenic diet and non-ideal oral hygiene. Prognosis could be improved with reduction in soda frequency and improved oral hygiene maintenance. Survival of the class II

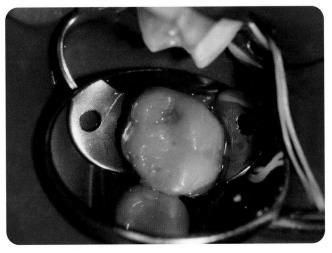

Figure 9.2.7. Final restoration

restoration is good due to the low to moderate caries risk and receptive acceptance of oral hygiene instructions

O. Complications and Alternative Treatment Plan

- If the patient had been classified as high risk, a stainless steel crown would be considered more appropriate. Likewise, if caries had extended to the pulp, requiring pulp therapy, a stainless steel crown would be the treatment of choice. Conversely, if the patient had excellent oral hygiene maintenance and the tooth could be isolated well, a resin-based composite could be considered as a restorative material

Self-study Questions

1. *A resin-modified restoration would not be appropriate for:*
   a. A low-caries-risk child
   b. A moderate-caries-risk child
   c. A high-caries-risk child

2. *The proximal walls of a class II preparation in a primary molar should:*
   a. Converge
   b. Be parallel
   c. Diverge

3. *The cavosurface margin of a class II preparation in a primary molar should:*
   a. Be beveled 0.5 mm
   b. Be beveled 1 mm
   c. Be beveled 2 mm
   d. Not be beveled

4. *Placing a primer adhesive prior to the placement of a resin-modified glass ionomer cement:*
   a. Increases the compressive strength of the glass ionomer cement
   b. Increases the bond strength to tooth structure
   c. Decreases the permeability of the glass ionomer cement

5. *A glass ionomer cement setting reaction occurs over:*
   a. Five minutes
   b. Ten minutes
   c. One hour
   d. Twenty-four hours

Answers are located at the end of the case.

Bibliography

American Academy of Pediatric Dentistry. 2011–2012a. Prescribing Dental Radiographs Reference Manual. *Pediatr Dent* 33(6):289–91.

American Academy of Pediatric Dentistry. 2011–2012b. Guideline on Caries-risk Assessment and Management for Infants, Children, and Adolescents, Reference Manual. *Pediatr Dent* 33(6):110–15.

American Academy of Pediatric Dentistry. 2002. Pediatric restorative dentistry consensus conference. *Pediatr Dent* 24(5):374–6.

Burgess JO, Walker R, Davidson JM. 2002. Posterior resin-based composite: review of the literature. *Pediatr Dent* 24(5):465–79.

Donly KJ, García-Godoy F. 2002. The use of resin-based composite in children. *Pediatr Dent* 24(5):480–8.

Waggoner W. 2005. Restorative dentistry for the primary dentition. In: *Pediatric Dentistry Infancy through Adolescence*, Fourth edition. Elsevier: St. Louis.

SELF-STUDY ANSWERS

1. c, A high-caries-risk child
2. a, Converge
3. d, Not be beveled

4. b, Increases the bond strength to tooth structure
5. d, Twenty-four hours

Case 3

Class II Resin Restoration

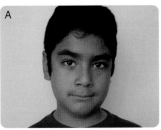
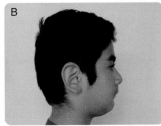

Figure 9.3.1a–b. Facial photographs

A. Presenting Patient
- 7-year-, 6-month-old Hispanic male
- Presenting for a recall examination

B. Chief Complaint
- Mom stated, "He is here for his check-up and he has some cavities"

C. Social History
- Patient is in first grade
- Patient is only child
- Parents are married
- The father owns his own plumbing company; the mother helps out with the business
- Socio-economic status is mid-level

D. Medical History
- Past history of rotovirus in December 2004. Patient was hospitalized for two days due to dehydration. No further complications
- Non-contributory medical history
- American Society of Anesthesiologists (ASA) I classification

E. Medical Consult
- Not necessary

F. Dental History
- Fair oral hygiene (brushes twice a day; supervised brushing, flossing)
- Tap water is fluoridated, uses fluoridated toothpaste
- High cariogenic diet
- Previous treatment was unable to be completed six months ago due to uncooperative behavior. Parents opted to defer treatment at that time

G. Extra-oral Exam
- Within normal limits

H. Intra-oral Exam
- Soft tissues are within normal limits
- Moderate plaque accumulation
- Oral hygiene is fair
- Early mixed dentition
- Tooth number 10 erupting; all permanent first molars present
- Occlusion: Bilateral class I molar relationship; bilateral class I canines; good spacing; overjet 1 mm, overbite 10%

I. Diagnostic Tools
- Two bitewing radiographs and a periapical radiograph of the mandibular right side (to evaluate possible pulpal or furcation involvement in tooth S) showed multiple carious lesions (Figures 9.3.2a–c).
- The patient may have a panoramic film taken at a future recall date

J. Differential Diagnosis
- N/A

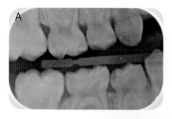
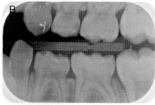
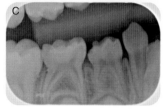

Figure 9.3.2a–c. Pre-operative radiographs

K. Diagnosis and Problem List

Diagnosis

- Dental caries

Problem List

- High caries risk
- Fair oral hygiene
- Poor diet
- Irregular use of dental home

L. Comprehensive Treatment Plan

- Establish a dental home
- Implement an at-home and in-office prevention plan
- Dental prophylaxis and fluoride treatment
- Treatment plan recommended:
  - Sealants on all first permanent molars
  - A(MO) resin restoration
  - B(DO) resin restoration
  - I(DO) possible pulpotomy and stainless steel crown
  - S(DO) possible pulpotomy and stainless steel crown

M. Treatment

Local Anesthesia

- Used 2% xylocaine with 1:100,000 of epinephrine
- Dosage for children is 4.4 mg/kg or 2 mg/lb

Rubber Dam Isolation

- Used a number 14 clamp, placed on tooth number 3, individual punched holes were used to isolate tooth A for treatment (Figure 9.3.3)

Cavity Preparation

- Cavity preparation is similar to a class II restoration for amalgam with modifications

- Using a number 330 bur, the cavity was prepared in the following manner:
  - Begin preparation of the proximal box, moving the bur in a pendulum motion from buccal to lingual
  - Once gingival contact is broken with adjacent tooth, check to see that the gingival margin is wider than the occlusal margin
  - After removing all caries, the axial pulpal line angle is slightly rounded, and a dovetail extension is made on the occlusal surface with the cavosurface margins beveled
  - The proximal box should not extend past the line angles; if so, then a stainless steel crown is indicated
  - Using a T-band matrix system, place the band around the tooth, with a wedge securing the band interproximally (Figure 9.3.4).

Restoration

- After placement of the matrix band and wedge, etch the tooth for 15 to 30 seconds with 35% to 40% phosphoric acid (Figure 9.3.5)
- Rinse thoroughly for 20 seconds and dry
- Apply a dentinal bonding agent, carefully following manufacturer's instructions (Figure 9.3.6)
- Apply resin composite material in increments, preferably no more than 2 mm of composite at a time. Incremental curing of the composite reduces polymerization shrinkage and ensures maximum polymerization (Figure 9.3.7)

Finishing

- A finishing carbide bur may be used to adapt the occlusal anatomy, if needed (Figure 9.3.8)
- Polishing can be completed with the use of enhancement points
- Use a sealant material to reduce occlusal wear and seal the restoration. The additional light curing will also help to obtain maximum polymerization of the resin restoration (Figure 9.3.9)

N. Prognosis and Discussion

- Ideally, a sealant on tooth 3 and a resin restoration on tooth B would have also been provided during the same visit, but the patient's level of cooperation did not allow for further treatment
- In this case, a resin restoration was performed instead of a stainless steel crown, because of the small size of the lesion and the fair patient cooperation. This patient is considered a high

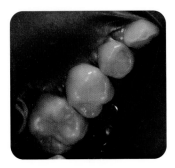

Figure 9.3.3. Rubber dam isolation

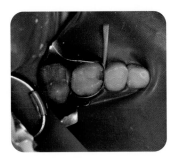

Figure 9.3.4. Cavity preparation and matrix placement

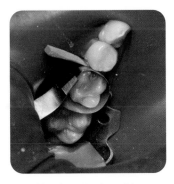

Figure 9.3.5. Etch with phosphoric acid

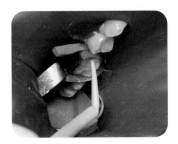

Figure 9.3.6. Placement of dentinal bonding agent

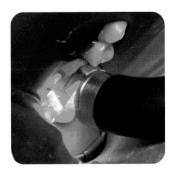

Figure 9.3.7. Light curing of resin restoration

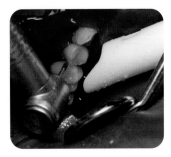

Figure 9.3.8. Finishing of resin restoration

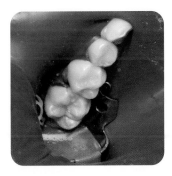

Figure 9.3.9. Final restoration

caries risk. However, having effectively instilled the importance of oral hygiene, recall examinations, good diet, and establishment of a dental home for this patient, resin restorations were determined to be the treatment of choice (see Fundamental Point 1).

O. Complications and Alternative Treatment Plan

- If the behavior of the patient would have been poor, making it difficult to isolate the tooth for a class II resin restoration, the alternative treatment would be a stainless steel crown

FUNDAMENTAL POINT 1

Guidelines for the Selection of Restorative Materials

- The American Academy of Pediatric Dentistry (AAPD) has recommendations regarding the indications and contraindications of restorations using resin-based composites. AAPD (2011–2012)

  Indications

- Small pit-and-fissure caries in which conservative preventive resin restorations are indicated in both primary and permanent dentition.
- Occlusal surface caries extending into dentin.
- Class II restorations in primary teeth that do not extend beyond the proximal line angles.
- Class II restorations in permanent teeth that extend approximately one-third to one-half the buccolingual width of the tooth.

- Class III, IV, V restorations in primary and permanent teeth.
- Strip crowns in primary and permanent dentition.

  Contraindications

- In cases in which a tooth cannot be isolated to obtain moisture control.
- In individuals who need large multiple surface restorations in the posterior primary dentition.
- In high-risk patients with multiple caries and/or tooth demineralization and who exhibit poor oral hygiene, and when maintenance is considered unlikely.

Self-study Questions

1. *In the cavity preparation for primary teeth, is the cavosurface margin beveled?*
2. *Are retention grooves placed in a class II preparation for primary teeth?*
3. *If the cavity preparation extends past the line angles, what type of restoration should be placed?*

4. *How long should primary teeth be etched?*
5. *Should the class II resin restoration receive additional light curing after polishing?*

Answers are located at the end of the case.

Bibliography

American Academy of Pediatric Dentistry. 2011–2012. *Guidelines on Pediatric Restorative Dentistry.* Reference Manual. *Pediatric Dentistry* Vol. 33(6), pg. 205–11.

Berg J., Donly K. 2011. Restorative Dentistry. In: *The Handbook of Pediatric Dentistry, American Academy of Pediatric Dentistry*, 4th Edition. Nowak AJ, Casamassimo PS (eds). 100–08.

SELF-STUDY ANSWERS

1. Yes
2. No
3. Stainless steel crown

4. Fifteen to 20 seconds
5. Yes

Case 4

Class V Glass Ionomer Restoration

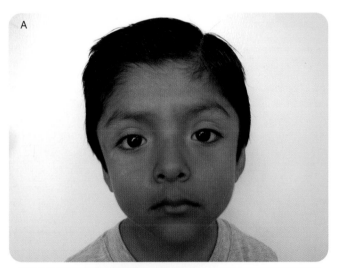

A

B

Figure 9.4.1a–b. Facial photographs

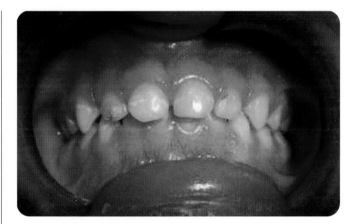

Figure 9.4.2. Pre-operative photo

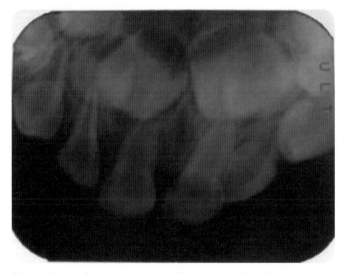

Figure 9.4.3. Pre-operative maxillary occlusal radiograph

A. Presenting Patient

- 3-year-, 8-month-old male
- New patient dental examination

B. Chief Complaint

- Parent states, "I am concerned the stains on his front teeth may be cavities."

C. Social History

- Patient attends preschool
- Enjoys playing with his friends and younger sister
- Parents are married and both work

D. Medical History

- Not contributory

E. Medical Consult

- N/A

F. Dental History

- First dental visit
- Optimal water fluoridation levels (0.7 ppm)
- Brushes teeth by himself
- High cariogenic diet
- Parent does not expect patient to be cooperative

G. Extra-oral Examination

- Within normal limits

H. Intra-oral Examination

- Moderate plaque accumulation
- Mild gingivitis
- Full complement of primary dentition
- Carious lesions on tooth D (FIL) and G (F)
- Facial decalcification on teeth B, E, and F
- Occlusion: Bilateral mesial step molar relationship, bilateral class I canine occlusion, midline aligned; 2-mm overjet, 90% overbite

I. Diagnostic Tools

- Maxillary anterior periapical radiograph (size 2 film) was obtained (see Figure 9.4.3).
- Bitewing radiographs were not indicated due to open contacts and visual absence of caries per American Academy of Pediatric Dentistry (AAPD) guidelines (AAPD [2011–2012a])

J. Differential Diagnosis

- N/A

K. Diagnosis

- Early childhood caries

L. Treatment Plan

- Tooth D (FIL) resin restoration
- Tooth G (F) resin-modified glass ionomer (RMGI) cement (see Background Information 1)
- Manage facial decalcification on teeth B, E, and F with a prescription remineralizing product such as those containing amorphous calcium phosphate

---

FUNDAMENTAL POINT 1
Anticipated Treatment Difficulties

- Patient cooperation due to age and parent's prediction of behavior
- Isolation of tooth as a result of proximity of caries to gingiva

---

FUNDAMENTAL POINT 2
Class V Preparation (Figure 9.4.4)

- Nitrous oxide conscious sedation was used for behavior management.
- Local anesthetic was not necessary for this patient.
- Cotton roll isolation was adequate.
- The cavity outline is kidney shaped and follows the extent of the lesion to provide retention.
- This may be done with a number 330 carbide or diamond bur.
- Removal of caries was done using a slow-speed round bur.
- The cavosurface margins of the cavity preparation must be 90° (butt joint).

Placement of Resin-modified Glass Ionomer (RMGI)

- Place a retraction cord, if necessary.
- Mix powder and liquid components of the RMGI thoroughly, following manufacturer's directions, and load into an appropriate syringe tip.
- The dentin is conditioned/primed (depending on brand used) according to the manufacturer's recommendation.
- Inject the mixed RMGI into the cavity preparation and condense with a hand instrument to eliminate any voids.
- The instrument may be dabbed in a bonding agent to prevent the RMGI from sticking to it and pulling the restoration out of the cavity preparation. It also reduces the surface roughness of the restoration.
- Contour and remove excess material.
- Light cure for approximately 40 seconds, placing the light as close to the restoration as possible without touching it.

Finishing of RMGI

- Finishing with a rotary instrument may not be necessary if the above steps were done properly.
- Use of a finishing bur at very low speed to reduce roughness is appropriate.
- The RMGI should have an unfilled resin adhesive placed over the final restoration surface.

BACKGROUND INFORMATION 1
Properties of Resin-modified Glass Ionomer

- Chemically bonds to enamel and dentin
- Releases fluoride
- Provides acceptable esthetics
- Less moisture sensitivity than resin-based composite

Indications for Class V Glass Ionomer Cement Restoration

- Difficulty isolating the tooth (less moisture sensitive than resin-based composite)
- Poor patient behavior (easy and fast)
- Moderate caries risk (fluoride release)

Croll and Nicholson (2002), Berg (2002)

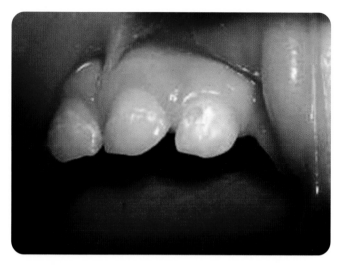

Figure 9.4.4. Class V cavity preparation

- Prevention Plan
  - Three-month periodic dental examination
  - Oral hygiene instructions
  - Dietary counseling
  - Use of fluoridated toothpaste and consumption of fluoridated water

M. Restorative Treatment for Tooth G

- Restoration with resin-modified glass ionomer (RMGI) cement (AAPD [2011-2012b]) (see Fundamental Points 1 and 2)

N. Prognosis

- The prognosis for this site to remain caries free is good due to the fluoride-releasing property of the restorative material, which reduces the chance of recurrent caries.
- High success for retention is expected because the restoration is not subjected to high occlusal force and it chemically bonds to the tooth structure.

O. Alternative Treatment

- Interim therapeutic restoration (ITR)

FUNDAMENTAL POINT 3
Indications for Interim Therapeutic Restoration

- Uncooperative patients that will be managed non-pharmacologically
- Patients with special needs
- Interim restoration for caries control
- Instances in which other restorative materials cannot be used

American Academy of Pediatric Dentistry (2011–2012c)

- Less invasive restorative technique without local anesthetic (see Fundamental Point 3)
- Gross caries removal with hand instruments (excavator and hatchet)
- Slow-speed rotary instrument with light pressure may be used to improve cavity design
- Restorative material is usually glass ionomer cement or RMGI

Self-study Questions

1. **What are the properties of RMGI?**
2. **What are the indications for class V glass ionomer cement restoration?**
3. **What are the indications for ITR?**
4. **How should an RMGI restoration be finished?**

Answers are located at the end of the case.

Bibliography

American Academy of Pediatric Dentistry. 2011–2012a. Prescribing Dental Radiographs Reference Manual. *Pediatr Dent* 33(6):289–91.

American Academy of Pediatric Dentistry. 2011–2012b. Pediatric Restorative Dentistry, Reference Manual. *Pediatr Dent* 33(6):205–11.

American Academy of Pediatric Dentistry. 2011–2012c. Policies on Interim Therapeutic Restorations, Reference Manual. *Pediatr Dent* 33(6):45–6.

Berg JH. 2002. Glass ionomer cements. *Pediatr Dent* 24(5):430–8.

Croll TP, Nicholson JW. 2002. Glass ionomer cements in pediatric dentistry: review of the literature. *Pediatr Dent* 24(5):423–9.

SELF-STUDY ANSWERS

1. Chemical bonding to enamel and dentin, release of fluoride, acceptable esthetics, less moisture-sensitivity than resin-based composite

2. Difficult tooth isolation, poor patient behavior, patients with moderate caries risk

3. Uncooperative patients who will be managed non-pharmacologically, patients with special needs, interim restoration for caries control, when other restorative materials cannot be used

4. Finishing with a rotary instrument may not be necessary if steps in placing restoration are done properly, a finishing bur at very low speed reduces roughness, place an unfilled resin adhesive over the final restoration

Case 5

Class V Resin Restoration

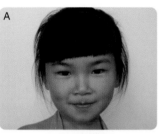 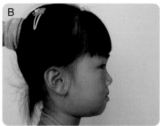

Figure 9.5.1a–b. Facial photographs

A. Presenting Patient
- 4-year-, 10-month-old Asian female
- New patient visit

B. Chief Complaint
- Mother states, "My daughter needs a check-up and is very nervous."

C. Social History
- Patient is in preschool
- Lives with mother
- Patient has a sister (6 years old)
- Mother is the primary caregiver and works full time
- Socio-economic status is lower-level

D. Medical History
- Patient was hypoglycemic at birth and was kept in the hospital for observation (see Fundamental Point 1).
- No medications
- No known disease and no history of allergies

E. Medical Consult
- Not necessary at this time

F. Dental History
- Prior to this visit the patient has not been to dentist in more than two years.
- Patient was fearful and anxious about the dental examination.

FUNDAMENTAL POINT 1
Hypoglycemia
- Obtain a complete understanding of hypoglycemia
  - When was the most recent hypoglycemic episode and has the patient experienced any complications from being hypoglycemic?
  - Has the patient been placed on a special or restricted diet?
- Be prepared to manage a patient that becomes hypoglycemic while in your care
  - A patient who is conscious can receive oral carbohydrates in the form of cake frosting. If oral carbohydrates are ineffective, medical assistance should be called to the scene. Fifty percent dextrose can be administered by an IV catheter if the patient becomes unconscious. However, if IV access is unavailable, glucagon can be administered intramuscularly. (Malamed 2000)

- Optimal water fluoridation levels
- Moderately cariogenic diet, including one and a half cups of juice daily.
- Toothbrushing without supervision twice daily.

G. Extra-oral Exam (Figures 9.5.1 a–b)
- No significant findings

H. Intra-oral Exam (Figures 9.5.2 a–e)
- Primary dentition
- Exfoliating lower central incisors
- Occlusion: 1-mm overjet, 10% overbite; generalized spacing in anterior, closed contacts in posterior; 2-mm diastema; mesial step primary molars, class I canines (see Fundamental Point 2)

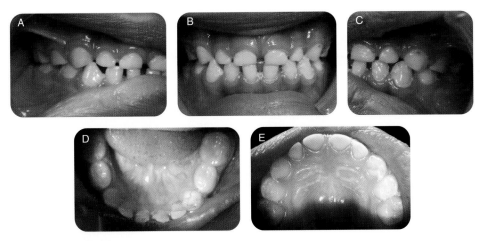

Figure 9.5.2a–e. Pre-operative photos

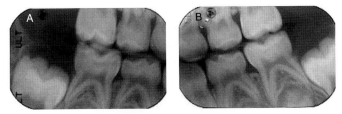

Figure 9.5.3a–b. Bitewing radiographs

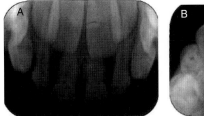
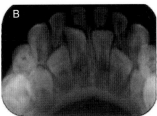

Figure 9.5.4a–b. A. Anterior maxillary and B. mandibular radiographs

- Soft tissues: Within normal limits
- Moderate plaque accumulation
- Oral hygiene is poor
- Multiple carious lesions

I. Diagnostic Tools

- See American Academy of Pediatric Dentistry radiographic guidelines (AAPD [2011–2012a])
- Two bitewing radiographs (Figures 9.5.3 a–b)
- Anterior maxillary and mandibular periapical radiographs (Figures 9.5.4 a–b)
- Radiographs show multiple carious lesions

J. Differential Diagnosis

- N/A

K. Diagnosis and Problem List

Diagnosis
- Multiple carious lesions
- Poor oral hygiene

Problem List
- High caries risk due to cariogenic diet, poor oral hygiene, and history of decay
- Generalized plaque accumulation
- No dental home

FUNDAMENTAL POINT 2
Orthodontic Evaluation

- Malocclusion: Orthodontic evaluation in primary dentition
    - Identify all anomalies of tooth number and size
    - Identify any anterior or posterior crossbites if present
    - Address the presence of habits along with their skeletal or dental sequelae

AAPD (2011–2012b)

L. Comprehensive Treatment Plan

- Establish a dental home and reduce apprehension for dental care
- Prevention plan
    - Dental prophylaxis
    - Fluoride treatment (5% fluoride varnish placed) (see Fundamental Point 3)
    - Review oral hygiene with parent and child
    - Recommend use of floss

- Three-month recall
  - Re-evaluate oral hygiene status and caries risk
- Restore decayed teeth (see Fundamental Point 4)
  - H-facial decay: Resin restoration
  - B-distal decay: Stainless steel crown
  - Address apprehensive behavior: Recommend use of nitrous oxide/oxygen
- Attempt to remineralize the incipient lesions with a remineralizing product such as those containing amorphous calcium phosphate
  - A-mesial incipient lesion
  - K-mesial incipient lesion
  - L-distal incipient lesion
  - T-mesial incipient lesion

M. Treatment

- Treatment (see Background Information 1)
  - Local anesthesia: 36 mg of Lidocaine with 1:100,000 epinephrine was administered
  - Rubber dam isolation: A clamp was placed on tooth J to achieve isolation (Figures 9.5.5–9.5.7).
- Behavior management was achieved with nitrous oxide sedation and tell-show-do technique

N. Prognosis and Discussion

- The prognosis for future caries is poor due to the patient's moderate cariogenic diet and poor oral hygiene. Prognosis could be improved with implementation of the proposed prevention plan. Efforts should be made to reduce the patient's anxiety to wean off the nitrous oxide and establish a comfort level with dental care.

FUNDAMENTAL POINT 3
Fluoride Varnish

- Due to the patient's high caries risk and young age, fluoride varnish was placed. Fluoride varnish may be substituted for the traditional topical fluoride treatment for the caries-active preschooler. Varnish may be applied after the prophylaxis and may be flossed through tight contacts (Soxman 2005). It is easily applied and enhances remineralization. Three yearly applications of fluoride varnish has been used effectively for children under the age of five (Featherstone 2006).

O. Complications and Alternative Treatment Plan

- Should the treatment plan be more aggressive to manage the patient's decay?
- Would daily use of a fluoridated mouthrinse be effective in remineralizing the incipient lesions?
- If patient lived in a non-fluoridated community would treatment differ?

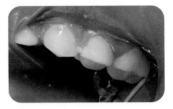

Figure 9.5.5. Rubber dam isolation

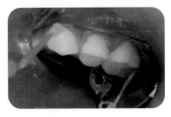

Figure 9.5.6. Placement of bonding agent

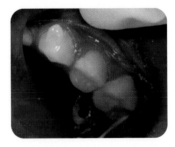

Figure 9.5.7. Placement of resin

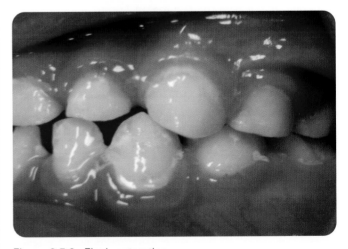

Figure 9.5.8. Final restoration

FUNDAMENTAL POINT 4
Selection of Restorative Material

- The class V lesion in this patient was restored with a resin composite. It was chosen due to esthetics and its resistance to wear. Composite resins are available in a variety of shades and opacities and their physical and mechanical properties are excellent (Waggoner 2005).

According to the Pediatric Restorative Dentistry Consensus Conference held in San Antonio, Texas, in 2002, a class V lesion in primary teeth can be restored with a resin-based composite. The tooth, however, must be adequately isolated to prevent saliva contamination (American Academy of Pediatric Dentistry 2002).

BACKGROUND INFORMATION 1
Class V Composite Resin Restoration

- Class V restorations are often needed on the facial of cuspids. The caries should be removed with a 330 bur until dentin is reached. The bur is then moved laterally into sound dentin and enamel to create the walls of the cavity. The pulpal wall should be convex, following the shape of the outer enamel surface. The lateral walls should be slightly flared near the proximal surfaces to prevent undermining of the enamel. A short bevel is then placed around the entire cavosurface margin (Waggoner 2005). It is important to place a beveled enamel margin and a butt cementum/dentin margin to enhance retention of the resin.

- In addition, several clinical steps must be taken to allow the resin to adhere to the tooth structure. Mechanical retention is achieved by flowing the water-tolerant primer into the surface of the dentin where it permeates into the spaces of the collagen that were created by the acid etch. The primer will then allow the hydrophobic bonding agent to bond to the wet surface of the dentin. The bonding agent then bonds to the primer and the composite resin (Berg 1998). The resin can then be finished and polished.

Self-study Questions

1. According to the AAPD caries assessment tool (CAT), what risk category would be assigned to a patient with evidence of radiographic enamel caries?

2. Which radiographs should be taken in a new patient in primary dentition that presents with closed contacts in the posterior teeth?

3. What is meant by the phrase "tell-show-do" in behavior management?

4. What is the concentration of fluoride ion in 5% sodium fluoride varnish?

5. Is local anesthesia always necessary for Class V restorations?

Answers are located at the end of the case.

Bibliography

American Academy of Pediatric Dentistry. 2011–2012a. Prescribing Dental Radiographs Reference Manual. *Pediatr Dent* 33(6):289–91.

American Academy of Pediatric Dentistry. 2011–2012b. Management of the Developing Dentition, Reference Manual. *Pediatr Dent* 33(6):229–41.

American Academy of Pediatric Dentistry. 2002. Pediatric restorative dentistry consensus conference. *Pediatr Dent* 24(5):374–6.

Berg J. 1998. The continuum of restorative materials in pediatric dentistry—a review for the clinician. *Pediatr Dent* 20(2):93–100.

Featherstone JDB. 2006. Caries prevention and reversal based on the caries balance. *Pediatr Dent* 28(2):128–31.

Malamed S. 2000. *Medical Emergencies in the Dental Office*, 5th edition. Mosby: St. Louis.

Soxman JA. 2005. Preventive guidelines for the preschool patient. *Gen Dent* 53(1):77–80.

Waggoner W. 2005. Restorative dentistry for the primary dentition. In: *Pediatric Dentistry Infancy Through Adolescence*, 4th edition. Elsevier: St. Louis.

SELF-STUDY ANSWERS

1. High caries risk
2. The radiographic exam should be individualized per patient; however, if the posterior teeth are in contact, the patient should receive selected periapical/occlusal views and/or bitewing radiographs.
3. The tell-show-do technique involves explanation, demonstration, and completion of a step
4. 2.26% fluoride ion
5. Local anesthesia may not be necessary in small Class V restorations; nevertheless, some form of local anesthesia may be necessary for rubber dam placement.

Case 6

Class IV Resin

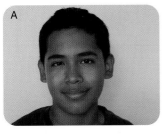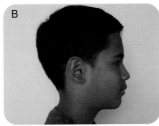

Figure 9.6.1a–b. Facial photographs

A. Presenting Patient
- 11-year-, 11-month-old male
- Trauma follow-up visit

B. Chief Complaint
- Mother states, "My son chipped his front tooth while skateboarding over a year ago. This tooth has never bothered him."

C. Social History
- Patient is in 6th grade
- Patient is involved in skateboarding, soccer, basketball
- Patient has a 14-year-old sister and 9-year-old brother
- Parents are married
- Father works full time; mother is a full-time homemaker
- Family recently relocated; no previous dental records
- Socio-economic status is low to mid-level

D. Medical History
- Mild, innocent heart murmur detected at one-month well baby check. Heart murmur has never been detected since the initial episode (see Fundamental Point 1 and Background Information 1).
- No medications

FUNDAMENTAL POINT 1
History for a Heart Murmur
- Obtain a thorough understanding of the status of the heart murmur
- Question on:
  - Documentation of heart murmur status
  - Follow-up evaluations of heart murmur
  - Any consults to a pediatric cardiologist
  - Any need for echocardiograms or chest films
  - Any symptoms experienced by the patient
  - Any medications that patient takes for this condition
  - Any need for antibiotic prophylaxis for subacute bacterial endocarditis
  - Any limitations or restrictions on any activities

Lessard (2005), Wilson et al. (2007)

E. Medical Consult
- Consultation with child's pediatrician confirms status of heart murmur as being innocent or non-existent. Pediatrician reports there is no need for antibiotic coverage prior to high-risk dental procedures.

F. Dental History
- Family recently relocated; no previous dental record available
- Usually routine six-month check-ups, but last visit was one year ago
- Sealants placed per mother
- Optimal water fluoridation levels
- Healthy, low-cariogenic diet

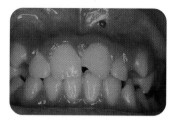

Figure 9.6.2. Pre-operative view

- Brushes teeth without supervision one time per day
- Flosses without supervision, on occasion
- No history of dental caries or dental restorations other than sealants
- History of trauma to tooth number 9 more than one year ago (never restored) (see Fundamental Point 2)
- Positive behavior for all previous care

G. Extra-oral Exam (Figures 9.6.1 a–b)
- Head and neck: Within normal limits
- Weight: 39.8 kg, height: 62 inches, BMI: Normal
- No signs of trauma to extra-oral hard or soft tissues
- No other significant findings

H. Intra-oral Exam
- Soft tissues: Within normal limits
- Late mixed dentition
- Maxillary right and left primary canines exfoliated recently
- Occlusion: 2-mm overjet, 30% overbite; adequate spacing both arches; class I permanent molars, permanent canines are erupting
- Mild plaque accumulation
- Oral hygiene is good
- Caries-free dentition
- Poor margins on three sealants: numbers 3, 14, and 30
- Tooth number 9 has an asymptomatic, non-mobile, uncomplicated crown fracture (Figure 9.6.2)

I. Diagnostic Tools
- Routine radiographs were taken within one year by the child's previous dentist, including bitewing radiographs and a panorex. Periapical radiographs had previously been obtained. These radiographs were requested, but were not available.
- Pre-operative periapical radiograph of tooth 9 was taken prior to restorative treatment; showed no pathology (Figure 9.6.3).
- Tooth number 9 responded normally to palpation, percussion, electrical, and thermal testing.

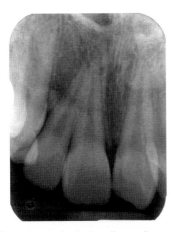

Figure 9.6.3. Anterior periapical radiograph

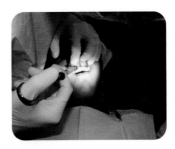

Figure 9.6.4. Administration of local anesthetic

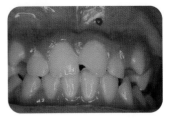

Figure 9.6.5. Pre-operative view of fractured tooth number 9

FUNDAMENTAL POINT 3
Mouthguards

- For preventing traumatic injury, custom mouthguards are more protective, comfortable, and retentive than preformed mouthguards. Therefore, they are more likely to be worn during sports. AAPD (2011–2012a)

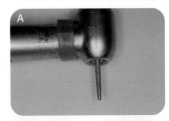
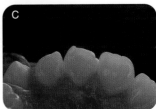

Figure 9.6.6a–c. Placement of a 1.5-mm chamfer (arrow) on the enamel margins with a number 1 DT diamond bur

J. Differential Diagnosis

- N/A

K. Diagnosis and Problem List

Diagnosis

- Faulty margins on sealants on numbers 3, 14, and 30
- Uncomplicated, crown fracture number 9 involving the mesial, incisal, facial, and lingual (MIFL) surfaces (more than one year ago)

Problem List

- Marginal defects on sealants on numbers 3, 14, and 30
- Uncomplicated, crown fracture number 9 MIFL
- Irregular dental home

L. Comprehensive Treatment Plan

- Establish a regular dental home
- Dental prophylaxis
- Fluoride treatment
- Review of oral hygiene (with parent and child)
- Re-seal numbers 3, 14, and 30
- Restore number 9 MIFL fracture with resin restorative material

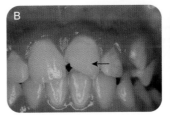
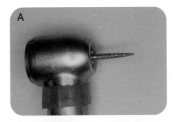
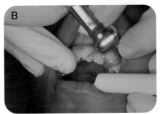
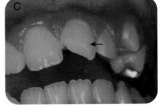

Figure 9.6.7a–c. Placement of a slight 1-mm bevel (arrow) on the chamfer with a number 1/8A diamond bur

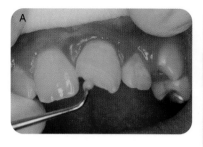

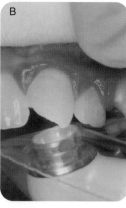

Figure 9.6.8a–b. Placement of a thin layer of glass ionomer liner on the exposed dentin

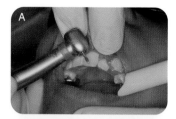

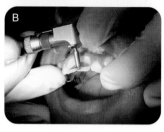

Figure 9.6.10a–b. Polishing of restoration

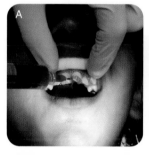

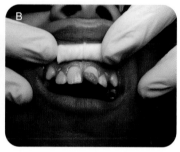

Figure 9.6.9a–b. Placement of a clear matrix band to prevent etching and bonding of adjacent tooth. Enamel margins were etched for 60 seconds with 35% phosphoric acid and thoroughly rinsed

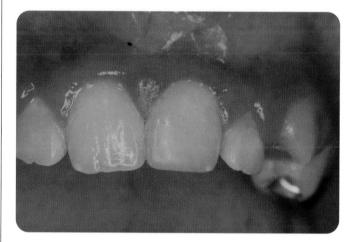

Figure 9.6.11. Final restoration

- Custom mouthguard to prevent further trauma because patient is involved in multiple contact sports (see Fundamental Point 3).
- Six month recall: Re-evaluate traumatized tooth number 9, re-evaluate oral hygiene status

M. Treatment (Figures 9.6.4–9.6.11)

N. Prognosis and Discussion

- The prognosis for maintaining the low caries rate is excellent due to good oral hygiene and history of no previous dental caries.
- The prognosis for the traumatized tooth is good due to the lack of sensitivity after one year. The tooth responds normally to palpation, percussion, electrical, and thermal testing.

- Moderate risk of traumatic injury can be reduced if parents and patient are compliant with mouthguard fabrication and use.
- Consider follow-up periapical radiographs at the six-month post-trauma check, sooner if symptoms develop.

O. Complications and Alternative Treatment Plan

- How would the management differ if the patient had a severe heart murmur and a previous history of infective endocarditis?
- How would the management differ if the patient had excess overjet and severe, lip incompetence?

Self-study Questions

1. *What type of radiographs are indicated for patient with a traumatized permanent incisor?*
2. *Following an uncomplicated crown fracture, when is final restoration recommended?*
3. *If a root fracture in the middle third of the root had occurred, what treatment would be indicated?*

Answers are located at the end of the case.

Bibliography

American Academy of Pediatric Dentistry. 2011–2012a. Prevention of Sports-related Orofacial Injuries Reference Manual. *Pediatr Dent* 33(6):63–6.

American Academy of Pediatric Dentistry. 2011–2012b. Guideline on oral and dental aspects of child abuse and neglect. Reference Manual. *Pediatric Dent* 33(6):147–150.

Lessard E, Glick M, Ahmed S, Saric M. 2005. The patient with a heart murmur: Evaluation, assessment and dental considerations. *J Am Dent Assoc* 136(3):347–56.

Wilson W, et al. 2007. Prevention of infective endocarditis: Guidelines from the American Heart Association: A guideline from the American Heart Association Rheumatic Fever, Endocarditis and Kawasaki Disease Committee, Council on Cardiovascular Disease in the Young, and the Council on Clinical Cardiology, Council on Cardiovascular Surgery and Anesthesia, and the Quality of Care and Outcomes Research Interdisciplinary Working Group. *J Am Dent Assoc* 138(6):739–60.

SELF-STUDY ANSWERS

1. Diagnostic errors are reduced when practitioners take two or more periapical radiographs following a traumatic injury. Each image should have a slightly altered beam direction.

2. Final restoration is recommended in six to eight weeks.

3. Stabilization with a splint for six to eight weeks or until mobility is reduced.

Case 7

Strip Crowns

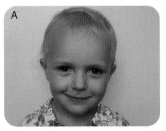
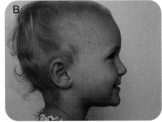

Figure 9.7.1a–b. Facial photographs

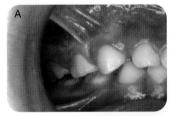
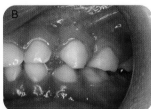
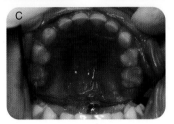

Figure 9.7.2a–c. Pre-operative right, left, and maxillary views

A. Presenting Patient

- 2-year-, 11-month-old Caucasian female
- New patient visit

B. Chief Complaint

- Mom states, "I think my daughter has cavities"

C. Social History

- Patient does not yet attend school
- Parents are married
- Socio-economic status is mid-level

D. Medical History

- Patient is American Society of Anethesiologist (ASA) class I
- Patient has never been hospitalized nor visited the emergency room for treatment
- No medications
- No known drug allergies

E. Medical Consult

- Not necessary at this time

F. Dental History

- Patient has never been to the dentist
- Parents have just recently initiated brushing child's teeth once daily
- High cariogenic diet
- Optimal water fluoridation levels
- Patient is very apprehensive and anxious

G. Extra-oral Exam

- Slightly convex profile (Figures 9.7.1 a–b)
- No other significant findings

H. Intra-oral Exam

- Primary dentition (Figures 9.7.2 a–c)
- Occlusion: Mesial step primary molars, right and left; no crowding
- Soft tissue: Within normal limits
- Moderate plaque accumulation
- Oral hygiene is poor
- Caries present in maxillary anterior and maxillary right first primary molars
- Patient very uncooperative for exam. Parent consents to treatment under general anesthesia.

I. Diagnostic Tools

- Two bitewing radiographs (Figure 9.7.3 a–b)
- Maxillary and mandibular occlusal radiographs (Figure 9.7.4 a–b)

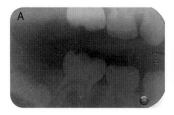
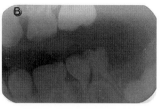

Figure 9.7.3a–b. Right and left bitewing radiographs

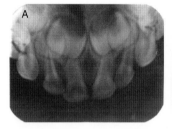
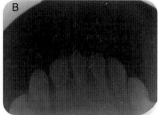

Figure 9.7.4a–b. Maxillary and mandibular occlusal radiographs

- Radiographs were obtained while patient was anesthetized
- Radiographs show multiple carious lesions

J. Differential Diagnosis
- N/A

K. Diagnosis and Problem List
Diagnosis
- Early childhood caries

Problem List
- Moderate to high caries risk due to moderate plaque accumulation, poor oral hygiene, poor diet, and caries history
- Multiple dental caries
- Very uncooperative and combative; patient requires general anesthesia for treatment

L. Comprehensive Treatment Plan
- Establish a dental home
- Dental prophylaxis
- Fluoride treatment
- Maxillary incisor strip crowns, stainless steel crown on maxillary right first primary molar
- Consider sealants on all primary molar occlusal surfaces
- Prescribe a remineralizing product such as those containing amorphous calcium phosphate
- Diet modification
- Three-month recall: Re-evaluate caries risk, re-evaluate oral hygiene status, review

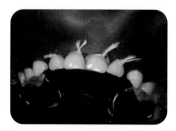

Figure 9.7.5. Absolute isolation before starting procedure

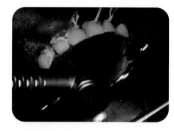

Figure 9.7.6. Preparation for strip crowns with a tapered diamond bur. Approximately 1.5 mm reduction is necessary

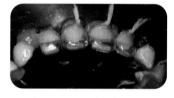

Figure 9.7.7. Fitting the strip crowns

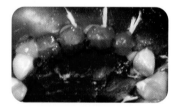

Figure 9.7.8. Etching of the teeth

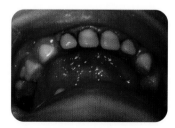

Figure 9.7.9. Strip crowns completed

oral hygiene and diet with parent and child

M. Treatment (Figures 9.7.5–9.7.9 and Fundamental Point 1)

N. Prognosis and Discussion

- If there is good compliance with the proposed prevention plan, then the prognosis for avoiding further caries is good

---

FUNDAMENTAL POINT 1
Strip Crowns

- The isolation of teeth is critical when placing strip crowns. Any contamination will have a negative effect on the acid-etch effectiveness, as well as the ability to obtain an adequate bond of resin to the tooth structure. When possible, ligation of a rubber dam around teeth to be treated can be achieved with dental floss or dental tape (Figure 9.7.5). Preparation of teeth for a strip crown involves incisal reduction of approximately 1.5mm with mesial and distal tooth reduction, which obtains adequate proximal space to fit strip crowns. Beveling of the facial and lingual incisal preparation provides the reduction necessary to fit strip crowns. A tapered diamond bur is ideal for preparing teeth for strip crowns. Following this general preparation, any decay that remains should be removed with a round bur (Figure 9.7.6)

- After the strip crown preparation is completed, a glass ionomer cement liner/base can be placed in areas where the preparation extends well into the dentin. At this time, strip crowns are selected, choosing the size that most closely replaces the original tooth dimensions. The gingival margin of the strip crown should be cut with scissors so that the original incisal height of the tooth is achieved and the gingival margin of the strip

crown adapts to the remaining tooth structure (Figure 9.7.7). All of the tooth structure and the glass ionomer liner/base is then acid etched with 37% phosphoric acid for approximately 30 seconds (Figure 9.7.8). The etchant is rinsed away with a water spray and the tooth is thoroughly air dried. An adhesive is applied, according to manufacturer instructions and light cured. It is helpful to place a small hole in the incisal edge of the strip crown so that composite can extrude when the crown is pushed into place over the prepared tooth. This relieves the potential for air voids to be created. Resin-based composite is placed intothe strip crown. (Highly filled resins provide excellent esthetics where margins of the preparation are not apparent through the restorative material.) The excess resin that extrudes through the hole can be easily removed when finishing and polishing. When the strip crown is fit into place, excess resin at the gingival margin can be removed with the tip of an explorer prior to photo-polymerization of the resin. The resin can then be light-cured from both the facial and lingual surfaces. Following polymerization, the strip crown is cut away and the resin surface is finished and polished (Figure 9.7.9)

Lee (2002), Waggoner (2002)

Self-study Questions

1. **What indicates the use of crowns rather than placing composites on anterior teeth in children?**
2. **List the different types of crowns for children**
3. **What type of radiographs are indicated for a patient in the early mixed dentition?**
4. **What are the three categories of information used to make a caries risk assessment as**

   defined by the American Academy of Pediatric Dentistry?
5. **Why is a hole placed in the incisal edge of the strip crown prior to the placement of resin-based composite?**

Answers are located at the end of the case.

Bibliography

Lee JK. 2002. Restoration of primary anterior teeth: review of the literature. *Pediatr Dent* 24(5):506–10.

Waggoner WF. 2002. Restoring primary anterior teeth. *Pediatr Dent* 24(5):511–16.

SELF-STUDY ANSWERS

1. Severity of the caries (patients with high caries susceptibility), extension, and caries risk assessment of the patient; restoration of carious primary molars where more than two surfaces are affected following pulpotomy or pulpectomy procedure; restoration and protection of teeth with extensive surface loss (attrition, erosion, abrasion); teeth anomalies; developmental defects; discoloration; patient's bite; appropriate cleaning and frequency of brushing; patient compliance; use as abutments for certain appliances (space maintainers); children who have extensive caries and must be treated under general anesthesia

2. Strip, stainless steel, open face stainless steel, prefabricated resin-faced stainless steel, acrylic

3. The American Academy of Pediatric Dentistry recommends that a patient with a transitional dentition should have a radiographic exam that includes posterior bitewings (if contacts between the teeth are present) and a panoramic radiograph or selective periapicals radiographs

4. History, clinical evaluation, and supplemental professional assessment

5. To avoid the development of air voids within the resin

Case 8

Stainless Steel Crown Restoration

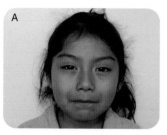
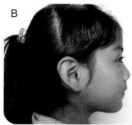

Figure 9.8.1a–b. Facial photographs

A. Presenting Patient

- 4-year-, 3-month-old female
- Patient presenting for restorative treatment

B. Chief Complaint

- Mother states, "My daughter has cavities and doesn't like the dentist due to extensive medical treatments and hospitalizations in the past"

C. Social History

- Patient is in pre-school
- Lives with both parents and 2-year-old brother
- Mother is the primary caregiver
- Socio-economic status is mid-level

D. Medical History

- The patient is American Society of Anesthesiologists (ASA) class III. Patient has complex cardiac anomalies, including hypoplastic left heart. Her oxygen saturation averages 85% on room air. She has a gastric tube for medication delivery and her physician recommends subacute bacterial endocarditis (SBE) prophylaxis
- Patient has been hospitalized numerous times for cardiac surgeries and other related procedures
- Medications: Captopril, Prevacid
- Allergies: Reglan

> **FUNDAMENTAL POINT 1**
> **Medically Compromised Patients**
> - Obtain all necessary medical consultations prior to initiating treatment (cardiologist, primary care pediatrician)
> - Obtain history of previous hospitalizations (general anesthesia experience, etc.)
> - Obtain medical clearance for general anesthesia
> - Determine need for SBE antibiotic prophylaxis; see: http://circ.ahajournals.org/content/116/15/1736.full.pdf (Wilson et al. 2007)

E. Medical Consult

- Medical consultation obtained from cardiologist. The patient was cleared medically for anesthesia. SBE prophylaxsis of amoxicillin 50 mg/kg recommended

F. Dental History

- Due to the patient's complex medical history, she was referred to another pediatric dentist for comprehensive dental care with general anesthesia in the operating room
- Radiographs have not been successfully obtained on an outpatient basis due to child's negative behavior
- Optimal water fluoridation levels
- Moderate cariogenic diet (excessive dairy product and juice intake)
- Mother brushes the patient's teeth once per day, but is afraid she is hurting the child

Oral Health and the Medically Compromised Patient

- The parents were informed of the importance of achieving optimal dental health in this medically compromised patient. Health care had focused on cardiac problems and the primary care pediatrician had informed the parents of the American Academy of Pediatrics, American Dental Association, and American Academy of Pediatric Dentistry recommendations to establish a dental home to maintain oral health as an important component of overall general health

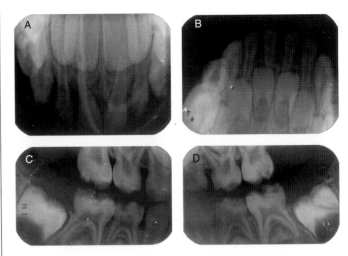

Figure 9.8.2a–d. Pre-operative radiographs

Extra-oral Exam

- No significant findings
- Convex profile

H. Intra-oral Exam

- Full primary dentition
- Occlusion: 2-mm overjet, 50% overbite; bilateral mesial step primary molars, bilateral class I canines
- Soft tissues: Within normal limits, excluding mild gingivitis
- Moderate plaque accumulation
- Oral hygiene is poor
- Generalized severe dental caries in all four quadrants

I. Diagnostic Tools

- Maxillary and mandibular anterior periapical radiographs and two bitewing radiographs show multiple carious lesions (Figures 9.8.2 a–d)

J. Differential Diagnosis

- N/A

K. Diagnosis and Problem List

Diagnosis

- Early childhood caries

Problem List

- High caries risk due to excessive juice and dairy intake, poor oral hygiene, and moderate plaque accumulation
- ASA III; complex cardiac anomalies

L. Comprehensive Treatment Plan

- Obtain appropriate medical consultations. Schedule treatment in hospital with general anesthesia due

FUNDAMENTAL POINT 2
Determine Need for Treatment Under General Anesthesia

- Due to this child's chronological and developmental age and the extent of treatment required, she would at least require sedation for successful treatment. With her medical history considered, this American Society of Anesthesiologists (ASA) class III patient is not a candidate for outpatient sedation, according to the guidelines of the American Academy of Pediatric Dentistry. General anesthesia in a hospital setting is required. See the guidelines at: http://aapd.org/media/Policies_Guidelines/G _Sedation.pdf

to extent of treatment plan, inability to cooperate, and medical history (see Fundamental Point 2)

- Panoramic radiograph will be obtained when the permanent incisors erupt to monitor growth and development
- Prevention plan
  - Dental prophylaxis
  - Topical fluoride treatment
  - Review oral hygiene (with parent and child) at initial and each subsequent visit to ascertain compliance with upgraded home care
  - Prescribe a remineralizing product such as those containing amorphous calcium phosphate
  - Three-month recall schedule

- Restorative treatment included: twelve stainless steel crowns for all canines, first and second primary molars, four prefabricated resin coated crowns for the maxillary anterior teeth (D-G)

M. Treatment

- Under general anesthesia local anesthesia was not used to avoid accidental post-op self-inflicted soft tissue trauma
- Rubber dam isolation with use of a W8A Ivory clamp placed on tooth K (Figure 9.8.3)
- Occlusal reduction 1 to 1.5 mm, using a number 330 bur in a high-speed handpiece
- Interproximal reduction 1 mm, using a number 1/4 DTX diamond bur to break contact. This is usually subgingival due to the broad, flat, and low contact between primary molars. (Figure 9.8.4)

- Select appropriate crown size
- Crimp the cervical margin of the crown as necessary to achieve a snug fit
- Cement with glass ionomer cement (Figures 9.8.5 and 9.8.6)

N. Prognosis and Discussion

- The prognosis for decreasing the occurrence of additional caries is poor due to poor oral hygiene, the underlying medical history, and excessive intake of juice and dairy products. Therefore, due to the patient's chronological age and caries risk, stainless steel crown restorations were planned for all primary molars, canines, and maxillary incisors to both treat the existing caries activity, but to also prevent the risk of recurrent decay in these teeth (Randall 2002, Seale 2002). Prognosis could be

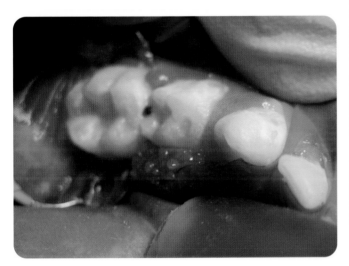

Figure 9.8.3. Rubber dam isolation

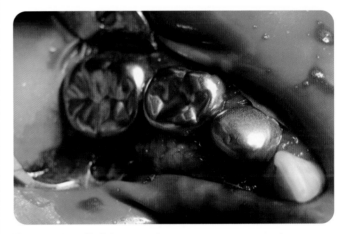

Figure 9.8.5. Stainless steel crowns post-cementation

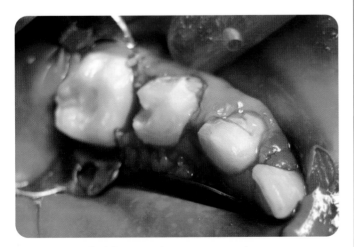

Figure 9.8.4. Stainless steel crown preparation

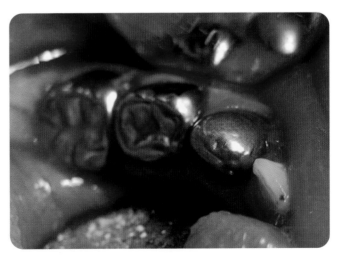

Figure 9.8.6. Stainless steel crowns completed

improved if parents and patient demonstrate good compliance with the proposed prevention plan

O. Complications and Alternative Treatment Plan

- How could management differ if the child were ASA I or II?

- How would management differ if the patient lived in a non-fluoridated community?

Self-study Questions

1. What are some important informational tools that need to be obtained when taking a medical history with a patient who is ASA III?

2. Why should this patient not be treated with outpatient sedation?

3. List three indications for stainless steel crown restoration in primary molars.

4. What type of radiographs are indicated for a patient with a full primary dentition?

Answers are located at the end of the case.

Bibliography

Randall RC. 2002. Preformed metal crowns for primary and permanent molar teeth: review of the literature. *Pediatr Dent* 24(5):489–500.

Seale NS. 2002. The use of stainless steel crowns. *Pediatr Dent* 24(5):501–5.

Wilson W. et al. 2007. Prevention of Infective Endocarditis: Guidelines From the American Heart Association. *Circulation* 116:1736–54.

SELF-STUDY ANSWERS

1. The nature of the disease must be clearly outlined. Appropriate medical consultations and a thorough review of previous hospitalizations and surgical/anesthesia history must be obtained

2. Children who are ASA I or mild ASA II are candidates for outpatient sedation. ASA III and ASA IV patients must be treated in a hospital setting with general anesthesia. See the following guidelines: http://aapd.org/media/Policies_Guidelines/G_Sedation.pdf

3. Extensive decay, large lesions, or multiple surface lesions in primary molars; high-risk children exhibiting anterior tooth caries and/or primary molar caries; children who require general anesthesia. See the following guidelines: http://aapd.org/media/Policies_Guidelines/G_Restorative.pdf

4. The American Academy of Pediatric Dentistry recommends that a new patient with a primary dentition should have an individualized radiographic exam consisting of selected periapical/occlusal views and/or posterior bitewings if the proximal surfaces cannot be visualized or probed. Patients without evidence of disease and with open proximal contacts may not require a radiographic exam at this time. See the following guidelines: http://aapd.org/media/Policies_Guidelines/E_Radiographs.pdf

INDEX

Italicized page locators indicate photos; tables are noted with *t*.

Clinical Cases in Pediatric Dentistry, First Edition. Edited by Amr M. Moursi.
© 2012 Blackwell Publishing Ltd. Pubished 2012 by Blackwell Publishing Ltd.

BMA